OUR STORIES

75 Years of the **NHS** From the People Who Built It, Lived It and Love It

EDITED BY

STEPHANIE SNOW

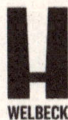

WELBECK

First published in 2023 by Headline Welbeck Non-Fiction
An imprint of Headline Publishing Group Limited

This paperback edition published in 2024 by Headline Welbeck Non-Fiction
An imprint of Headline Publishing Group Limited

Cataloguing in Publication Data is available from the British Library

Paperback ISBN 978 1 8027 9348 2

Offset in 9.35/13.99 pt Baskerville MT Pro by Jouve (UK), Milton Keynes

Printed and bound in Great Britain by Clays Ltd, Elcograf S.p.A.

MIX
Paper | Supporting
responsible forestry
FSC
www.fsc.org   FSC® C104740

Headline's policy is to use papers that are natural, renewable and recyclable
products and made from wood grown in well-managed forests and other
controlled sources. The logging and manufacturing processes are expected to
conform to the environmental regulations of the country of origin.

HEADLINE PUBLISHING GROUP
An Hachette UK Company
Carmelite House
50 Victoria Embankment
London EC4Y 0DZ

www.headline.co.uk
www.hachette.co.uk

This book is dedicated to all the voices
of our NHS, past, present and future.

Contents

Chapter 5: 1980s

Chapter 6: 1990s

Chapter 9: 2020s

Chapter 10: Reflections

Foreword

ADAM KAY

A few years ago, I was doing a press junket in the United States and was asked "What's so great about the NHS?". I stumbled around for a good answer – it slightly felt like I was being asked what was so great about food or air. This seemed particularly absurd, in the land of the nothing-for-free. I pointed out that the availability and affordability of healthcare is constantly polled as number one of all concerns worrying American citizens. I talked about healthcare bills being America's number one cause of bankruptcies, affecting hundreds of thousands of families every single year. I said that I live in a country where nobody is bankrupted because of hospital bills, and not a single person worries if they'll be able to afford their medical care. I described the NHS as our greatest single achievement as a nation – free at the point of service, based on your clinical need, never based on your bank balance. A place where no receptionist ever takes a swipe of your credit card. But I couldn't quite get to the heart of what's so great about the NHS.

This is the book I wish I'd had in my pocket.

It is an extraordinary, personal first-person history of the NHS, told from its very first days and from every possible angle. From Joan Meredith campaigning as a young woman in the 1940s for "Medical Care For All" to Antonette Clarke-Akalanne hearing about the NHS at school in Barbados in the 1960s and flying over to train in Derby. There's Sonya Baksi, a doctor who fought to legalise abortions, Derrick Stephens, a hospital chef, and

Jonathan Blake, one of the first people diagnosed with HIV in the 1980s. No one can tell their stories better than they can, and I urge you to read them. Each is an interesting snapshot of a life interacting with the health service, but cumulatively they are an important portrait of 75 years of the health service.

As I sat down to write this foreword, I attempted to tot up the number of times I could think that the NHS has saved my life, and the lives of my family and loved ones. I couldn't. Its value and importance are almost impossible to quantify.

Happy birthday, NHS. We love you. Here's to the next 75.

Introduction

Capturing the voices of *Our Stories*

STEPHANIE SNOW

For 75 years the NHS has interwoven with the lives and work of all those who live in the UK, providing healthcare and at times employing as many as one in every 25 people of working age. Each day millions of us across Britain's cities, towns, rural communities and islands seek healthcare from the vast, complex web of round-the-clock services staffed by millions of nurses, porters, receptionists, cleaners, pharmacists, doctors, students, paramedics, chaplains, managers and many others. The cradle-to-grave arc around our lives has become watertight since 1948. Over 97 per cent of babies are now born in hospital, compared to around 33 per cent in 1948. The number of people dying in hospital has also risen over this period. It is impossible to overstate the importance of the NHS in our national life. It is part of British DNA. It embraces our shared experiences of being born, growing into adulthood, working, building families, living in communities, suffering illness and disease and, finally, dying. It encapsulates what it means to be human, and its history is the story of our lives over the past 75 years. The public and social value of the service is deep and enduring; for people in the UK, the NHS is more than a healthcare system. It represents compassion and equality. And despite the complicated histories of long waiting lists, failures in care and persistent issues of racism and discrimination, it stands in our imaginations as the very best example of humanitarianism.

Our Stories is the first book to tell the story of the NHS through the voices of patients, staff, policymakers and ordinary people from the Scottish isles to Cornwall, from the Welsh valleys to Belfast, and beyond. It reveals the rich, personal stories embedded in the contours of the historical landscape of the NHS across England, Wales, Scotland and Northern Ireland. What has been the value and meaning of the NHS for our lives and communities? How has the NHS shaped us, and how have we shaped the NHS? And what of its future?

The people in this book respond to these questions by telling their stories of birth, life, work, illness and death, from the 1930s through to the present. The NHS is a vital, living thing in people's lives. Every story encapsulates a unique relationship. Patricia Miller speaks of having the NHS in her DNA. Hughie Erskine believed the NHS ran through his blood. For Geoff Adams-Spink, the NHS is a well-loved but slightly dysfunctional family member. The stories are shocking, poignant, reflective, tragic and joyous: Norman Sharp's landmark hip replacement in 1948; Paula Wiggs's sudden liver failure at the age of 32; Yvonne Ugarte's loss of a child to meningitis followed by the birth of a baby conceived with IVF; Lionel Joyce's anguish at how little we really know about mental health.

The stories are full of courage, creativity, ambition, reflection, frustration, fulfilment and love. Love for the endeavour of improving life for everyone. And love for the NHS as an expression of our shared humanity. But these stories are not fairy tales. Our interviewees' love for the NHS weaves through their deeply reflective critical assessments of its strengths and weaknesses and the changes that are needed to improve health for us all. They look forward to the future with fear and hope.

My own path to bring these stories into being began in 2006. An opportunity came up to research NHS history. Professor John Pickstone, my then boss at the Centre for the History of Science, Technology and Medicine, zealous in his quest to apply scholarly skills to contemporary dilemmas, was keen to explore the successive NHS reorganisations in Manchester. I had just completed a long stint of research and writing on the introduction of anaesthesia to medicine in the nineteenth century. The NHS seemed like a refreshing change. It was also a chance to make sense of my own NHS story.

I had lived through my husband's long journey from medical student to consultant. I had tested him in his revision for never-ending exams; lived with a skeleton in the corner of the living room; cooked meals for his team when they were on call at Birmingham's Accident Hospital; drunk sherry at the Royal College of Surgeons after he passed the fellowship exam first time; was familiar with NHS camaraderie and dark humour; valued the constant supply of hot water for baths in NHS accommodation; witnessed the satisfaction of good patient outcomes and the mental haunting that followed tragic deaths or surgical complications; borne the frustration of the perennial pressures of capacity, funding and staff shortages; and seen the stress and exhaustion when services and people were overstretched. Patients and their stories became part of everyday conversation. They expressed profound gratitude for their care through boxes of apples, chocolates, wine and many, many cards, often handmade by children.

I also had my own patient experiences: a period spent in an infectious diseases unit after returning from Hong Kong with a raised white cell count; chronic urinary tract infections; one traumatic hospital birth; and two amazing home births, with the same midwife attending each. My brother had trained in medicine, the first in our family to do so. As a junior doctor he attended the Kegworth air disaster, when a British Midland Boeing 737 crashed into an embankment on the M1 and later, as a cardiologist, worked in Bristol during the inquiry into high rates of death in children undergoing cardiac surgery. I knew the NHS through these many different facets already, but from 2006, I began to look at it as a historian.

That first study of NHS reorganisations in Manchester was followed by work on the experiences of BAME NHS staff, the introduction of new stroke treatments in the 1990s, and the history of Guy's and St Thomas' in London. I worked in collaboration with other historians, clinicians and social scientists. From the outset I was struck by the goodwill of people towards the work, people who were willing to spend hours being interviewed and sharing personal archives. We developed strong links to local NHS organisations and leaders. Manchester Primary Care Trust had an far-sighted medical director in the late 2000s – Professor Rajan Madhok – who funded some of the local studies and was keen to use history to inform policymaking and practice. I had always been interested in how the NHS was a space where matters of life and death interweaved through the mundanities of working life – the tragi-comic elements of operating theatres and clinics, the chaos of A & Es, bulging waiting areas bringing people together from all walks of life, the common sense and kindness that prevailed as patients faced their fates, and patient-staff and staff-staff interactions as acts of solidarity in the shared experience of life.

This is what I was capturing in interviews on the ground. But when I looked to archives and other sources to extend the work beyond leaders and clinicians, there was very little material. Contemporary historical work on the NHS focused on policy and politics. Most of the people who had built and developed the NHS since 1948 did not feature in the historical record. *Our Stories* could not have been written in 2006 because there were no sources. My conviction that we were missing a huge chunk of NHS history and a key strand of post-war British history led me to begin the NHS at 70 project.

With support from the National Lottery Heritage Fund, NHS at 70 began in 2017, with the aim to create the first digital archive of NHS history by recording the stories of patients, staff and the public in 10 localities across the UK. In each location we trained volunteers from all walks of life as interviewers to capture this oral history. To ensure the archive was as diverse and representative as possible, we worked in partnership with the NHS and other health organisations, national and local charities, and community groups to recruit interviewees.

By March 2020 we had trained over 150 volunteer interviewers in oral history methodologies and collected more than 800 interviews with people aged from 18 to over 100. As the scale of the Covid-19 pandemic and its significance for the NHS revealed itself, we suspended face-to-face interviews. But we also realised that we had an extraordinary opportunity to capture the unfolding of Covid-19, and thereby leave a valuable historical footprint of one of the defining events of the twenty-first century. In July 2020 we were successful in gaining funding from the Arts and Humanities Research Council to partner with the British Library to create a national collection of Covid-19 testimonies. This also allowed for the deposit of the NHS at 70 interviews, alongside the Covid-19 interviews, to form the collection *Voices of Our National Health Service*. It stands as one of the largest health-focused oral history collections in the world and is now a permanent resource at the British Library.

By building a history of the NHS through the voices who have lived it, I hope to create a new and more complex, vivid portrait of the institution and the ways in which it mirrors the wider social, political and economic changes across the UK since 1948. It should help us to shift from asking questions about *what* happened to *how* and *why*, to explore what those changes meant for individuals and communities, to consider how they are remembered, and to reflect on what that means for the present. Oral history has always been a powerful method of capturing voices from communities that have often been overlooked in more traditional historical methods. Rather than answer a prescribed list of questions, oral histories like these focus on the broad life stories of interviewees, who are encouraged to speak to events and moments of personal significance. The interview process supports and encourages interviewees to share the meaning and purpose they have attributed to their experiences and the ways in which this has shaped their lives over time.

The value of testimony goes far beyond remembering dates and facts – it inspires us to imagine, and that is the key to historical engagement. 'History has to be burned into the imagination before it can be received by the reason,' noted the nineteenth-century historian Lord Macaulay. Listening to people share special and personal moments from their lives enables us to imagine and connect to different times and places. It helps us better understand our own experiences and place in history, and begin to see the larger patterns that cut across periods and issues. Through meeting the past, we can move beyond the personal to the collective – and look forward to the future.

The creation of the first NHS oral history collection *Voices of Our National Health Service* has truly been a collective endeavour involving more than 130 interviewers and over 2,400 interviews. Some of the subjects were interviewed once, others on multiple occasions. Some of the interviews are relatively short; others continued for several hours. The passion people feel in recording their experiences and reflections for future generations is embedded in the testimonies. The Covid-19 collecting work and the shared sense of living through a pivotal historical moment added urgency and meaning to these more recent interviews: 'This project is essential to help us understand the past and learn for the future'; 'It's so incredibly important that we write the history of what's happened so that people in the future can look back and see the experiences as they were lived and felt'; 'It is important that those of us who are involved in the NHS are able to leave a legacy for those coming after us'; 'I am part of the family of the NHS, and I believe that I have a role to play to let the world know what happens in the NHS'. Many interviewees have expressed their ambition that their testimony should be used, not just to celebrate and understand the NHS's past, but to shape its future – and the future well-being and health of us all.

All the interviews used in *Our Stories* come from *Voices of Our National Health Service*, and I would encourage you to visit the collection to discover others.[1] Selecting a handful of stories from this vast collection has been an almost impossible task, and the ones chosen have been greatly shortened from their original length. The aim has been to give as wide a range of narrators and perspectives within the limits of a single book as possible. In some stories, material has been combined from several interviews. In others, the material has been reordered to give more coherence for the reader. Speech in real life is also full of additions – like 'actually', 'really', 'you know', 'I mean, like, I think' – so, for the same reasons, these 'fillers' have mostly been edited out. However, I have retained interviewees' phrasing or syntax to showcase the uniqueness of their story in their own words. At every point the intention has been to edit people's speech to allow their thoughts, reflections, and experiences to shine through the written text as brightly as they do in the recordings.

The seventy-fifth anniversary of the NHS in July 2023 prompts reflection on its future, and much of it will follow well-worn and contested political and economic tracks. But *Our Stories* brings fresh voices to the conversation that convey the deep public meaning of the service: its inextricable associations with the saving and improving of life itself, and the consistent public passion for the principles of a universal health system that is free at the point of use for all citizens. The survival of a premature baby; intensive-care treatment during pandemics; recovery after psychosis; daily insulin to keep diabetes at bay; a hand held while a life fades away – it is impossible to express the social value of healthcare in more transactional forms such as budgets, cost-benefit analyses or performance targets.

Nevertheless, as many of the voices in this book acknowledge, the resources for health spending are finite and we need to continue to work within these as well as urgently address the continuing inequalities in health. The first 75 years of NHS history show us how each decade has brought innovations in treatments and therapies that provoke new ethical and moral dilemmas about balancing the spread of resources against different health needs, and this will likely continue. Like Joan Meredith, who stood on the streets of Nottingham in the 1940s campaigning for a national health service that would provide care to all, we do not know how things will change in the future. But the experiences, thoughts and feelings shared by the voices in *Our Stories* span the past 75 years, and offer a fresh and vital point of reflection from which to look forward and prepare us to meet the challenges that lie ahead.

The beginning of the NHS

It was 1930s interwar Britain – rife with social unrest, economic recession and severe poverty. Rampant infectious diseases like tuberculosis (TB) and polio had no cure and were life-threatening. Heart disease, strokes and cancer, for which there were limited treatments, were the main causes of death. Infant and maternal mortality rates were high. Occupational diseases and disabilities from industrial working environments like mines, steelworks and factories were common.

Hospitals struggled to finance new medical technologies like X-rays. And many institutions, particularly those caring for older people or those with chronic sickness and mental illness suffered staffing shortages. Concerns about population health, especially that of babies and mothers, and the fitness of men to fight wars, had been growing since the turn of the twentieth century. The British Army had rejected over 70 per cent of men volunteering to fight in the Boer War in 1899 due to poor health. And in 1936, 59 babies out of every 1,000 live births died before they were 12 months old.[2]

But healthcare was 'make do and mend'. In 1911 the first milestone towards a comprehensive healthcare service was reached when the Liberal government, led by David Lloyd George, introduced a National Insurance scheme. The scheme provided health insurance for the lowest-paid workers and required contributions from employers. Workers gained sickness benefits and access to medical care, including treatment for TB in a sanatorium. They also gained unemployment benefits, though dependents' care was not included, nor was dental care covered. Subscription schemes run by local hospitals or charities were popular with those who could afford the contributions. But many people, particularly women and children, were left without healthcare.

Health services were a jumble of hospitals of all shapes and sizes, general practices (mostly run by sole GPs) and public health functions. Hospitals fell into two main groups: voluntary hospitals and municipal hospitals. Voluntary hospitals had been set up by groups of local benefactors in cities and towns, relying on private funding through charitable donations. A few London hospitals, like St Bartholomew's and St Thomas', had medieval origins, but most developed from the 1700s onwards. They provided care for accidents and acute but non-infectious diseases. As medical knowledge grew, specialist hospitals were built, focusing on specific conditions or parts of the body, including maternity; eyes; and ear, nose and throat. Outside cities and large towns, smaller cottage hospitals, often run by GPs, provided care to rural populations. Some of the largest voluntary hospitals included medical and nursing schools; the growing importance of science had led to the expansion of research- and laboratory-based clinical work in these institutions. Municipal hospitals, run by local authorities, provided care for infectious diseases, mental health and chronic diseases and many had been established as workhouse infirmaries under the Victorian Poor Law. Public health functions, such as mother and baby services, which included health visitors and district nurses, were also provided by local authorities.

The start of the Second World War in 1939 proved an unforeseen catalyst in establishing a comprehensive health service. Fear that Britain would be overwhelmed by high numbers of civilian casualties led to the establishment of the Emergency Medical Service (EMS). Hospitals were grouped in regions, which enabled blood transfusion and specialist services, including orthopaedic fractures and plastic surgery, to be developed across the patch. The EMS created a snapshot of hospitals across Britain for the first time. Over 80 per cent of hospital beds were in municipal hospitals run by local authorities and overseen by Medical Officers of Health. The remaining 19 per cent were in the voluntary hospitals, which were administered by boards of governors. Voluntary hospitals had been struggling to keep afloat as the costs of new medical technologies such as X-ray machines outstripped the income they received from health subscription schemes and donations. Nevertheless, the public viewed these hospitals as prestigious, whereas municipal hospitals were associated with the stigma of the workhouse and reviled conditions like mental illness, old age and physical disability.

At the height of the war in 1942, William Beveridge, Liberal politician, economist and social reformer, produced his recommendations for a comprehensive social welfare programme that is the basis of the welfare state as we know it today. He said citizens should be able to access state support 'from cradle to grave', including a comprehensive national health service, without being charged for treatment. Public opinion polls confirmed the enthusiasm of the British people for these plans. The political response to Beveridge's recommendations was less positive because they were more radical than many in the Conservative government expected. Nevertheless, a 1944 White Paper set out plans for a new health service that would be centrally, rather than locally, governed.

Commitment to a new comprehensive system of healthcare featured in both Labour and Conservative manifestos for the 1945 general election. But the unexpected landslide victory of the Labour Party under the leadership of Clement Attlee catapulted Aneurin Bevan into the spotlight as the new minister for health and housing. Bevan's vision of what a national health service should look like and how it should be funded produced the NHS of 1948. Britain would still have had a national health service if the Conservatives had won the 1945 election, or if another politician had been appointed as health minister by Attlee. But it would have looked and felt very different.

Bevan grew up in the mining community of Tredegar in the South Wales valleys. His father was a miner and his mother was a seamstress. Bevan entered the colliery aged 13, becoming deeply involved in the working-class struggles for better wages and working conditions. After periods of unemployment, he became a union official and led the miners in the 1926 General Strike. He was a member of the Tredegar Cottage Hospital Management Committee and in 1929 was elected as Labour MP for Ebbw Vale. His lived experiences as a young miner and activist in the harsh social conditions of the South Wales valleys were critical in shaping his vision of what a national health service should provide, how it should be financed, and by whom. Four of Bevan's nine siblings had died. He watched his mother struggle with household budgets. And when Bevan was aged 28, his father died in his arms, choked to death by pneumoconiosis, a lung disease caused by the inhalation of coal dust.

Bevan's vision was for a health service that would make treatment and care available to everyone, regardless of their ability to pay. The anxiety caused by the need to pay directly for healthcare was cruel and hindered recovery: 'No society can legitimately call itself civilised if a sick person is denied medical aid because of lack of means,' he argued.[3] If people were fearful of the costs, then they would delay seeking medical attention, which could create more sickness and even permanent disability. Mothers were most likely to suffer because they put their own health needs after those of their families. For Bevan, the essence of a satisfactory health service was that everyone was treated the same, regardless of whether they were rich or poor. For that reason, financing the health service out of national taxation was the best and fairest means of ensuring all citizens enjoyed equal access to healthcare when they needed it. A service that provided care which was free at the point of access was a massive contribution to the civilisation of society, he asserted.

Translating this vision into reality proved challenging. Bevan did not have a blank canvas to build a health service from scratch; he could not simply commission new hospitals, set up new services and train a fresh workforce. Instead, he had to take the people, the structures and the services which already existed and fashion them into a national service. From a twenty-first-century perspective, it is hard to appreciate the resistance Bevan faced.

Vociferous opposition came from Conservative MPs, fearful of the long-term economic and social burden for the state; the British Medical Association, lobbying on behalf of doctors who did not want to become state employees; local authorities, which wanted to retain control of municipal hospitals; and voluntary teaching hospitals, which resisted the loss of independence. The NHS Bill in March 1946 set out how the new service would be created from existing services. Hospitals would be nationalised; GPs, dentists, opticians and community pharmacists would contract into the service; and public health functions, including health visitors and ambulances, would remain with local authorities. The minister of health would have overall responsibility, distributed through regional health boards, to: 'promote the establishment ... of a comprehensive health system designed to secure improvement in the physical and mental health of the people ... and the prevention, diagnosis and treatment of illness'.[4] Its key principle was that every citizen had a right to healthcare.

Bevan cajoled, compromised and persisted. His work experience from the trade union, of bringing opposing sides into consensus, stood him in good stead. Hospital doctors were offered higher salaries and retained their right to do private practice. Voluntary teaching hospitals were taken out of regional structures and linked directly to the Ministry of Health. GPs remained as independent small businesses, contracting into the NHS. Few would have had the stamina and tenacity to persist in the face of such opposition, as Bevan himself later reflected: 'I sometimes wonder whether a person of a less belligerent personality would have started the scheme at all. A certain amount of aggressiveness was necessary to push aside many of the resistances which would have prevented the scheme from being started at all.'[5] But, finally, the 'Appointed Day' for the launch of the new Service – as designated in the 1946 National Health Service Act – arrived.

'This Day Makes History', declared the Ministry of Health's advertisement in *The Times* newspaper on Monday 5 July 1948. 'Insurance and assistance to help in all the changes and chances of life, a free national health service for all – these are the great landmarks in British social progress which we have reached this month ... The better health resulting from the health service will help us answer the call for MORE AND MORE PRODUCTION', it concluded. It was the beginning of a new era in British history – and the history of healthcare across the globe.[6]

Chapter 1:
1930s–1940s

'I remember this country without a health service. It cost two and six to call the doctor. You didn't call them unless it was absolutely essential because we were in the hungry thirties.'

LORNA FINLAY

'The doctor said he would do this operation on the kitchen table.'

JOAN PEARTON

'I remember her having very bad boils on her fingers. My aunt suggested that the insurance man was very good at cutting these. It was a "make do" healthcare.'

CATALINA BATEMAN

'We followed the progress of Aneurin Bevan very closely because my grandmother was so proud that her husband had been connected with him.'

MEGAN FOX

'It was exactly the same as when the NHS come in, in 1948. We already had it in Tredegar before that.'

PHILIP PROSSER

'Remember, we hadn't viewed a better health service, necessarily, we just wanted one that was free that everybody could have because we had no idea of what lay in front of us.'

JOAN MEREDITH

'At that particular time, a lot of the surgeries were very poorly furnished, poorly cleaned and poorly staffed.'

BRIAN LASCELLES

'I do remember exactly what he looked like, sitting up in bed with his pyjamas and this shock of grey hair.'

JUNE ROSEN

'Park Hospital, because it was all relatively new and shiny, seemed to be just the ticket.'

EDMUND HOARE

'Tuberculosis was a widespread disease in those days. I was up in the sanatorium for several months.'

RUTH EDWARDS

'Off I went, with my shiny shoes and half a crown in my pocket, on the 5th July 1948 to the Royal Victoria Infirmary.'

ETHEL ARMSTRONG

'I owe my life to the NHS. I could never have paid for the treatment that I've had, and the attention. It was a marvellous thing. It included everybody. It was one of the biggest things that's happened in my lifetime. Even makes the war look small fry.'

NORMAN SHARP

LORNA FINLAY

Lorna grew up in the 'hungry thirties' in Northern Ireland. Her mother's fear that she would be 'inspected' by health visitors was shared by many, but rapidly settled once the new service was up and running.

I remember this country without a health service. It cost two and six to call the doctor. You didn't call them unless it was absolutely essential because we were in the hungry thirties. Nobody had any money in Northern Ireland, least of all the country people, of which I was part of. I remember the midwife coming to deliver my brother. It cost two and six for the delivery. The district nurse had a free house, paid for by the council, and you could go and knock on her door. Every village had a district nurse and she would treat you for free. We were known as panel patients – my father had National Insurance when he was sick, but he didn't get it for the family. I have a receipt from the old infirmary in Derry where my mother spent three nights. She got free hospital treatment but she had to pay for board and lodgings, eight shillings and sixpence for board and lodgings. My father was earning between £2 and £3 a week, so it put a hole in that week's earnings.

I had surgery in Omagh Hospital when I was about eight. I was there for six weeks and I only saw my parents once during that time. We lived outside Strabane; Omagh was a long way away – nobody had cars and there was a very poor bus service and my parents could ill afford the bus fare. There wasn't any care taken of children separated from their parents. I have memories of pining for my mother while I was there, but I don't feel I was damaged in any way.

TB was rampant around where I was living. There was no vaccination at that time, and most people around me had a shed in the back garden and whoever had TB in the family was isolated in the hut. If they were very ill, they went to Forster Green's in Belfast or to another TB hospital. They got a food allowance since TB is a disease of poverty, but an enormous lot of them died. Infectious diseases were also rampant. When we went to school in the thirties, most of us just got scarlet fever, measles and chickenpox, and went to bed for a few days. Vaccination in earnest didn't start until much later.

Although it was a period of great poverty in Northern Ireland, I was never hungry. I had a very stable, religious family background and there was no smoking, no drinking. Whatever money my father had was spent on the family. Everybody helped everybody else. All children's clothing was recycled – adult clothing would be cut down to make a skirt for me, for instance. My mother was a dressmaker and absolutely everything was recycled.

We lived in the country and because we had our own vegetable garden, we had our own potatoes and our own hens, so we had eggs. We didn't have luxuries, but we were not starved. It may have been called the hungry thirties, but I cannot remember ever being hungry. Cake was something you got at Christmas. You didn't get any pocket money, except Granny might have given you a penny now and again.

When my mother was told there was going to be a health service coming to help her with the development and the health of the children nought to fives, my mother's attitude was, 'Goodness me, I hope they don't come to me!' and 'We're not going to know when they're coming. I hope I have the beds made and the sheets on!' She saw health visitors as an inspector.

Aged 95 at the time of this interview, Lorna can remember her childhood 'much better than what I did yesterday'.

JOAN PEARTON

Joan was born in the district of Derker in Oldham, Lancashire. 'It was what I would call a middle-working-class area,' she remembers. Joan's family was among many who accessed healthcare through subscription schemes. Operations performed at home saved the additional cost of a hospital stay.

A man used to come to our house every Friday evening, just before teatime. Called Mr McCandlish. Very nice man. He was very jovial. He used to sit down, and there was a black book waiting for him with a shiny shilling on top – on the sideboard, near where he sat. He used to take the shilling, put it in his bag and write in the book. And he was known as 'the doctor's man'. He used to come and spend, say a quarter of an hour talking about things in general. And I used to look forward to his visits. So this would be the mid thirties.

We had a terraced house. It was brick-built with a yard, which had an outside lavatory. Later, we had a bathroom put in. We didn't share outside facilities. And we had decent-sized rooms. I was an only child until I was six and a half, when my brother was born. My mother worked in the mill from being 11 years old. She worked part-time and part-time she went to school. She married at the age of 20/21 and after that, she didn't work. My father worked at Ferranti's, an electrical engineering company in Hollinwood. He was foreman of the tool department. He rose to be a manager eventually. Other men in the area used to go off, suited and booted to offices of various kinds. I know of one or two who had very good jobs, say in the town hall or places like that. They were what my mother called 'people who will work and play', by which she meant that they would have their wages, whether they were working, or on holiday, or maybe ill.

I didn't even go to a hospital when I needed my tonsils and adenoids removing. I was around four. I remember having had very sore throats. And the doctor said that I needed my tonsils and adenoids removed. Furthermore, he said that I didn't need to go to hospital. That he would do this operation on the kitchen table. Which seems very strange these days. I distinctly remember us having a deal table in the kitchen. And my mother scrubbing it one Sunday morning. That was the first that I knew that something was going to take place. In our kitchen, we had very good light, because apart from the big windows, there were windows over the top of them that jutted out. The table had to be pushed under the windows so that it was in a good light. In the morning, the doctor who was going to do it, and his partner who was going to administer the anaesthetic, arrived. And I can remember being put onto the table. And the doctor saying to me, 'Do you like perfume, Joan?' And I said, 'Yes.' And as I lay down, and they put something over my face, I can distinctly remember saying, 'But I don't like that!' Nonetheless, it did its work. I woke up some time later, wailing that my throat hurt. I was given an ice cream cone, which, I must say, did alleviate it somewhat – temporarily. I remember feeling very sorry for myself, but I recovered from it normally. Though looking back now it seems very strange to have surgery done at home.

Joan was interviewed by her daughter, Zoe Harwood.

CATALINA BATEMAN

Catalina's parents met when her Chilean father was in England breaking in horses for the army. They married just before the end of the First World War and returned to Chile.

I was born in Punta Arenas, Chile. The outermost part of the Earth. My father decided that he would buy a farm in Australia and start there. It was so far away from the community that most of the children went to school on horseback. But the worldwide depression came in the thirties, and he had to leave because he was foreclosed on his farm and he couldn't pay the mortgage.

The family returned to Manchester when Catalina was 11.

My mother was very run down after this unhappy experience. My father had worked his passage back to South America to try and get work. I remember her having very bad boils on her fingers. My aunt suggested that the insurance man was very good at cutting these. It was a 'make do' healthcare. We did manage to scrape together the sixpence for the Manchester Saturday Hospital Fund, and that covered the family if you needed to go into hospital. It was a fair amount then.

The schools in Manchester were closed when war broke out in 1939. The whole school was evacuated to Blackpool. Because there hadn't been any enemy action in Manchester, the education committee brought children back again. I contracted pneumonia. That was before the wonder drugs. It was very serious. My father, who joined up again in the air force, was sent for because I was so seriously ill. He got compassionate leave. I was too ill to move. My uncle sent for a specialist from the Manchester Royal Infirmary and he said I was not to be moved from the settee I was already lying on. So I survived thanks to his advice and my mother's care. She'd never nursed anybody before, but she made a good job of it.

I always wanted to be a nurse. I had been accepted provisionally for entrance to Manchester Royal Infirmary. But once I'd had this very severe damage to my lung, they weren't interested in damaged goods, so I was out on a limb. After a long convalescence in Wales with my aunt, I was accepted at Altrincham General Hospital, which was a smaller hospital nearer my home. The doctor gave me a certificate to say that if I felt it was too much, I was to leave, but I never had to have a day's illness after that. I was very successful at nursing, I felt. Really in the right place.

There were then two different types of hospitals. There were the council hospitals, which were like Crumpsall and Withington, which were run by the health department in the towns. But most of the smaller hospitals were voluntary hospitals, which were run by contributions from the public. Altrincham was an extremely busy hospital because we had heavy industries, very severe agricultural injuries and some terrible car accidents with shards of glass. When RAF Burtonwood became a US Army base our theatre was very busy with their members who came into Altrincham. There was trouble between our men on leave, or civilians who didn't like the Yanks. They had nice uniforms, but I did resist their tights and nylons!

The D-Day soldiers were injured in their hundreds, standing on mines and so on. It wasn't a shock to me, having seen such awful heavy industrial injuries – it was the sheer number. We went down to Victoria Station to collect men from the trains with adapted buses, perhaps six stretchers on a line instead of the seats. Just prior to the war, there had been the Spanish Civil War, and a lot of Manchester men went to fight. One of the Spanish consultants had learned his skills in that conflict. There were two skin units, to try and replace some of the damage that had been done to those bodies, and we had his experience to work on, which was a big help really. The army did have some antibiotics. We were a little ahead of the times, as the Americans taught us to use drips.

Antibiotics were seen as 'wonder drugs', and by 1943 the US had produced enough penicillin for it to be supplied to Allied army forces who came to the UK to support the war effort.

Manchester Corporation had a public health department, which I thought was wonderful. Preventive medicine was their mantra. I was accepted for the health visitor's training in 1948. It was all part of the healthcare, but the

Town Hall district nurses and health visitors were more for the community. We specialised in school children, and the diseases then were very marked. Rickets, lack of sunshine, TB. There were hospitals and convalescent homes around Manchester built specially for their care. Styal, now a prison, was one of those marvellous buildings in which children had convalescence in little houses. It was a complete village; it had the church, and facilities for teaching as well there. We had terrible skin lesions from things which are now treated by modern drugs. Every clinic had a bath and a bath attendant, because scabies before DDT treatment was rife. It lent itself to bites on the scalp. They became infected and that's when children became ill. Now, that's where our bandaging skills came in, because we shaved the child, put special ointment on those terrible sores and finished it off with a capeline bandage, which was a great skill in those days. Bandaging was one of the skills of the older, pre-war nurses. It was a skill because you needed to make your bandages in a certain way in order for them to stay on. Hygiene was the thing in any of our treatments. It was a very professional business doing a dressing. Special trays were set and we washed and sterilised our own instruments. There was no disposables in those days. Dirty bandages – that was all that was thrown away, or burnt in the boiler room.

Catalina was asked at the end of the interview what would improve the lives of older patients. 'I would like to see more community nurses provided, because I think most people prefer to live in the community they belong to. People do need more help in home care. Rather like my home, which is sheltered housing with a little extra care if needed.'

MEGAN FOX

Megan has deep family connections with the Tredegar Medical Aid Society through her grandfather Edward Hughes.

My grandfather Edward Hughes was a member of the Query Club, which was formed by the founder of the Medical Aid Society: Walter Conway. And Conway gathered around him a group of men with like views about the costs of the Medical Aid for people that just couldn't afford it. My grandfather worked very hard with them there and, of course, Aneurin Bevan was there and his brother, Billy Bevan, and a lot of men of like feelings who wanted to improve the conditions of the working people here in Tredegar, especially the miners. My grandfather suffered the same eye problems that Aneurin had; I think it's called uncontrolled eye movement. He died young, my grandfather.

My father died as a result of working underground in the Number Nine pit here in Tredegar. He suffered severe injuries which resulted in his death a couple of months later. I was five months old. I had a sister of two and a half, and we went back to live with my grandmother, who was then a widow. My grandmother had seven children and she reared them with help from my mother, who went back there to live with us two in a three-bedroom house. It was a very warm and loving environment to be brought up in. My grandmother always used to make sure that my mother went out and voted. They would go out together and they voted up in one of the local chapels. When we were children, we used to go up skipping and singing, 'Vote, vote, vote for Aneurin Bevan, chuck the Tories out the door!', until the officer in the chapel used to come out and send us going. We followed the progress of Aneurin very closely because my grandmother was so proud that her husband had been connected with him. My mother and I used to go and listen to Aneurin if he came to Tredegar during the elections. We've heard him over the recreation ground, we've heard him in the circle and we saw him countless times walking around, you know.

I was a polling clerk in one of the polling stations, the last one in Tredegar down in Bedwellty Pits. We had to catch the colliers' bus to get down there in the morning, the officer and myself. I was the clerk and it closed at 10. Aneurin had gone around all the polling stations within the area – Rhymney, Ebbw Vale, Tredegar – and Bedwellty Pits was his last one before going home. He came in and – I can see him now, with a grey overcoat – and he was so tired. He said, 'Thank you for being here, how did I do?' 'Oh, you did very well,' we said. With that, there was a shout, 'Don't close the door!' and Aneurin knew who it was. It was an old farmer from down where Bedwellty Pits was. And he said, 'Oh, come on Perkins, you're always last!' And that was the last time I saw him. It was wonderful. I went home and told my mother and gran, you know, oh, they were ever so chuffed that I'd seen and talked to him and shook his hand. But oh, he was tired.

Aged 82 at the time of interview, Megan takes huge delight in her grandfather's involvement in the Tredegar Medical Aid Society. 'Little things keep coming back, you know, when you speak about it, and I'm ever so proud.'

PHILIP PROSSER

Philip was born in Tredegar in 1939 and speaks of the importance of the Tredegar Medical Aid Society.

I was born in the Royal Oak pub, Dukestown, Tredegar. And I was born with club feet. At the time, my father was paying into the Medical Aid Society. So I was taken then to one of the top orthopaedic doctors in Wales, Nathan Rocyn-Jones. That was the start of my treatment for quite a few years. When the NHS came in 1948, I was transferred over to the NHS. My last operation was when I was 18 years of age, which was in the Royal Gwent Hospital in Newport. And since then, I played sport and done all these things, but I do get trouble now, which is natural.

The Medical Aid in Tredegar at the time was if your father, or any of your family, if they were paying into the Medical Aid, you were entitled to all the free things that were going on. If you wanted to be taken to Newport, or taken to Bristol, for treatment, they'd pay for you to go. It was exactly the same as when the NHS come in, in 1948. We already had it in Tredegar before that. People, as long as they paid in their contributions, they were allowed to have glasses, teeth taken out. The whole family were cared for, just by a donation. A couple of pence in each pound.

We know that Aneurin Bevan took the idea of the Medical Aid Society. There was a chap there called Walter Conway. He was brought up in the workhouse and was the secretary of the Medical Aid Society. Aneurin Bevan just took the idea himself to Parliament at the time, but it originated from Tredegar. We've got a plaque down in a museum commemorating Walter Conway as a boy brought up in the workhouse. It was a big sort of thing, that, you know.

In recent years Philip has had two knee replacements and treatment for prostate cancer. 'Over the years, from when I was born right up till the prostate cancer, I've been treated well.'

JOAN MEREDITH

Joan lived in Carlton, Nottingham. Her father was a gentleman's tailor and outfitter and her mother assisted in the shops. The family could afford healthcare, but Joan's awareness that other people didn't enjoy those benefits led to her campaign for a national health service.

I have a memory of my father telling me that I was fortunate because we could afford a doctor if any of us were ill, but other people couldn't. We weren't particularly rich and I think I was about 10 or 11. So, it might have been about the time my younger brother was born because I know there was a doctor there, and a midwife. I don't think a lot of people, on the whole, could afford a doctor. I've always valued that understanding. I don't know how I got roped in to campaign for the National Health Service, but my dad saying that was probably the reason I did. What I can remember vividly is my cold hands and my cold feet from carrying this banner, which said something like, 'Medical Care For All'. I can remember trying to write the banner. Remember, we hadn't viewed a better health service, necessarily, we just wanted one that was free that everybody could have because we had no idea of what lay in front of us. I think at that age, I'd only want people to have what I had. We didn't have any other vision of it.

I belonged to an organisation, the Young Christian Workers, that did want to help people – and do that through politics, by influencing our local representatives as well as MPs, because we wanted to change the world. We wanted to have some kind of equality and particularly for poor people, because at the same time as the National Health Service, we were also worried about the poverty of children. How I became politically active and how I came to read some of Karl Marx, I really don't remember. It's funny, a Catholic reading Karl Marx, but Karl Marx was different in those days. We hadn't got the examples of what Russia had done with Karl Marx, and other countries. If you look at the way he enabled and looked at society as it was then, they were getting hold of something very attractive. So I wasn't tainted by what became of communism because it was at the beginning.

People used to go round these streets in a lorry and the speaker – whether it was the local councillor or the MP – they spoke from the back of a lorry because that was a good platform. I remember standing in these cold streets with this banner. And also in the middle of Manchester, there is a square where you get political people speaking. I remember heckling speakers. It was great fun, you see, but it strikes me now that we were rather more politically aware, if naïvely, in a way, because my mum sent us to do some things for people as well. My mum would send you out to take dinner for someone. In the shop, she let people pay credit – something that would be quite common in those days for a family business.

Joan continued her campaigning with Action Against Poverty in the 1950s and became a social worker, advocating for early intervention and family support. She died aged 96 in 2021.

BRIAN LASCELLES

Brian's father was a GP and the family moved frequently between practices when Brian was a child.

Before the health service, doctors used to start as assistants, with a view to taking over the practice. Or if somebody had died in a single-handed practice, it would be a death vacancy, which were much in demand because you could go in as your own boss and build the practice up. Practices were bought and sold on the basis of paying the widow of a death vacancy, for instance, about two and a half times the annual income of the practice. My father moved from Worthing to Pinner and from Pinner to Watford, building up the practices which had been run down by the previous ancient or sick doctor.

In 1947 we moved to a surgery on the site of an old monastery on the borders of the City of London and Spitalfields Market in the East End. We had an entrance for patients into a waiting room, a consulting room, a little dispensary and a door out of the surgery. The rest of the house was private. It was a three-storey house, and we used to have postgraduate students from Bart's Hospital who came to do the odd evening surgery as a relief. And it was a relief. When you were working 24/7 single-handed, you did need to have some assistance. We had very good quality doctors who knew how to run things properly. At that particular time, a lot of the surgeries were very poorly furnished, poorly cleaned and poorly staffed. We were very lucky to be on the edge of the City of London with Bart's Hospital on the doorstep. Basically, I never left Bart's. I was living in the area, a student at the hospital, and then qualified and was sending my patients to the hospital. I regard that as a very fortunate occurrence.

I should mention that my father was against the NHS. He went into this surgery they had in 1947. He had 18 months of build-up to the coming of the National Health Service. The hospital doctors on the whole were in favour of it but GPs felt that, as they were independent professionals, they could decide how to run their practice. They didn't feel they wanted interference. But eventually he came round to the idea that the NHS was a good idea.

Before the NHS came in, it was all on a private basis, except for people who were on the so-called 'panel'. The panel was the safety net for people who couldn't afford to be private patients and so they were treated free and a small, nominal fee was paid by the government to cover the cost of this. The practice was evolving all the time. New appointments were coming as well as the National Health Service. In fact, we subsidised the health service in a fashion because the practice was run 50/50 with private appointments and private patients, and the rest was paid for by the NHS.

Brian's father was not unusual in opposing the NHS, and pockets of opposition among doctors continued well into the 1980s. GPs remain as independent contractors – GP partnerships are contracted into the NHS to provide care.

JUNE ROSEN

June was a small child when the NHS was launched in 1948. Her father was a Manchester City councillor and the family hosted Bevan the night before he launched the NHS at Park Hospital, Trafford.

My grandfather was a GP. He'd been a surgeon on the Western Front in the First World War, but not demobbed [demobilised] till 1920, because he'd had to look after the wounded. He went into practice when life was very different. He went out with a horse and brougham carriage and a high silk hat, even though he lived in an area of complete deprivation – a very, very poor area of Leicester during that time. GPs did everything. They sewed people up, they set limbs, they delivered the babies. It had to be something very particular that took you to hospital. He had a pharmacy where he made up his tablets and all medicines, and I remember sitting on the side and watching him putting the tablets in boxes. Everything was wrapped up in beautiful white paper and sealed with sealing wax, and put on the hall table for people to take away. Whether they were panel patients or private patients, everybody got the same.

He had a speaking cube outside the front door because nobody had a phone. It was hooked on the side of his bed as patients could come in the middle of the night. People could speak to him and he could go off on his call. He had one afternoon a week off. Otherwise, he covered it all. He never went to the cinema or to the theatre without somebody coming over on in the middle of the play and saying, 'Could you please go and see somebody?' My mother said they never sat down to Christmas dinner without him disappearing. But that was his life. I know it moved my mother very much politically. The living conditions were absolutely horrendous: mould, rats, vermin, no sanitation. This was my grandfather's patch. And I know that he was much loved as a doctor.

Where did your father's political interests come from?

My grandmother, I think, would have liked to have been Mrs Thatcher, but she was the wrong generation. She canvassed for Winston Churchill before the First World War, and she loved it. I suppose she gave that to her children as well. So my father was a very young councillor in Ancoats in the thirties and forties, very different to now. It's apparently the best place to live in England, it certainly wasn't then. The people were fantastic, but the conditions weren't. In the twenties and thirties, there was no legal aid, and he was a solicitor, and he ran legal aid. Anyone who was poor in Manchester could go and get his advice – no win, no fee. So he was very involved. My parents moved to Urmston in the spring of 1943. It was a lovely place to live. Great community, there were quite a lot of green spaces and nice parks. And of course, Park Hospital, which is now Trafford, was the local hospital. My father was a Manchester City councillor and he was very involved with the Labour Party. And we very often had cabinet ministers to stay, because it was wartime, or just after the war, and we had a spare bedroom, which was very handy. I don't think they ever brought their ration books, and how my mother managed to feed them, I'm not quite sure. But it meant that we had people coming in and out who were very interesting people. When I was eight, Aneurin Bevan came to stay the night with us because he was going to launch the NHS.

I remember my parents talking about it, and how it would be a very momentous occasion. I was told we had somebody important coming to stay. My mother said, 'We're going to take our guest breakfast in bed, and you can come with me.' So we took a tray upstairs. I do remember exactly what he looked like, sitting up in bed with his pyjamas and this shock of grey hair. Aneurin Bevan, of course, had seen deprivation in the Welsh valleys that I don't think people can imagine today. He was so intent on getting the health service set up. And he felt that in time, it would cost less to run, rather than more, because people would have such a different baseline of health. My mother, a doctor's daughter, told him it wouldn't work, much to my father's amazement. He said, 'How can you say that?' She said, 'Well, people are people, and the more they have, the more they will want.' Nobody at that time could possibly have envisaged the sort of developments that we now have. New hearts, new lungs, new hips, new knees, cancer treatments. But of course, she was right, wasn't she? When she was a very old lady, in her nineties, she said, 'You know, when I meet your father in the next world, the first thing I'm going to say is, "I told you so."'

I think my parents felt the NHS, it was all part of making the world a better place. I remember my mother saying that after the war was a wonderful time to be in politics – we really felt we were going to build the new Jerusalem. It was a very heady time to be involved to put everything on its feet again.

June went on to have a long career in the NHS. She trained as a physiotherapist, moved into management by sitting on NHS Trust Boards and provided complementary therapies to patients in the Christie Hospital. She shares her reflections on the future of the NHS in Chapter 10.

EDMUND HOARE

Edmund worked for 26 years as consultant at Park Hospital, later Trafford General Hospital, where the NHS was launched in 1948. He's fascinated by the hospital's history, especially its intertwining with the roots of the NHS.

It's an interesting history because Park Hospital was always a public institution – it was never a voluntary hospital. When the health service came, it was probably the most modern hospital in the Manchester area. Park Hospital was built in the 1920s as a proper district general hospital. Built to deal with acute patients, with radiology and pharmacy and all the things that you'd associate with a hospital. It had proper wards and the idea was that it was going to provide comprehensive care for the local community, which was Urmston and Davyhulme. West Manchester was beginning to build up, so this was the hospital that would serve this new area. It was built by the Poor Law, but not like a Poor Law hospital, which usually had big blocks and was a bit forbidding, with a high number of long-stay patients and that kind of thing. The Poor Law was abolished in 1929 and all the Poor Law hospitals became the responsibility of the local authority, so Park Hall became the responsibility of Lancashire County Council.

At the beginning of the Second World War, the British Army took it over because they needed some facilities. It took casualties from Dunkirk and also the Norwegian campaign. Later in the war, the Americans took it over because in 1944, in preparation for D-Day, Americans were flooding over to this country. At the end of the war, it was handed back to Lancashire County Council. So that was in 1945. Then in 1948, that was where Aneurin Bevan formally opened the NHS. I can only speculate as to why he chose it. I mean, Manchester was obviously industrial, it was Labour, socialist. Rochdale was the foundation of the co-operative movement, so they probably were all factors. The last thing you wanted to do was to open it in London because, after all, London was where all the posh people were and where all the posh teaching hospitals were. This was a national health service, not a London health service, so it had to be out of London. Park Hospital, because it was all relatively new and shiny, seemed to be just the ticket. It was, if you like, the new broom. This lovely new hospital which was going to be a National Health Service hospital. Bevan wouldn't have wanted to do it at Manchester Royal Infirmary because that was a voluntary hospital – and that was also where all the posh people went and posh surgeons worked.

Edmund worked at Park Hall from 1976 until 2002. 'I had a wonderful sequence of medical secretaries. Part of the thing was that they were all local girls. They lived a mile from the hospital. The nurses often were all trained in the hospital, had families and relatives who lived nearby. So there was a sort of sense of responsibility of looking after your own community and that I think made a big difference.'

RUTH EDWARDS

Ruth lived in the old mining village of Garndiffaith in Torfaen, South East Wales, and was interviewed in the cottage where she had been born 90 years before. She began work in a public health laboratory in the run-up to the NHS and contracted TB through working on TB specimens. She was lucky enough to recover after a long stay in a sanatorium.

I took a job with the old Monmouthshire County Council, which was responsible for public health. I went to work in the public health laboratory as a trainee technician. Part of my job was to examine the specimens from the local sanatoria caring for TB patients. The upshot was that I contracted pulmonary tuberculosis from my work. I went there before the end of the war, which would have been about 1945, and I was taken ill in 1949.

Tuberculosis was a widespread disease in those days. You couldn't think of any family which didn't have it or know somebody who had it. Housing conditions were so small and cramped and overcrowded – that was one of the main causes. I was caught in the early stages of the disease. I was sent away to a sanatorium, Llangwyfan near Denbighshire, a long way from home. We were put in wooden huts and the treatment then was bed rest, bed rest and more bed rest and fresh air. All the windows were open, even in the most bitter winds. We were of a generation to remember the drugs like slippery elm and calf's foot jelly and red and green medicine. That was about all people had. The new drugs, like streptomycin, hadn't been brought in there. I was up in the sanatorium for several months. There were young girls more seriously ill, who we later heard had died, and about the only treatment that was possible was a pneumonectomy – the removal of the lung, or part of the lung. I was sent home, fortunately, without any surgery. I had a long, gradual recovery and frequent check-ups in the chest clinic, and it was deemed to be much better.

While Ruth was working in the laboratory, the NHS began.

Aneurin Bevan started a tour of hospitals and other institutions to inaugurate the National Health Service. One of the hospitals he came to was

Llanfrechfa Grange Hospital, which was then a hospital for the mentally handicapped. My friend Betty Martin and I went there. At that time it was a fashion to collect people's autographs. I went up to Aneurin Bevan and asked him if we could have his autograph. 'Certainly.' A photographer from Newport, Happy Snaps, photographed us. That's how we met Aneurin Bevan. He asked us where we came from, which department, and we told him, and then he went on to speak about the beginning of the National Health Service. I was very young and we were a bit gullible. We were interested in people like film stars and getting famous people's autographs, and the importance of his impact on society didn't really grab me at the time, I must admit – except that we knew something was happening to change it. I didn't have much of an impression of Aneurin Bevan and I didn't know much about him. He wasn't too lofty that he couldn't talk to us. He did ask us where we were from and what we did. And that always has stuck with me.

Ruth died only three months after recording her story in May 2018. In her interview, she said: 'I know some of the things I say will be cut out, but I hope somebody will keep some of it.'

ETHEL ARMSTRONG

Ethel grew up at a time when women didn't have the same opportunities as men. She began as a cadet at one of the large asylums for people with mental illness and on the day the NHS was launched, she began training as a radiographer.

I lived in a terraced house. Two very hardworking parents who were talented people but, in the thirties, never had the opportunities that I had. My father's Aunt Lavinia, who was always called Auntie Veen, ran a doctor's GP service from her little two-bedroomed terrace house. It was absolutely immaculate. Her kitchen was kitted out and the GP would make up all the medicines. A cough bottle, or a rubbing cream for your back. It might cost you a shilling. Patients waited in her front room and Auntie Veen lived in the small dining room at the back. For that, she was paid rent. And that eked out a living and she did that for the best part of 20 years. So I was part of the two-tier health system.

I was quite bright and got a grammar school place. I was desperate to do dentistry or medicine. But in those days, if your parents couldn't keep you for six years till you qualified, there was no way that you could do either of those because there was no grants. I had a wonderful headmaster, Mr Carr, who said, 'You've got every qualification to get you into any university, Ethel, but I'm afraid the two state scholarships will go to two boys who both want to follow their father's footsteps. One wants to go into dentistry, one's toying with either law or medicine.' The state scholarships went to the boys because it was always assumed that they would stay in their career till the day that they retired. So in 1947 the headmaster said, 'I can get you a place in healthcare because there's something going to happen. It's on the cards for a year's time. I can get you a place as a gofer, where at least you would learn the ropes. It opens a door for you to get experience. Even if you can't do medicine, it will at least partly fulfil what the rest of your life is going to be about.'

I was offered a place at St Nicholas's in Gosforth, the largest mental health establishment in the north-east, and I thought, 'Oh, I don't really want to do that.' Mr Carr said, 'Look, do that for 10 months and I'm sure that something will come up around about the middle of next year.' He said, 'I want you to do that because you will learn the basics of protocol, code of conduct and dress code.' So I learnt the ropes of what you can and can't do, if there was going to be this wonderful new system. You spoke when you were spoken to. And you always turned up with shiny shoes, which is one of my trademarks, shiny shoes.

I just wanted to be part of that world. I had no idea where it was going to take me. Because at 17, believe it or not, I had never put one foot inside a hospital door. It was absolutely new. But it was the only pathway that I could see. Mr Carr said, 'You've got to dip your toe in the water. I don't want you to waste the enthusiasm that you've got at the moment.'

Beginning at St Nicholas's, that really was scary. I went on the bus, with shiny shoes and half a crown in my pocket that was my bus fare to get back home again. I saw these big gates and this long drive. I saw people suited in their tweed. It was a hot day and I thought, 'Poor soul, he's got a big tweed jacket on.' These were the inpatients. A lot of them had been incarcerated in that situation because they were shell-shocked. Some of them from the First World War. Their families didn't know how to deal with the terrors, the nightmares and the constant shaking. So they were incarcerated and a lot of them stayed there till they died. The first thing that I was given was a large key on a chain, because every door was locked. There was a long corridor that had seven doors and every one had to be locked. There was a colony there for Down's Syndrome children whose parents didn't know how to look after a Down's child and didn't know how to get the best potential. Now I see so many Down's children and, I mean, they're obviously Down's children, but they're doing jobs, there's no segregation of them at all.

I was in an office with 10 ex-servicemen and grew up very rapidly. We didn't have computers. The only one that had a typewriter was the chief's private secretary. You learnt the importance of record-keeping, filing, proper names, proper data, you know. I would do lots of filing, send out acceptance letters when families asked could they visit their son, or their daughter or whoever. There was only one small wing then for voluntary patients. Most of the patients in the main building had been sectioned and they were there for treatment. I did whatever job came up. There was a laboratory and a very nice gentleman there would tell me what they were doing with these specimens and why they were doing it. I crammed a lot into my 10 months. Plus the fact that I was quite a talented singer in those days and they used to have concerts for the staff, to raise funds for the patients. I was always roped into that. Then they discovered that I was quite a good table tennis player and I was then co-opted onto the men's team. The staff were like a large family. They were good fun to be with, but they were caring and compassionate and kind. I was totally hooked on healthcare, but used to worry about these people that had been in there for so long. 'That can't be right,' I used to think. Mental health was a bit like the 'cancer' word then. In the village, you know, elderly ladies said, 'Oh, poor Mr So-and-so, he's got the big C.' The word 'cancer' was mentioned as though it was a dirty word. And now, thank God, I've seen so many changes in 70 years. I remember with a lot of affection those days. A scary world, but everybody did their best to make it less scary. But – you didn't take things for granted. You always made sure that the doors were locked behind you.

After 10 months I had a note from Mr Carr: 'I've got an appointment for you. They are taking students in the department of radiodiagnosis and I want you to go. I've spoken to one of the consultants who's a colleague of mine. He, too, is a Quaker.' Off I went, with my shiny shoes and half a crown in my pocket, on the 5th of July 1948 to the Royal Victoria Infirmary [RVI] in Newcastle. The consultant said, 'We would like you to join the Queen Elizabeth Hospital in Gateshead. That's where you will get concentrated, good, practical work done.'

Your lectures were done at the RVI. It was hard going in the beginning because juniors did all the jobs. After you'd done your anatomy and your positioning and radiography, which is very exacting, you had to do photography and go into the darkroom. It was all wet processing of film. There was nothing automated. You flew by the seat of your pants. You had a steel rule in your pocket and a straight eye. Radiotherapy was a specialised thing and there was none of the modern equipment that takes away all the nasty side effects, like the skin burning, that the old machine used to have. It was a learning curve. You did all your anatomy in the medical school with a couple of the consultants. There'd be a cadaver laid out on the table and you had to identify parts. Quite honestly, you know, up till then I don't think I had ever even taken a bone out of a piece of meat.

The department opened at half past eight in the morning till five o'clock, and then you were on call with nobody apart from the night porter. That was your eight o'clock at night till eight o'clock in the morning shift, and you had to live in. You had to know how to handle a really badly injured patient coming straight on a trolley from casualty. Then you would go home and wait for your next call.

I qualified in 1951 and was appointed as a junior radiographer at the Queen Elizabeth at £21 a month. I had £17 a month to take home because they deducted meals and laundry for my white coat that had to have every button put in properly. My superintendent was a Scot. She'd never married. She was a delightful tutor and taught me a lot of things I value today. When I qualified, she said, 'The first and most important duty' – and I thought, 'Oh, I'm going to hear words of wisdom here' – 'is that your Chief's coat is always clean, straight from the laundry, well-aired on the radiator and has every button put in. You have to un-starch his sleeves, and do remember to un-starch each pocket, particularly the one where he keeps his pens.' That is the best advice that I've ever had, because if your Chief came in and he'd hit traffic and then he had to try and un-starch his white coat because he couldn't get his arms through the sleeves and he couldn't get his pens in his pocket, oh dear, that was a bad day. He'd go around banging this and banging that. Give him a clean coat with the buttons in and his sleeves open, with pockets he could put his pens in – that was a happy day.

After two more years I was offered a senior post and then I was acting superintendent. In those days, married women who managed to get a super-intendentship were very rare indeed. They were always given to men, who were usually from the military. For a female, I'm very proud to say that in my working career of 42 years, I was head of department four times.

Pneumoconiosis [lung disease caused by inhaling dust often in an industrial workplace] was high and tuberculosis was absolutely the scourge. Whole families were admitted to sanatoriums way out in the wilds. You staffed those with two juniors and you. You were a totally self-sufficient unit. They all had to have routine chest X-rays. If one in the household was picked up with tuberculosis, then the wife had to be screened, the children had to be screened. If they had got a suspicion or confirmation of early tuberculosis, then the men would go into the men's ward of the sanatorium, the women would go into the women's ward, the children would go into the children's unit. They'd be incarcerated, bed-rested for 18 months. Everywhere was freezing cold. The windows would be almost at right angles, and the wind used to whistle in. Treatment was bed rest, fresh air and good food. After the Second World War, we had rationing until the fifties. So milk, eggs and cheese, that was part of your recovery treatment. When the first drug treatment came out, the tablets were as big as horse pills and were called PAS [para-aminosalicylic acid]. That did eliminate a lot of the long-stay patients for tuberculosis who could be managed at home. I think now of the number that I used to X-ray regularly for update and review that had had one lung totally removed. The whole of that side was caved in. It was quite mutilating surgery.

In 1956 Ethel's husband – 'my true North' – was offered a job in London, where Ethel also found work. We'll join her next in the 1980s, when she becomes involved in pioneering breast screening.

NORMAN SHARP

Aged five, Norman became severely ill with septic arthritis, which caused permanent damage to his hips and joints. His story bridges the coming of the NHS and the value of innovations in orthopaedic surgery driven by the Second World War. In November 1948 he underwent one of the first hip replacements on the new NHS. Doctors did not involve patients in decisions about their treatments at this time, which meant that Norman had no idea of what had been done to him, or that he was making history.

In 1930 I started school aged five, a perfectly normal kid, and I'd only went to school a couple of weeks and I became poorly. And I had to go to bed. Mother had to call the doctor. And after a few days, I was blue around the groin. And doctor said, 'Well, you'll have to get Norman to a hospital, Mrs Sharp.' But the ambulance took me to the workhouse, which provided care for very poor people, because the workhouse was the only place that had a sick room for the children.

Middlesex County Council took over the workhouse the same year that Norman was admitted and changed the name to Hillingdon County Hospital.

I was very poorly. They said I'd got septic arthritis and it had gone to the hips, and of course, that attacks the cartilages, and so when you move your joints there's nothing to grease them, so to speak. And that was very painful. I can remember a wound at the top of the right hip that they used to come around every day and syringe out. When anybody came near the bed, it seemed to start me crying. They decided that everybody should walk on the other side of the ward when they had to pass my bed. Those days they had screens at the top of the ward and the bottom of the ward, and they used to have to fetch them from one end or the other, if they were doing any treatment at the beds.

The doctor told Father there's nothing more they could do and he would have to put me on open order. That meant that your days were numbered. It meant that parents could come and visit you any time of the day or night, and bring you your last wish. Father said, 'Is there anything you'd like, my lad?' I said, 'I would love some fish and chips, Dad.' And when I'd eaten them, he said, 'Did you enjoy that?' I said, 'Oh, lovely, can I have some more tomorrow?'

Remembering the struggle that his parents would have had in finding the money to buy him the fish and chips reduced Norman to tears. Contrary to the doctor's predictions, Norman did not decline and was put on a treatment regime of massage, sunray and electrical therapies.

Mother used to push me to Hillingdon Hospital, three miles in the pram, three times a week for massage and treatment. The sunray treatment was first and that was like a big lamp, about two-foot diameter with two sticks of carbon. You laid on the massage bed in the nude, and they put the lamp down on you and that was nice and comfortable. But you were only allowed about 10 minutes of that, and then you had a massage all the way up the legs and the back. Mr Woodcock was a blind masseur. He used to get his watch out and feel the face and say to me, 'It's half past 10, Norman, that's in the morning.' Then we'd come to the electrical treatment and that was a little box, two wires coming out of it, and the wires had a brass pad on each end of the wire. They'd put one brass pad on your thigh just above your knee and tie that on with a wet bandage. And then they'd put your foot into a bowl of water and throw the other pad into the bowl of water. You got this tingly feeling. I could turn the knob up and increase the pulses to what I could stand. The treatment stimulated the muscles and after they'd been massaged were all nice and free, and limp. You could imagine – because you wouldn't experience it – how your legs would feel good, as if you've done a long run.

Norman was sent to the country branch of the Royal National Orthopaedic Hospital (RNOH) in Stanmore, which provided specialist care for children suffering from tuberculosis in bones and joints.

The first thing they did was to put me in a plaster of Paris cast. Us kids called it a 'full spiker'. You can't sit up or anything, but you just look down from your neck and you see the toes sticking out and then it's plaster all the way up your legs, up your tummy, to your chest, to about the nipple line. And of course, plaster don't move. The first few days you just don't know what you're going to do with yourself. I got my sister to send up a big 12- to 14-inch knitting needle. When you got that knitting needle slid down inside the plaster cast, and you found the itchy spot, oh, that was beautiful! The knitting needle was your best friend. We used to have a lot of fun, the kids. It wasn't all doom and gloom.

The time came for the plaster to come off after about 12 weeks. That was another operation. The man came with the shears, like tree croppers today – and he'd put these croppers down the side of your toe and start nibbling away at the plastic. And, of course, the first problem was the ankle, he had to get round the ankle to get up the leg. That could take a long time because he'd have to just crop the plaster away, and after a few oohs and aahs, he'd get round the ankle and come up your shin, your leg. And then, of course, the next problem was the knee. So he gets around the knee and then once he'd done that, he would start off under your arm, up your chest and start going down. And he'd meet up. The hip wasn't too bad because that doesn't protrude. The inside of the leg was very difficult because he had a job to get the shears in to get up the inside. Eventually the plaster cast was in two sections. You can't move, you've got no strength after 12 weeks, you just laid there. I can see it clear as crystal. I was so uncomfortable because the beds, they were hard those days that I couldn't rest. So the Sister had the bottom half of the plaster brought back to the ward. They cleaned it all out and relined it with gauze and cotton wool, and they placed me back into the bottom half of that plaster cast. And of course, I was comfortable then because that had been my home for 12 weeks and it fit and everything. They allowed me to have that for two or three nights. Then they had to teach me to walk because the plaster cast had done its job. It had fused the hips so I had no hips. I wobbled along like a duck, from the knees.

Norman was discharged out of Stanmore after 18 months with a caliper (splint) to support his leg and, aged six, returned to school.

I went back to school and, in the morning playtime, I went over to the toilets, which was a little brick place out in the playground, all open, no roof or anything; it was just three walls. You went in and had your wee. I had a caliper on – that's a splint on my leg – and this other kiddie was in there and he started taking the mickey out of my caliper and me walking. So I punched him on the nose and he went howling back into the school. The teacher got wound up then, and so they sent me home. And they said, 'I'm sorry, we can't let you come to this school, Norman, because we're frightened you're going to get knocked over.' Nobody was going to knock me over – I was a tough little kiddie. But the fact that I'd hit this chap and they thought, 'Well, if he hits him back with the caliper on ….' So I couldn't go to school. The School Board man comes round, and after a while they said, 'He'll have to go to a special school.' They called them crippled schools then – they wouldn't use the term today. And my mother said, 'He's not going to a cripple school. He's been 18 months in hospital. He's not going away again, I don't want him to go away again.' So my dad said, 'Well, all right then, if that's what you wish, then he won't go.' And it went on and on for weeks and months, and they were going to send my father to prison because I wasn't going to school. And he found out that if he could get me into a private school, I wouldn't come under the jurisdiction of the county. And there was a girls' private school across the road. So he got me in there. So I went to the girls' school.

I had no pain. I was walking from my knees. I couldn't run or anything, but I made those legs work hard. I got friendly with the other boys in the village and got friends. We'd go down the river paddling in the little stream and we'd go up to the closes with the swings and the slides. I joined in everything that they did. When they climbed a tree, I climbed the tree, but I used to go up like a monkey with me arms and just rest on my legs, and up to the next branch. But, yes, I did everything that the boys done. I used to like wrestling with the kids, because if I could pull them to the ground, I was their equal.

In 1939, aged 13, Norman went to the London branch of the Royal National Orthopaedic Hospital in Great Portland Street for more treatment.

Dr Rocyn-Jones, he straightened one of my legs. They broke the thigh halfway along and that was another plaster job. But I only had one leg in plaster then and that was on for 11 weeks. They used to have tapioca for pudding, and I couldn't abide tapioca. And the Sister come back in and she says, 'You've got to eat it, it's the food, and you've got to eat it.' And she started picking up this tapioca in the spoon and trying to work it into my mouth. And so I took a mouthful and I spat it all over her.

On 31 August 1939 these men in black caps and black suits came around, saying, 'Everybody out, everybody out!' So Father had to come up to London and fetch me because I'd just come out of a plaster a couple of days and I couldn't walk. On the Sunday, September 3rd, the war was declared. That's why they emptied all the hospitals – for the wounded servicemen. At 11 o'clock the sirens all went and everybody was stood at the front garden gate looking up for the bombers.

Norman served an apprenticeship as a toolmaker, working at the gramophone company HMV's factory in Hayes, which developed and manufactured radio equipment during the war. At 21 years old, he says, 'I was one of the boys. Used to go up to London, to the Hammersmith Palais de Danse – and that was all right until about 1944, when the Americans come over. Then we give up. We just didn't have the nylon stockings or the chocolate to attract the girls.'

I was agitating for an NHS when I first started work. I worked next to a chappie that was rather keen politically in those days, because he would tell you he was a communist. And of course, Russia was our friends back in those days, so there was no risk about talking about them. Those days it was all, 'Everybody's in it together.' And he learnt me a lot when I started work. There were quite a lot of us and we used to go into Hayes Park, near the factory site, and have a meeting. We talked about the people that can't afford care, whether there should be this and there should be that, and people should be able to get a doctor when they need one and things like that.

The NHS was all free and nobody had to struggle and worry where the next bottle of medicine was coming from. My mother was one of the first beneficiaries. She got a hearing aid. She had a big bag that she used to carry the batteries in, and then a wire going up. She used to put it under her blouse, round her neck, into her hearing aid.

In November 1948, out of the blue, Norman was called back to Stanmore.

Professor Seddon came to visit me. 'Young man,' he said, 'I'd like Mr Newman to see you. He's just come back from America on a new idea they've got.' The next week Mr Newman came in and said, 'I think we can help you.' He said to the Sister, 'I'll do the first one next week and the second one three weeks later. He'll be on penicillin three days before, and two weeks after the operation, and M and B [a sulphonamide that treated bacterial infections].'

I just assumed that he was going to do the straightening on my left leg. I knew it was something special because as soon as Professor Seddon was mentioned coming to see me, it was a big flap in the ward. I came back from the operation, and the first thing I did was felt down ... Where's the plaster? I couldn't feel a plaster. And I thought, 'My goodness me, what's this, no plaster? I've always had to have plaster.'

Three weeks later I went down again. I still didn't know what they were doing. After the second op, they brought the X-ray machine to the bed. That was the first time I knew what they had done. I saw these two cups on my hips. That was the first time I'd ever heard about cups. And that was after the second op. Because doctors didn't discuss with you, you see. They only talked amongst themselves. They never discussed with the patient what they were going to do, or anything like that, like they do now. I think today you'd get every detail. But those days, the patient wasn't involved.

Norman had undergone the first hip replacement ever done on the NHS on 1 December 1948, with the second hip replacement completed on 22 December 1948. The septic arthritis he'd suffered as a little boy had damaged the lining of the joints. During the operation Newman inserted cups made of Vitallium, an alloy developed in the US in the 1930s, between the head of the thigh bone and the hip socket.

The chappie opposite me was an elderly chappie, Jimmy. I said to him, 'What's all this about then like, Jimmy?' So he told me what they were and he said, 'I'll send you over a magazine.' He had a magazine in his locker that was all about these cups. It told you that they'd tried these new cups out in America. I didn't know it was pioneering surgery. It was just I'd had a couple of cups put in. My knees were stuck together all my life. I couldn't get two fingers between my knees. When I woke up, I could get five fingers or more, my whole hand between my knees. That's the first time I can remember ever parting my legs and that was the marvellous thing. I just felt good. But I wasn't allowed to walk on them for six months. I had to go to the pool and exercise. The ward orderly pushed me down to the pool in the chair and lifted my legs in. They put a chute into the pool, lifted me onto the chute, and I slid down the chute into the pool!

We had a pilot come in from a plane that had crashed in Italy. He was a big noise. He used to get these stewardesses to bring in a case full of food, because food was still on ration. When the Sisters had gone home at night, he'd get the food out – tomatoes, sandwiches and that. And I said, 'Oh, we need a drink with all this.' So I go round the ward and make a collection. Then, in my wheelchair, I'd go out of the hospital. I found a pub. I spent all this money. There was a tray in the bottom of my wheelchair. The landlord used to come out and put all the bottles in the tray for me. I'd have a blanket over so nobody could see. I'd go back and we'd have a party. The nurses went off at about eight o'clock. Once the Night Sister had been round, we'd say, 'Little parcel for you on the table, Sister.' Then she'd go, 'You behave yourself, you boys.' We wouldn't see her all night then. And we'd have this party. Of course, it soon got notorious. All the nurses then started to come into our parties. This is in 1949. It couldn't happen today. We had control of the kitchen, so all this food that this pilot used to get in – steaks and tomatoes – at 10 o'clock we used to start doing a fry-up. It could well have been Butlin's, we had so much fun. I got my brother to bring in the gramophone and a load of records, and I had it on the side of my bed there, the old wind-up gramophone. One of them at the end of the ward would shout, 'How about a bit of music, Norman?' 'So what do you want?' 'Oh, "Twelfth Street Rag".' So I'd play a record for them and then they'd start picking the tunes, and we'd have a dozen records or so.

So you had beer, you had food, you had women – and you were DJing?

I'm not ashamed of it, but I did instigate rather a lot when I think about it!

I was in Stanmore for six months or more. And then they sent me to Farnham Royal Recuperative Home. It wasn't long before we had parties there as well! I was just as fit as a fiddle and there was nothing wrong with me. I was in no pain. I've never even taken an aspirin for my hips. I've never been to the doctor's. The last person to inspect my hips was Mr Newman, the surgeon himself, in 1949. It was definitely Mr Newman's courage that won through, because he wasn't encouraged by the other doctors. They all said, 'Oh, he's too young' and everything. He had a bit of resistance. But Professor Seddon said, 'Norman was a good case.' Professor Seddon was the big man at Stanmore and his word was it. He said to Mr Newman, 'That's all right.' So the other doctors just had to sit back, tongue in cheek.

On his return home Norman was invited to a neighbour's wedding. While in hospital he'd learnt how to play the piano, as the wards he'd stayed on had pianos.

I went up on the stage and I sat at the piano and started playing and got the kids around me. This young lady came up and we started talking and it turned out she was a nurse at Stanmore. She'd started a few months after I'd left. We just hit it off. And we got married and hence four boys, grandchildren and lots of great-grandchildren.

I owe my life to the NHS. I could never have paid for the treatment that I've had, and the attention. It was a marvellous thing. It included everybody. It was one of the biggest things that's happened in my lifetime. Even makes the war look small fry.

Norman suffered no more problems from his hips for the rest of his life. In 2019 he entered the Guinness Book of Records for having the world's longest-lasting hip replacement. Interviewed when he was aged 94, he said, 'I've still got the pictures in my mind of when I was five years old, they're as clear as crystal. And I feel that should be given to the benefit of other people to learn and understand how it was years ago.' He died in August 2021 and donations from his funeral were given to the Royal Orthopaedic National Hospital at Stanmore.

At the end of the 1940s

The NHS was the first health system in the world to offer free and comprehensive state-provided healthcare to the whole of the population. Millions of people who could not afford to pay for healthcare, including women, children, the elderly, the disabled and the unemployed, were able to seek treatment after 5 July 1948. The public take-up of services was rapid and exceeded all expectations, with patients flocking to see GPs and to get dental treatment and spectacles. Dentists fitted over 33 million artificial teeth over the first nine months of the NHS, as people who had suffered poor dental health for decades sought treatment.[7] More than 33,000 prescriptions for surgical boots and appliances were issued in the month of November 1948 alone.[8] The creation of the NHS met the aspirations of campaigners like Joan Meredith, who wanted everyone in society to have the same access to healthcare that she and her family enjoyed.

A universal health system also meant that everyone could benefit from the most recent scientific and medical advances, including new drugs and innovative surgical techniques. The NHS was established at a point when science and medicine seemed truly to be conquering infectious diseases and extending life. Diseases with high mortality rates, like TB, could be cured with antibiotics. Smallpox and diphtheria were preventable thanks to vaccines. New surgical techniques enabled chronic painful conditions – such as arthritis in the hip – to be treated by the insertion of artificial joint replacements. Norman Sharp's story exemplifies how the NHS changed people's lives by giving them access to the very latest treatments, regardless of their financial resources. He was in his early twenties when he had two hip replacement operations in December 1948 to treat a painful and disabling condition he had lived with since the age of five. He was freed from pain and disability for the rest of his life. Without the NHS it is unlikely that he could ever have afforded the treatment – and little wonder that he believed he owed his life to the NHS.

Norman's gratitude was multiplied millions of times over by other patients who benefited from care during the early months of the NHS.

Contemporary surveys show that by 1949, the British public viewed the NHS as an institution which embodied national pride and values, affirming Aneurin Bevan's claim that a universal comprehensive Service that separated access to care from payment was a mark of a civilised society. In practice the NHS was introduced through three separate Acts of Parliament covering England and Wales, Scotland and Northern Ireland. But it quickly became known and talked about as a single system, a fact that reveals the deep relationship that was developing between the public and the NHS, and the ways in which the NHS would become so much more than a health service.

In 1948 and the years immediately following its introduction, the new NHS embodied the post-war hope and optimism for a better future for all citizens, regardless of class, politics, religion or geography. The first challenge it faced in the 1950s was that of building a larger workforce and expanding its services.

Chapter 2:
1950s

'Most people got polio, it affected their legs.
Mine ... affected my arm. I can't use my left arm.'

KEN MURRAY

'We became like mothers to them. We all had our favourite.'

SYLVIA NEWMAN

'There were 10 medical schools in London.
I was turned down by eight of them.'

SONYA BAKSI

'Winston Churchill, the prime minister ...
said there were jobs waiting. It was like an invitation.'

TRYPHENA ANDERSON

'We had to call ourselves Mr Carroll and Miss Margison.
We weren't allowed to mix.'

BRIAN AND PAT CARROLL

*'Everything is against you when you are getting
a footing in a foreign country.'*

DIPANKAR DATTA

*'So they banned my mum and dad from seeing me.
Can you believe that?'*

PATRICIA

*'If a patient is crying ... we sit at the edge of the bed
and hold the patient's hand.'*

ANTONETTE CLARKE-AKALANNE

*'We used to like it really when they cried because
they was showing some sign of recovery.'*

MARGARET BATTY

*'Volunteering ... took a lot of your time up,
but you were doing good for other people.'*

HAROLD MERCER

KEN MURRAY

Ken was born into a working-class family in Gateshead in 1946.

I contracted polio in 1948 aged two. My sister told me I was really ill with high temperatures. She can remember the doctor coming and giving me a pencil to hold. Tried it with one hand, then tried it with the other. I could hold it in this one. But I couldn't hold it in that one. [*shows interviewer which one is which*] I was in an iron lung for a number of years. My parents were only allowed to visit me once a month. That was through glass; they could only stand outside. My siblings weren't allowed to come. The hospital used to have a balcony and when you were in bed they used to push you out on the balcony, doesn't matter what the weather was. As I got older I was allowed to come home at weekends. My sister used to say that I was always crying for the nurse. The iron lung was part of the treatment for polio because it helped you to breathe and get oxygen. Most people got polio, it affected their legs. Mine didn't. It affected my arm and it stopped at my right elbow. I can't lift my arms up. I can't use my left hand. I've got restriction in my right hand, right arm. Muscle wastage in both arms. When I was younger, I had real bother with my chest breathing, bronchitis, because my chest is very narrow. I was always frightened of dogs when I was older. And I wondered why, because we've never had a dog. My mother told me that while I was in hospital, my arms were suspended up in a bed, and a dog got into the hospital and jumped on the bed. And that's why I was frightened of them.

I was a spoiled brat when I came out! I went to the Cedars School for handicapped children. I was now aged nine or 10. My father was very staunch Catholic. [*laughs*] I'm laughing because it was harvest festival time and you had to take in fruit and vegetable to school. I remember coming home singing, 'Bringing in the Sheaves'. My father clouted me across the back of my head – 'Stop singing Protestant songs in my house!' I used to go to the hospital twice a week to have electric treatment through my muscles to try and stimulate them. They were like a pencil with an electrode on the end, and they used two of them, like when you were in the lab when you were a kid and used to dissect a frog and touch parts of the frog to see how its nerves work. They give me a splint and this thing was like a false arm. It was like a gadget that went on your arm and you could lift it up and it would lock and you could lift it again, it would lock in different positions. But it was no good. It used to rip every shirt I had. It was funny, you talk about the NHS expense, they used to send an ambulance for me, two guys, for one person, twice a week! After a while they did nothing and I just got on with my life, basically.

My parents said I wasn't getting educated, so they sent me to an ordinary school, which was an eye-opener. A very rough school, but I was quite happy there. I left when I was 15 and went to work at Armstrong Whitworth in Gateshead metal industries. The only education I can remember in hospital was very minimal. The most education I got was my parents. I can't hold a pen properly, so I write like this [*shows interviewer how he writes*]. I adapted the way of working for me. I had to learn to fasten my clothes, I had to learn to put them on, to take them off. Couldn't fasten shoe laces, still can't – it's one thing I cannot do, fasten bloody shoelaces! [*chuckles*] The job I had was office work. You used to have to wear a tie. I remember my father teaching me how to put a Windsor knot in with one hand, and I can still do it.

If you went for a job it's like, 'Does he take sugar?' attitude. Basically, he's good at his job. But the point is he could be sick, he could do this, he could do that, and we would lose more time. Therefore, we're better off employing somebody else. That was an attitude that you lived with in those days. In the 1990s I was on a management staff committee which met once a month … with the board of directors of NEEPCO [North Eastern Electric Power Corporation]. The Disability Act came in and, of course, I've been registered disabled for a long time. There was a real nice man, a real gentleman. He said, 'NEEPCO's policy was that they would treat everybody who was disabled as able-bodied and they would have the same rights.' 'Can I ask this question?' 'Yes.' 'Two people go for a job, one's in a wheelchair and one isn't. The one in the wheelchair's got more qualifications and more experience than the able-bodied person. Who do you give the job to?' 'Chap in the wheelchair, obviously.' 'How does he get in the building?' 'Sorry?' 'How does he get in the building? You haven't got any ramps or steps. There isn't a toilet available for a wheelchair. You couldn't employ them unless you spend thousands on alterations. Do you employ him?' He just went, 'Mmm, we will have to look at that.'

I contracted what's called PPS – post-polio syndrome – about two years ago. Not much known about post-polio syndrome. The Americans did some work on it. It's like polio, again. Getting over all the infections is a lot harder but that could be to do with age as well [*chuckles*]. It can be fine for two weeks, it can be fine for two months. The only way I can explain it in words is, it's like having a 48-inch chest inside a 38-inch frame. It's hard. It's painful. You can't fix it. I go to the doctor. He just shakes his head, 'There's nothing I can do.' 'Alright, I'll send you for some tests.' I just want them to know how to manage it. At the moment I manage it with CBD oil. And it works for me. Might be in my head. I don't know. But I take it every day. It doesn't kill it the pain, but it helps.

Ken was born at a time when severe epidemics of polio left many children crippled with permanent disabilities. Mass routine vaccination programmes for children had been introduced with the NHS for diphtheria, TB, smallpox and whooping cough. In 1956 a polio vaccine was introduced, which was later replaced by a live-attenuated vaccine delivered on sugar cubes.

SYLVIA NEWMAN

Sylvia was one of many young girls who joined the NHS as cadet nurses straight out of school.

My mother said I would make a good nurse. When I was 16, I finished my exams at school in July '49, and by August 15th, I started my nursing career. My mother had got the application form, and it was to work on a premature baby unit at the hospital in North Shields. 'Why do you want to be a nurse?' It was a very simple interview from the matron. The reason they used cadet nurses was to work on the premature baby unit. There hadn't been one before the NHS, and it was one big room with six cots and two incubators. We took babies who were under five pounds in weight. In 1949 the viable age of a baby was 28 weeks.

Can you remember your first day as a cadet?

Yes, vividly. I was really wanting to start, and yet anxious. The uniform was green check. We didn't wear aprons; you just wore the uniform. I was greeted friendly by the Sister and partnered up with one of the other nurses, and she showed me how to feed babies, and how to look after them, and explained about the Oxygenaire neonatal incubator that allowed oxygen and carbon dioxide levels to be measured and adjusted. Then I went up to the dining room for breakfast. All the meals were free at that time. One of the ward maids said, 'Oh, you'll get used to this, don't worry.' She realised I was a newcomer. But that's what they were like in the hospital; they were quite friendly.

The Ward Sister was very good, she was like a mother to us. I wouldn't say she was a disciplinarian, but she knew we had standards to maintain, and she kept us right with whatever we did. We wore a gown and a mask to go into this nursery for feeding. The cleaners had to be in earlier, and they oiled the floor so that dust didn't fly around. But we didn't have very good arrangements for sterilisation. Each bottle had to be made up separately for the babies. We had to sterilise bottles and teats by boiling them. There was no pre-packed tubes, or anything like that. We were taught to tube feed as well. About four or five months after I had been there, they managed to arrange to have a milk kitchen with a steriliser and a fridge there for bottles, so we could make bottles up and store them.

You weren't allowed to go on the other wards, because of risk of cross infection. We didn't have many deaths. There was one spell when there was an outbreak of vomiting and diarrhoea among babies, and we lost babies then. We became like mothers to them. We all had our favourites. And we tended to keep to the same babies so they weren't crossed over all the time. If you fed the baby in cot number two, another nurse would look after others. It was a very relaxed atmosphere. The unfortunate thing is the mothers were never allowed to handle their babies. There were long windows, and the mothers could just look in, which would be totally unacceptable now, but that's how it was then, for the risk of infection. Even when babies died, we had to lay them out.

It was always a nice day when the baby reached five pounds and could be dressed in their own clothes and handed to their parents. There was no teaching to the parents, no preparation for them to look after these babies when they got home. They would obviously be visited by a health visitor, but we didn't do any of that teaching. It was a very happy ward to be on, and the Sister looked after us very well. We never felt that it was difficult; we enjoyed it. Your salary was £7 a month.

Sylvia began full nurse training at the age of 18.

The first day, we all had to go and report to the matron. You were called 'pinkies', because your uniform was pink and you wore starched aprons and starched caps. Because you were a resident in the nurses' home for three months, you had to hand your ration book in. Every week, you were given two jam jars, one with your butter in, one with your sugar ration. I can tell you, the butter was probably rancid by the end of the week, because you just kept it in your bedrooms.

The matron said, 'You're starting your training, and I wish you well. Take an interest in everything that you're taught.' The first week was spent in the classroom with a tutor. You were then allocated to whichever ward. Lectures usually came in the evening, because the Ward Sisters weren't keen on letting you off for an afternoon lecture. We did have one or two in the afternoon, and they were always the consultants. Every week you went into the class-room for a Saturday morning, and you got more lectures then, and tests.

The nursing hierarchy consisted of the matron, the assistant matron and the Home Sister. There was one Ward Sister per ward, and she had senior staff nurses. We did have probationer nurses, perhaps three or four, in train-ing. Then there were the domestic staff. Ward cleaners, who – they did the floors, sweeping and that kind of thing. The ward maids, they did things like clean the lockers, and wash the beds and served the meals.

State Enrolled Nurses (SENs) only did two years training, and there was a limit ... they couldn't administer dangerous drugs, things like that. Some of these male nurses who were SENs had been in the forces and had worked with the medical corps in the Far East or wherever the war was going on. A few of them remained as SENs, but others took the extra year's training and became State Registered Nurses (SRNs). So after the SENs came the auxiliary nurses. They were hands-on. They did the bedpans – and it wasn't only handing them out, it was cleaning them. And the same with sputum mugs used to collect phlegm that patients coughed up. That was a job I hated. I shudder now when I think about it. That was the hierarchy of the nursing profession.

As a student you did give bedpans out, you did bathing. When the consultant did the ward round, it was your job to drag the screens round the patient. And when the consultant came, you were the one that had to expose the patient, wherever she was going to be examined. You were taught all of that. If it was chest examination, you cover them up to the waist. If it was abdominal, you would expose them from the armpits down, and all this kind of thing. You were learning, because the consultants didn't go out of the room to discuss. I always seem to remember them discussing at the edge of the bed. The only record at the end of the bed was a temperature chart – you didn't have records. I was more nervous of the consultant. Because it was a bit like the *Doctor in the House* film. They were the hierarchy.

You were always in awe of the consultants because you revered them, you really did. We were really subserving, even to the doctors. Some of them were junior and hadn't been in hospital as long as we had. At the end of the three months, you had learned quite a bit on each ward. There were no intensive care units in those days. The ill patients were in the first two beds on the ward, and if they were terminally ill, they were in a side ward. And there was nothing like chemotherapy then. Cancer patients were treated just with tender love and care, nursing care.

At the end of the third year, it was your finals. The day I sat my examination it was June 2nd 1951 and it was Derby Day. I was leaving the house. My dad said, 'Does anybody want to have a horse on the Derby?' I looked down this newspaper, 'Never Say Die'. I won £2, which was a lot then. In the final exams you were asked to do things like set a tray if the doctor wants to take a blood specimen, or set a trolley for putting in a blood transfusion. They questioned you while you were doing it. You had to wait six weeks for your results. That was nerve-wracking. They came to matron. You had to all queue up to go in. She congratulated you and allocated you to a ward.

There were no kidney units, or specialist units for any particular disease or complication. One of the things that did materialise quite quickly was the opening of the Ear, Nose and Throat unit about 1951/2. It was all fitted out and they had their own theatre. Because everything was free, lots of mothers had their children have their tonsils out. Whether it was necessary or not, I don't know.

The children's ward was very small, only had about eight to 10 beds. They were mostly children, who were maybe asthmatic, or a fracture patient. Those children seemed to be in for weeks. The visiting time was very sparse, only on a Sunday afternoon for an hour. That's the only time they saw their parents, so that wasn't very good. Their parents would bring treats in for them, but they were all centralised in a cupboard, so that all the children got the same. We might have let them have one little thing that their mum had brought in, but mostly, they were shared out, because some children didn't have anything brought in. So it was to just keep them all the same.

Sylvia specialised in midwifery before leaving to get married in 1959. She was asked to return in 1964, even though she was married with children. In 1984 she became deputy director of maternity nursing for North Tyneside, and eventually retired in 1996. She continues to value her early time as cadet. 'You got an insight into hospital life. It was like a bit of a grounding. You learnt discipline. You respected your seniors.'

SONYA BAKSI

Sonya's paternal grandparents were Jewish refugees from Poland, and her maternal grandparents came from Germany and Lithuania. Her father won a place at Guy's Medical School in London and later met Sonya's mother at a hunger march in Stamford Hill. Both parents were passionate about improving health, and took the children on their travels. 'We went round all the hospitals in East Germany, we went round Hungary. There was such hope. There was such belief in how health could be improved. If you work from the bottom and look at the factories and look at the children and look at the housing and look at the food. This was the orientation that my parents had because they had been denied all these things in their own upbringing.'

I went to a girls' grammar school. All our teachers were women. None of them were married because of the marriage bar in the 1930s. If you were married, you weren't allowed to teach anymore, because the teaching jobs had to go to the men. All my life, I've grown up with quotas. There was a quota in the schools with scholarships. Only one in six could be Jewish. So 36 girls in my class, six Jewish, 30 not.

My brother wanted to be a doctor, and my father didn't want him to be a doctor. My father wanted me to be the doctor – and I didn't want to be the doctor [*laughs*]. I think he wanted women to be doctors. There were 10 medical schools in London. I was turned down by eight of them. When I went to the one that my father trained at, they always ask you, 'Have you any connection to school?' 'Just my father.' 'What was his name?' 'Samuel Lefkovitch.' That was the end of the interview. Another interview, they said, 'What position do you play on the rugby field?' 'I don't play rugby.' They looked up from my papers and saw that I was a bloody woman [*chuckles*]. That was how it was. When I got to University College London, they said, 'Do you have any connection with the school?' 'Yes, my brother is studying here.' They took me in.

One of the older medical students took us around. He stopped in the room with all the corpses, knowing that most of us would be seeing a corpse for the first time. He stood there to tell us what books to get. And he did it on purpose. Everybody's beginning to feel queasy and thinking, 'How can I do this?', you know? When we had our first anatomy lesson, and they pulled the sheets off, there was six of us around our table. 'Who's gonna do the first cut?' I had to do it. Nobody else wanted to do it. Somebody had to do it.

I found the training very difficult. I remember coming home crying after seeing a Maltese diabetic patient who was going blind, and how lonely he was on the ward. My father said to me, 'You've got to learn to care and not to care.' Afterwards, I used to say, when I'm teaching, 'When the patient comes into your room, nothing in the world exists except the patient in front of you. And when the patient leaves the room, he doesn't exist anymore. Otherwise, you can't cope.' The whole world is the person in front of you when they come. And when they've gone, that's it.

It was five long years. The time that I really felt I was doing proper work was obstetrics. We lived in, and we did the deliveries. My father died three months before I qualified. It was a very hard time in my life. Being obsessive, I went through every medical exam paper and did little short answers for how I would approach the questions. There wasn't anything that came up that I hadn't done a short answer on. I walked out of all my papers an hour early. They were three-hour papers. My friends thought, 'Poor Sonya, she's having such a tough time. And now she's gonna fail.' But, of course, I didn't. I passed and I got a job in my teaching hospital, which is kudos, especially for a woman. When we graduated, the men were called 'Doctor' and I was called 'Miss'. For the first year I was not allowed to use the title 'Doctor'.

Sonya was to become active in the abortion law reform movement in the 1960s.

TRYPHENA ANDERSON

Tryphena was born in a small village in Jamaica in 1933 and came to train in nursing in the NHS. Britain had suffered shortages of nurses and auxiliary staff since the 1930s. The new NHS needed more staff, and a solution was found through recruiting people from British colonies and former colonies, in the first instance from the West Indies, including Barbados, Jamaica, Trinidad, Saint Kitts and the Windward Islands.

People came out to Jamaica like Winston Churchill, the prime minister, and Enoch Powell, and said there were jobs waiting. It was like an invitation. England was recruiting especially for nurses in the West Indies. At that time, in Jamaica, although you have a British education and you've got some exams under your belt, where were the jobs? When the invitation was put out, parents who had a piece of land, or who had a bit of money or some timber that could be sold, they were willing to sacrifice this for one person or more to go to England, have a proper profession or work in industry. At the same time, you're committed to sending money back home because your fare has to be paid for so somebody else could come.

I had a friend that was working at the general hospital and she asked the matron, should I have the interview in Jamaica. Matron was crafty: 'No, come and be interviewed here.' They made an appointment for me to go to the Labour Exchange on Castle Boulevard in Nottingham. I was interviewed there and I was accepted.

During training you didn't just go on the wards, they'd take you to places connected to medicine, like where Boots used to make the insulin from the animals. And we went to visit where Florence Nightingale lived in Derbyshire.

My aim was to be a health visitor from the start. All you need, if you are white, was SRN [State Registered Nurse] maybe just six months, or three months midwifery and you're in; but I'm Black. My mother always said, 'If you want to get on, you've got to get more than they have.' So, I've done three specialities, that means I've got psychiatric, got general, got midwifery. When I passed my psychiatric exam, I went into matron's office: 'You've passed, Nurse.' I gave such a beaming smile. 'Yes, Nurse, you've passed, but your troubles have only just begun. Because before, somebody was responsible for whatever mistake you made, but now you're going to be responsible for yourself and somebody else's mistake. How do you like that?'

Tryphena became the first Black health visitor in the UK in 1996. She worked for the NHS for over 30 years.

BRIAN and PAT CARROLL

Mass radiography screening campaigns were one of the NHS's successes. Chest radiography – X rays – was used to detect TB in patients well before the NHS, but once antibiotics proved an effective treatment, attention focused on detecting TB in the population at large. Brian and Pat worked together on a mass radiography unit in Manchester. Brian was born in Longsight, Manchester, and during the Blitz his family moved to Moss Side. Pat came from Cheshire: 'I'm not a Mancunian. I have to make it clear. I was born in Wilmslow, grew up in Disley. So I'm a Cheshire cat.' Brian went into the RAF as a photographer and was 'directed into radiography' when he came out. Meanwhile, Pat had joined the NHS.

How did you meet?

Brian: [*laughs*] I was X-raying people coming through. She was interviewing them.

Pat: I was taking their details before they went through for X-rays. It was a mass miniature radiography unit based at Monsall Hospital in Manchester, but we covered all of Manchester and Salford over two or three years. We didn't have a van like other mass radiography units. Everything was moved by a pantechnicon van. Every fortnight the X-ray equipment, the generator, the office equipment was loaded up and taken to our next survey site. It was screening for TB, lung cancer, heart disease.

Brian: By the time we got to it, the original target – TB – had more or less disappeared. We started finding lung cancer. So that was a new beehive.

Pat: There weren't, at that time, power-assisted steering vehicles. We were X-raying at big companies that had a lot of drivers, and finding drivers of these whacking great heavy vehicles that had a heart problem they didn't know about. The idea was to try and eradicate TB. We had GP referrals, we had the general public that could come in and the results were sent to their own home, we had the National Service boys. Part of the medical for the lads going into the forces was to have a stamped chest X-ray. They would come to us on Monday morning for their X-rays. Always great fun. They were quite a larky lot.

Brian: Absolute havoc. We put up these partitions to form dressing rooms and what have you. And large arrows pointing the way through. By the time we'd finished, they were all pointing at the ceiling!

Pat: We went to factories, drill halls, church halls. We had big companies that would send all their staff to the nearest place where we were doing a survey. Everywhere we learnt about what people made, or what they did. 'Are you one of the confectioners that makes those little pineapple boats?' 'Yes, we do.' And the next day she sent someone across with a little tray of these pineapple boats, so that was lovely.

It went like clockwork. We put all our stuff into two filing cabinets. Then we had big beaver-board screens that we used to create dressing rooms, with big pieces of wood for feet. That was all manhandled onto the van by the removal company. The X-ray equipment was supervised by Brian – the portable darkroom, the generator, X-ray machine. The removal men were a regular crew. As long as the electric kettle came, it was fine. We could have a brew!

Patients came to the desk and we would fill in a card with your name and your details. Have you had any recent X-rays? Did you have any specific problem, or had you had pleurisy? Anything like pneumonia that would show up as scarring. It would help the medical director when he was looking at the film. People would just take off their belt, or any jewellery. As long as there's nothing metal from your waist upwards, you didn't have to take anything off. If there was something on the miniature radiography that made the doctor say, 'I'd like another look at that', we'd invite that person to come back for a large film. Friday was set aside for large film, and people would get stripped to the waist. If they were a lady they could wear a chest cover. A large plate X-ray was done, which would show things in greater detail.

Brian: It did surprise us, though, when we were working in Salford, we'd ask them to come back to Manchester and have a large film just to clear it. And at least a dozen of them said, 'Oh, they couldn't come back.' 'It's only down the road at Lewis's department store.' 'Oh, I never been there. Never left Salford.' It was staggering, wasn't it?

Pat: When we went into Lewis's, they'd put out a whole row of Ercol chairs for the people to wait. Then they sold them in the sale. [*laughs*] But they hadn't had a lot of use, really. It struck us as being quite funny.

Brian: What about the undertakers? [*chuckles*]

Pat: It was the Co-op funeral service that we're screening. This chap looked at me as I was filling in his card. 'Oyster satin', he said. 'Pardon?' 'Oyster satin for you, my dear, in your coffin. You'd look good in oyster satin.' 'Thank you for that information!'

Brian: Nice of him.

Pat: We did go to a factory. The lovely girls that came all had bits of fluff and cotton around them. It was a very long building, a low ceiling. They were chattering with themselves. And we couldn't hear what people were telling us. So I stood up: 'Ladies, can you please keep the noise down? I can't hear what people are telling me and we don't want to make any mistakes, do we?' 'Oh shut up and sit down, ye old cow!' That was the only time we ever got any verbal.

Brian: We had a fortnight every year in Strangeways Prison.

Pat: Some of the prisoners would help unload. In those days, Strangeways had male and female prisoners. We had to walk along the corridor with clanging iron gates at each end and set up in this huge room that had a concrete floor. A trustee would make tea and coffee for us, and he wore a red armband. A prison officer would bring people down in fairly small groups and they would be treated in exactly the same way as members of the general public. The women were brought through separately. They had to strip to the waist, and we provided chest covers for them to wear. When we were clearing away from one of the visits, some of the boards were missing. The lads that helped take stuff from the X-ray area to the van were laughing around the corner. They produced these boards. 'We're just doing it to see if we still could!'

Brian: You'd ask them their occupation and they often said 'self-employed'.

Pat: We had a portable darkroom. And when we went to the prison, female prisoners had to wear a chest cover. And this lady came forward, didn't she?

Brian: If you have a chest X-ray, you go face up, chin up, arms behind you, right? But when you did that with this lady, you could see she had a rather inappropriate tattoo on the back. Oh, dear … [*chuckles*].

Pat: Brian had to send the female radiographer into the darkroom: 'Mrs Bate, you must go in the darkroom and don't come out until I say.' Because the tattoo was more or less pornographic, wasn't it?

Brian: Oh, aye, it was pornographic.

Pat: We X-rayed the Manchester City football team. You would have heard of Bert Trautmann, who played for City. The lady sitting next to me was interviewing him prior to his X-ray. 'Oh, Miss Margison, this poor young man has broken his neck.' 'Yes, Bessie, but it's Bert Trautmann.' We didn't ask for any autographs; it were very professional. We closed for an hour at lunchtime. Brian and I'd take a packed lunch and we'd sit and have our lunch together.

What do you remember about first meeting Brian?

Pat: The first survey I went on was at The Wood Street Mission. I had to go down into the basement – and there was a great big skip that had all the white coats in that we wore – and find myself a white coat that fitted. They were all laundered at Crumpsall Hospital. You just found one that would fit best. It was very hit-and-miss. Brian was there, chatting with the darkroom tech who had come down to collect some more film. That was when I first met him. 'Well, he looks a very nice young man in a white coat.'

We had to be discreet. Everyone was called by their surname – there were no Christian names at all. Even though we worked together every day, it was just surnames. We thought it was quite good fun, actually. We'd been going up together for quite a little while, being very discreet, and the medical director must have found out that two of his staff were going out on dates. He issued an edict that the technical and clerical staff were not to mix. Well there were only five of us on the unit. That was really quite difficult to do. So we just had a little quiet chuckle about it, and we carried on regardless. The senior admin lady was really a little bit disparaging about it. Everybody else was delighted.

Brian: We had to call ourselves Mr Carroll and Miss Margison. We weren't allowed to mix, as it were. We had a Victorian doctor, didn't we?

Pat: Running the unit, yes. Very correct, very proper. We had to pay deference. In those days, if anybody was older and had the senior position, you would show due respect. We were all pretty well groomed. The white coats were done for us, so that was easy. But sometimes the coats had been starched to such an extent that you couldn't pry the sleeves open. One Monday morning, trying to get these white coats open properly, Brian put his hand in to go down the sleeve and the whole sleeve came out – it was starched to unbelievable levels!

Brian: It was quite a happy little bunch.

Pat: I left in '63 and went to work at St Mary's Maternity Hospital. The medical records officer interviewed me and offered me a job and a higher grade than the one I'd applied for. 'Yes, that sounds very interesting.' 'It's just a formality, but I do have to send you down to the secretary of the United Manchester hospitals. Go down by taxi and take this letter with you.' He looked at me up and down. 'Walk across the room. Yes, you've got decent legs, you'll do.' He had to give it his say-so. He was probably, 'Why do they keep sending all these people down to me if they think they're suitable?' and a bit fed up. I thought it was absolutely hilarious. I was in patient records. It was a training hospital, so you had quite a young crowd. It was a lovely atmosphere. That was clerical work. All of the ledgers were written up by hand, in ink. The records, the information taken from the case notes for research, I did all that in longhand. There was nothing computerised at all. It was all paper.

Brian and Pat married in 1963. Brian joined a German-based company with X-ray equipment and worked there for 30-odd years, witnessing the introduction of CAT scanners (1970s) and MRI units (1980s). The difference between the new technologies and X-rays was 'astonishing', said Pat. They were first interviewed in 2018; Brian died in 2019 and Pat has done further interviews since. She said, 'People aren't generally interested in what happened 50, 60 years ago. It's rather nice to think that we can still contribute something.'

DIPANKAR DATTA

Dipankar came to the UK in the late 1950s and was one of the first doctors of Indian origin to be appointed consultant in the NHS. Through the 1950s the spread of people coming from overseas to work in the NHS expanded to include Indians and Pakistanis who had suffered through .the horror of Partition, which created modern-day India and Pakistan (comprising West and East Pakistan, the latter of which became modern-day Bangladesh).

I was born on 30 January 1933 in undivided India, part of which now belongs to Bangladesh. In those days there was no health service in India, and without the voluntary organisations like in the United Kingdom, the poor people had no health service at all. My father was one of the top physicians. It was mainly my father who wanted me to become a doctor. Physics was my love, but I had to divert to doctor. I studied medicine in Calcutta, which is now known as Kolkata. I was very unhappy and reluctant to continue. For the first six months, I didn't read anything, though I had all the books, because I was planning to leave medicine. Then when the exam came, I had no alternative but to read and take the exam. I qualified in 1957 and ultimately liked medicine very much. I came to United Kingdom for a postgraduate degree, because the opportunity to have postgraduate training and education was very little in India.

My father, being a Victorian, he wanted me to get accustomed to all the big places. Which was the worst thing you can do. If you are going to learn clinical medicine, it is hands-on. But though I was an adult, I did not disobey my father. It was a great burden to him; he was funding me with money from India. I got used to many of the big hospitals in London: St George's, Hammersmith, Queen Square, Institute of Neurology. I was not studying. I was just going around very miserable. Everything is against you when you are getting a footing in a foreign country with a totally different weather and food and people around you. You are lonely and depressed before you recover and can put your mind to study – it takes several months.

The postgraduate education was not very well-structured, even for the local boys and girls, forget about the foreigners. As a very junior in London, there was hostility because we are nobody. You've got no footing in the hospital, you are really a nuisance, you're coming around and looking for some knowledge or experience, but you are not part of the system. The consultant is trying his best. But it's not very easy to be friendly with 20 people around you because he has got a job to do.

My first job was in the Windygates area of Fife, Scotland, as a senior house officer in a chest unit which had 64 beds: 32 tuberculosis and 32 non-tuberculosis chest beds. There was another doctor from India before me and he introduced me there. I found the staff very friendly, and very grateful to have somebody there to look after them. The consultant was not there most of the time and many staff were not too well trained. Some didn't even have postgraduate degrees. I was the only doctor, and I was on call every day, seven days a week. If I had to take weekend off, I had to take permission from a consultant. But that's the way we worked and gave service to this country.

The burden of chest disease was very high from the industrial lung disease and tuberculosis. We saw a lot of tuberculosis in the UK, which was surprising to us because you are coming from India – a tuberculosis country. Because there was a lot of poverty in southern Scotland, there was a very high level of chest disease and coronary heart disease. There were people who worked in the mines, or were smoking heavily. Every house was burning coal for cooking and heating, so the pollution was very high.

After that, I was almost aimless. I didn't know where to go, what to do. I was determined to do general medicine, but was being pushed all the time to do geriatrics or psychiatry. The best boys and girls of this country were competing for four main branches of general medicine: medicine, surgery, gynae/obstetrics, and paediatrics. The son of the soil gets preference. This is true all over the world. So we were the interlopers trying to get into that top discipline. My wife, who was Scottish and graduated from Glasgow Medical School, was against going to practise the American or Canadian type of medical practice, so that helped my mind to decide I was going to stay here and keep on fighting.

I wanted to do cardiology, but I didn't get the chance to get trained up, so I took gastroenterology and hepatology, and trained myself. I worked hard and read every day for one hour in the library after lunch. Instead of gossiping about golf, I used to go to the library, and people used to think that I was being unfriendly. 'Well, I'm not, I don't enjoy talking about golf.' To become consultant, you had to be senior registrar in a teaching hospital, and it was impossible to infiltrate there, because their own boys and girls were competing. You are always fighting against an unwinnable situation. I'm not the best product of India, but when I became a consultant in general medicine in Hairmyres, I was the first foreigner to be appointed as a consultant in general medicine in Scotland, and probably the fourth or fifth in the whole United Kingdom. I was one of the luckiest people.

Doctors were going around like God, and if they made some mistakes, it was hidden. In spite of all the knowledge and experience and good intention, you are going to make mistakes. It's like an aircraft: millions of miles they travel without any problem, then suddenly one goes – so making mistakes is never going to be eradicated from human activities. People didn't believe that doctors made mistakes, or hid truth; now, they know that they do, like all human beings. Conceit is part of the human character and it is not only present among the politicians, it is present in all professions. And if a doctor was too conceited, he wouldn't refer the patient to somebody else who may know better than him. And we really did not behave with the patients with much time and kindness and compassion. There was a little bit of dictatorship in the attitude, not just among the doctors, but also among the nurses. That has gone, or is going, now.

If my waiting list was big, more than four or six weeks, I used to hold a special extra clinic on Saturday. If I told the Sister that my clinic was too big and could she please arrange it, she would do it, or ask the staff nurse to come along and administrator would allow it. Nowadays, it will not be allowed. Not only would you not have a staff nurse or Sister agreeing to have an extra clinic, the manager would not allow it because it implies more expenditure. So that sort of attitude and professionalism we had has gone. Many have become nine-to-five jobbers.

Now retired, Dipankar reflects, 'NHS has had a great impact on my life, because we could not have practised medicine the way we have practised here. I have been lucky to go to the top and I have a lot of happy memories.'

PATRICIA

Patricia's ear mastoid problems began as a small child.

I could remember always feeling ill. Always being around the doctors. People poking around in my ear. It was just going from bad to worse. Aged five, I had penicillin injections every day. I used to dread it and I was so sick of it. I thought, 'Well, I'll get around this.' I put cotton wool in the plug holes so they won't be able to get the plug in, but course they found out. I must have had a sore throat because when my mum took me down to the hospital in desperation, and they kept me in, the first thing they did was take my tonsils and adenoids out. I can remember being wheeled into the operating theatre and people around me, and then the rubber ether mask. It was absolutely terrifying. I was absolutely terrified. The other memory which has scarred me for life is my mum and dad used to come and visit, and then I'd get upset. So they banned my mum and dad from seeing me. Can you believe that? 'Oh, she's getting too upset, so don't come again.' One day I saw them peeping from behind this screen at the entrance to the ward. I just went mad. I got out of bed and started to run. They disappeared because they were scared; they didn't want to upset the staff. I can remember running all over the hospital, then somebody must have caught me and took me back. Can you imagine? I only realised it relatively recently, you know, when you look back over the pattern of your life – I must have had what they call abandonment issues. Especially being an only child focused upon by mum and dad and my aunties and grandma.

It was three months in hospital. The only reason they sent me out was because there was an outbreak of measles and whooping cough. I had both at the same time. Dr Barnes used to come and see me every day. 'You could do with going on holiday, some fresh bracing air.' So we went to Fleetwood, and it was bitterly cold!

The outpatients part was quite small. Just one room. Four rows of seats on either side, two doctors' offices and a dressings clinic in the middle. You wouldn't be given an appointment; you'd just be told to go on that day.

Sometimes we'd be there all day. Rows and rows of people. Everybody moved up as somebody else came out. There were people knitting, and the whole of life was there. The toilets were outside – just one toilet for everybody. But what an incredible place. What service you got. From aged five to 11, I'd go there. They'd clean the ear and put these dressings in. It was always a problem. I had another operation when I was 11. In a ward with six or seven ladies. It was very quiet, very organised. I used to help making the beds and play at being a doctor. They used to come around with newspapers, you know, and at home I was never allowed to look at the *News of the World* or any scandal sheet. I very daringly got the porter to get me a copy. I felt so guilty. But read it from cover to cover! At the Women's Voluntary Service, there was this really glamorous lady. She had red hair, nicely made up, and she and her friend used to serve tea and biscuits. I remember her vividly from when I was five, and she was still there when I was 19.

I've spent a lot of time in hospital over the years. And now you get these young people sitting there saying, 'I've been sitting here for 10 minutes.' And you've got the doctors apologising for the waiting. I'd think, 'How dare you?' But is that just the irritation of an elderly person? I don't know.

It was to take until the 1970s before children were given full access to their parents while in hospital and, like Patricia, many children continued to experience deep distress.

ANTONETTE CLARKE-AKALANNE

Antonette was born in the island of Barbados in the Caribbean in 1941 and decided to apply for nursing in England after listening to a talk about training opportunities while at school. Like Tryphena, Antonette learnt of the opportunity through the NHS's recruitment drives. The 1948 Nationality Act granted citizenship to people from Commonwealth countries, which allowed them to enter Britain freely.

When I was a little girl, I used to play with my dolls. It was always a nursing game. I was the doctor. I gave the injections. I wanted more and more to become a doctor. But my family couldn't afford the cost of training, so my option was to be a nurse. At the age of 18, I applied to our general hospital in Barbados to train as a nurse. While I'm waiting to hear from the general hospital, Enoch Powell, minister of health at that time, invited the Caribbean people to come and train as nurses. At my school this gentleman came from England who talked about the benefit of doing nursing in England. I thought this was a good idea, so I took up the offer from a hospital called Derby City Hospital, which is in the Midlands. I came over to England at the age of 18, and after I was here for six months, my mother sent me the letter from the general hospital in Barbados. But obviously, it was too late. There was no way that I was going to leave what I started in England and rush back to Barbados. I was an ardent Catholic. I'd be at church all the time with my mum and I sung in the choir. I actually wanted to become a nun. When I came to England, as a nurse, I still wanted to be a nun – to finish my general nursing and go back home to the convent. But I met my late husband, so I got married.

It was very exciting. I had a very sheltered life. My sister and I were never allowed to go dancing. We were never allowed to go and see a film, except if it was a religious film. Looking at it as that girl of 18, coming to England was an opportunity. I could probably do what I want! But time got nearer, that fear come in. My mother organised with a seamstress to make the clothes that I would come to England in. I had a beautiful pink woollen suit, skirt and top with a white blouse. I had some pink shoes, a lovely felt pink hat, and a pink handbag. I must have looked a sight in England! I must have looked a sight! I flew over. Many of the other girls went by boat to England. But my father said, 'I don't want you going by boat, because Jamaican men …'. He had ideas about the other Caribbean islands. The hospital sent me an itinerary about how to get from Gatwick Airport to Victoria Station for the train up to Derby. In Barbados, most white people are rich. So I had the thought in my head that in England, all the people would be rich. It was quite an eye-opener. I sat on the bus from Gatwick and I am seeing English people cleaning the road. And I'm thinking, 'Well, I didn't expect that!' [*laughs*] 'The rich people in Barbados, they don't do that!' Sister Burns was the head of the nurses' home, and she looked after all the girls. You couldn't be married or have a child. If any of the girls got pregnant, they were out. That was the end of their training. It was like coming from home to home. If any of us were ill, she looked after us and she advised us and so on. The first morning I went on the ward, but it was only an introduction because we had to do the Preliminary Training School before we did any hands-on work. I was the only coloured nurse, but a group of other nurses were all Irish – so because I was a Catholic as well, I got on really well with them.

The wards – wow! – it was eye-opening. The wards were long in Derby City Hospital. Twenty beds up one side, and 20 down the other side. You had a sluice room, it's like a dirty room. You go and wash the bedpans, take your specimens to test with a Bunsen burner. Urine for protein and sugar and so forth. We had a clean room, which was a surgical room, if patients had an injury or needing dressing change, and so on. The steriliser room was where you had the autoclaves [steam sterilisers]. The syringes were made of glass and the needles were made of steel. The junior nurses would wash the needles and push the stylet inside the needle to take any blood or debris outside, then those needles would be steeped in sterilising solution. The glass syringes will be washed out and put in gauze and put in big drums into the autoclave. If a patient had a drip, it was made of rubber and the bottle was made of glass. I put that rubber drip under the tap, and wash out the blood or solution, shake it out, make sure that it was coming out clear, put it in this drum, and you put that in the autoclave. I can remember the smell of urine and lots of antiseptic.

All the services were under the matron. Matron could come and tell the maid off if she didn't clean the floor. We nurses had to put all the wheels of all the beds in one direction. We were taught how to make the beds, and all the ends of the beds had to be a certain way when you look from one end of the ward. It was like a military ward. It was wonderful. Everything was perfect.

What was the relationship like between the nurses and the patients?

Oh, it was so different. We could help the patient emotionally. If a patient is crying, or in distress, we sit at the edge of the bed and hold the patient's hand and listen. 'I'm here. What's wrong?' We came into nursing because we were caring people. It was a caring environment. We got paid because we have to live and eat. But most of us nurses at the time went in because of philanthropic reasons. Basically, the salary was so poor. When I first started here in England, I got £1,000 a year. Can you imagine that? I lived in a nursing home, I didn't have to pay for my food, I didn't have to pay for my uniform, and the washing was free. So £1,000 a year at that time was really good. Now, it's different. It is a job – you go into it because you earn a certain amount of money. And if you don't think that money is good, you let me go and get a different type of job, man.

Antonette's recent experience of hospital care was distressing. 'Nowadays, you cannot sit at the edge of the bed. Nowadays, nurses is more interested in how that machine work. I've experienced it myself. I went into hospital and I'm thinking, 'Shit, good lord, I would like to die first before I ever come in here. You know, it is so different. There is no emotional attachment anymore.'

MARGARET BATTY

Margaret came from a family with strong links to nursing and medicine.

I started at just over 17 at the Royal Hospital for Sick Children in Edinburgh, and did three years there. My grandmother, my aunt were both nurses. An uncle was a doctor, so nursing seemed a very obvious thing for me to go into.

The hospital took burnt children. They had a plastic surgery ward, and it was the only burns unit in Scotland. That was my first ward experience, which, as a 17- or 18-year-old, was quite an experience, you know. The patients were on slings above beds with a hole cut out in the canvas for a bed pan to go underneath. They would be wrapped in saline bandages, and they would have saline baths, where they would weigh the bandages to see how much fluid had been lost. Everything was done on fluid balance charts because that's what killed a lot of the patients, the lack of fluid. They used to do the most horrendous operations, when you did your stint in theatre, you know, where they would take flesh from the thighs and the buttocks and put it onto their hands.

We used to like it really when they cried because they was showing some sign of recovery. They would come in pale. I've never forgotten, really, one little boy called Alex – and he had drunken bleach and he was completely burnt. His oesophagus down to his stomach was completely burnt and they had to put in more skin grafts on the oesophagus. He had a tracheotomy, but we all remember and talk about him nearly every time we meet. He survived and he's now a grown man with children. He was such a cheerful little chap, you know, would get the others throwing paper aeroplanes at each other and all things like this. He was a remarkable kid. There was a happiness about some of the situations. I think that's why we've all stayed so close together as a group, because you became a little family and looked after each other within the hospital hierarchy. The pay was shocking. I think my first pay as a student nurse was £8, 10 shillings a month. Out of that you had to buy textbooks and stockings and your accommodation, but all your food was provided. It was very strict as well. You were to be back by 9.30, but we used to bribe the boiler man with 10 woodbines to let us climb in the boiler house window. Ten woodbines was the going bribe.

Margaret, like so many nurses of the time, remembers nurse training as a very special time. 'I formed the strongest bond in my life with those girls that I did that training with, and now in my eighties, I'm still friends with all of them.'

HAROLD MERCER

Harold served in the RAF as rear gunner during the Second World War, flying Halifax Bombers. He was demobilised in 1947. A lifetime of volunteering led to him being a North East finalist for the Pride of Britain Awards in 2019.

I was visiting Preston Hospital, which was half hospital and half workhouse. I can remember the old scrub tables in what they called the dining room, and a group of people sitting round these tables. I happened to know one of the chaps. 'Oh, hello, Harry.' 'What are you doing here?' 'We're the League of Hospital Friends organisation and we work for proceeds to buy extra amenities for the patients in the hospital. Would you like to join us?' That's how I became a member of the League of Friends in 1957, and I did 60 years of service as chairman of North Tyneside League of Friends.

Preston Hospital was still half workhouse until about 1960, and the NHS took it over completely. I can still see those old gentlemen. They were all in the same type of worsted wool suits they had in those days, and were all the same colour. I can picture them to this very day walking out of what was then the workhouse and sitting on Preston Road beside Christ Church. They had no home, so they ended up in the hospital as a workhouse, really. That was their life. They had nowhere else to go. They ended up at St Nicholas's in Newcastle, a hospital for mentally ill patients and it later became Preston Hospital completely.

Preston was a very ancient hospital and the equipment wasn't really up to standard. That was one reason we raised funds to help to bring better equipment into the hospitals at those times. We raised many, many, thousands of pounds over the years. Coffee mornings, concerts, dances. Anything that raised money, we took part in it. Took a lot of your time up, but you were doing good for other people and, after all, that's a part of life – helping other people.

Preston was one of many hospitals across Britain with old buildings in desperate need of refurbishment. But there was no money to build new hospitals until the 1960s, and it

was a matter of patching up and making do. The only significant upgrade of the 1950s
was the building of over 700 operating suites for surgeries.

I could arrange concerts with the Salvation Army band and songsters choir.
I would say, 'I'll get the band to come and give a concert, and all you've got
to do is help organise the seating arrangements and that sort of thing.' At
that time, I wasn't a member myself – all my family were members. The
only reason I wasn't a member was because I had gone to the Methodist
Church to be with my wife at the same church. I didn't think it was right to
have two churches in one house, so I left the Salvation Army, which was a
great blow to my mother. We were still going to church and doing the same
things exactly as I did before, except I didn't wear a uniform; I just went to
church in the civvies as you normally do.

All the money went into the funds to buy extra comforts and extra equipment. When the first cancer things were talked about, we gave a donation
of £100 to start them off, which was a lot of money then. We would also
help the patients because some wouldn't have any pyjamas or any soap, so
we made little boxes up with soap and toothbrush, toothpaste. Just the small
things that people need in a hospital.

People seemed to spend quite a lot of time in hospital. I think patients in
those days were experimented on, really, with new medicines, which today,
people take for granted. I was in Sanderson's Hospital for three months
with my leg in the air. Not allowed to get out of bed at all. I got so used
to it, it became part of my life. I had a tape recorder and a few tapes and
every morning the girls [nurses] would say, 'Come on, Harry, put the tapes
on. We love the music!' They were popular songs of the day. I spent a lot
of time amusing the nurses with the music. Nursing in the fifties and sixties
was more wholesome. They were dedicated to the job. They weren't there
for wages. They were there because they wanted to help. You got very good
patient care. You felt as though you were the only one being looked after.
They gave the whole of their time to you for the 10 minutes or whatever –
the focus was on you, then, you know.

Harry had been born into a family of nine in North Shields, North Tyneside, in 1922.

His first brother died before he knew him, and he also lost a sister to illness.

Life was very hard for most people in those days. There wasn't a lot of money going around and people lived on very low wages because, although there were quite a number of shipyards on the Tyne, the wages weren't very high. Most people had to make do and mend in those days, which meant if you had clothing, they were sort of patched up, darned, woolly jumpers which had to last you a long time.

I had a sister who was about three years older than myself. I was only three at the time myself, but I can picture that little girl, lovely blonde hair. Every morning she would come down and run her hair under the tap in the backyard. Because there was no water inside houses in those days, you had one tap in the house and that was in the backyard. My mum would come and shout at her, 'You mustn't do that, you'll get your death of cold.' But she still carried on doing it. When she was about five, she took ill and died. I can picture that little white coffin in what we called the front room, waiting for the hearse to come. The horse came along with the hearse, and they took this little white coffin away and I never saw her again. Everybody else went up to the cemetery except my eldest sister, who stayed to look after me. People say you cannot remember things. I say, 'Well, I remember as plain as the nose on my face.' I still think about it now. It tends to bring a little tear to my eye. A lovely little girl. I had two sisters after that, so I had company.

There was always one person in the street people looked up to if they had little illnesses, colds, etc. They would come down to my mum's. 'Such-and-such has got a bad cough, or they're not feeling well, can you come up and see?' Even people falling ill and dying, she would go and take care of the situation. If it was an illness she could take care of herself, she would do so. She would arrange to go to the doctor and get tablets. But remember, in those days, nothing was free. They had a system, I think it was sixpence a week you paid, and that covered you for most little illnesses, colds, flu and that sort of thing. We were all in the sixpence arrangement with the doctor. The whole street would be in it. That was my mum – if she could help anybody, she would do it. Even if it cost her a lot of hard work, she would stick in and do it.

We had three little rooms: a kitchen, a little bedroom and a big bedroom, which was used as a front room as well. My mum made a shop out of the front room and baked bread and buns for the men as they were going to work. They came past our house to go down to Smith's Dock, which was a shipyard builder in those days. She would get up, five o'clock in the morning, bake bread – and it was all ready for the lads as they came out. The room was also used as a bedroom at night. My dad was what they called a 'skipper' on the river. He would take fresh water to the ships on the river. They called them 'water men'. He was in the dock one day and he was knocked into the dock by the crane – about a 60-foot drop. He was really badly injured; he never got back to full-time work again. They did manage to give him a job as a gatekeeper in the smaller dock, but he lost his main income. So my mother had to go out to work instead. She used to get up at four o'clock in the morning, go down and clean the offices of the shipyard, just to feed us. Everybody in the street was a friend. You could knock on a door and say, 'Mrs So-and-so, you know', and would run a message for her, just for a slice of bread and jam.

Growing up at a time when people had to make do and mend and help each other, giving back to the NHS was a natural outlet for Harry's concern for other people.

One reason I volunteered was because I needed help myself from the hospital, so why not give a little bit back in the form of raising funds towards special equipment that they needed? Our ideal is to help the patient and put them at their ease before they even see any doctors. Just do a little friendly chat, you know – and it's surprising; you sometimes get a whole family's history in two or three minutes. You can picture how they live at home by how they talk to you. We help put them at their ease, and I've done that since 1957. I think we've become part of the hospital. You know, the volunteers are really part of the hospital now. Without the volunteers, I think, the hospitals would be struggling. Although we don't get paid, we get paid by our own satisfaction of helping people. That's our wages. But now we have rules and regulations we have to stick to. We have to be careful how we speak to people, and you never touch people. At one time you could shake hands.

Now, under these rules that the government have about touching people, we have to be very careful. Even getting on the buggy, officially, you're not supposed to help them on and off. But what do you do if it's an old person who gets on? Surely you can give them a little bit of a hand?

It's not the same world, I'm afraid, to me. Perhaps I'm old and living back in the old days when everybody helped one another, or was willing to help other people. Have a little chat and have a bit of a laugh. Now, you've got to be so careful of what you do and what you say and, as I say, as far as touching people, that's out of it altogether. I'm still enjoying every minute, and I'll be back, probably in a couple of weeks' time, on the door again, meeting and greeting, making people welcome. Making them feel as though they'll get the help.

Interviewed in 2019 aged 96, Harry was still meeting and greeting patients at North Tyneside General Hospital. He died from Covid-19 in 2020.

At the end of the 1950s

The pinch points and pressures on the NHS that were to shape its history were well established by the end of the decade. Issues of rising costs; staffing shortages and modernising infrastructure in the context of a growing, ageing population; expensive new treatments; and a rise in patient expectations are as familiar to us now as they were to people in the 1950s. It was a long-established assumption that a state-provided health service would eventually lead to reduction in demand and, thereby, costs, as people's health improved. But not even Bevan had anticipated the levels of need across the population.

The annual cost of the NHS was extremely difficult to estimate. Figures for the NHS in England and Wales ranged from £132 million in the 1944 White Paper to £152 million in a financial memorandum to the 1946 NHS Bill.[9] In the event, the costs greatly exceeded these estimates with the actual spend of the NHS's first year of operation standing at £373 million.[10] The costs of prescription medicines were especially high and led to the introduction of a one-shilling prescription charge. Bevan supported prescription charges but argued vehemently against charges being imposed for false teeth and spectacles and he resigned in protest from the Labour government in 1951. Two years later, concerns about NHS costs led the Conservative government to commission a committee of enquiry, chaired by the economist CW Guillebaud in 1953. Unexpectedly, the Guillebaud report published in January 1956 was positive. No extravagances or inefficiencies were found and, indeed, it recommended more funding for hospital modernisation.[11] Just as in pre-NHS times in the charitable hospitals, volunteers like Harold Mercer continued to support health services by fundraising for items that were not funded from core budgets, such as visitor refreshment facilities and new equipment.

Recruiting enough staff to support the new NHS's development was one of the major challenges of the decade and a harbinger of the perennial staff shortages which have dogged NHS history ever since. Britain had suffered shortages of healthcare staff, particularly nurses and auxiliary workers, since the 1930s, and already relied on staff from Ireland and Central and

Eastern Europe. The problem was exacerbated by the wider post-war labour shortage. Established at a point when the British Empire was breaking up, the NHS looked to enlist staff from British colonies and former colonies, particularly those in the Caribbean and South Asian subcontinent. Britain was anticipated to be a land of opportunities and promise, and people from former colonies were granted full citizenship through the British Nationality Act of 1948. But the first generations, including Tryphena Anderson, Antonette Clarke-Akalanne and Dipankar Datta, experienced racism and hardships, particularly around training and career development, that made it difficult for them to progress and achieve their aspirations. It is quite possible that without the contribution of these overseas staff, the NHS could not have continued to develop as it did.

The tenth anniversary of the NHS was celebrated with a debate held in the House of Commons. Despite the ongoing pressures of costs and staffing, the NHS had established itself as a valued British institution that united political opponents. The NHS 'is regarded all over the world as the most civilised achievement of modern Government', proclaimed Aneurin Bevan. The disappearance of TB was compelling evidence of the benefits of a universal health system: 'To some extent, it is due to higher standards of nutrition and better housing … and also to new drugs. But the main point remains: all those drugs and medical facilities would not have been available under the old system … The new knowledge would be there, but it would not reach the people needing it.'[12] Bevan continued, in his contribution to the debate. The benefits of the NHS were to continue through the 1960s, as new drugs and technologies led to more complex diseases and conditions being treated than ever before.

Chapter 3:
1960s

'I was the first one at the hospital to introduce free visiting. I asked parents to come in when their baby's feed was due so that they could feed their baby.'

JUNE HEWETT

'I was appointed the first ever male assistant matron at Crumpsall Hospital in 1966. Each day brought different problems, different aspects.'

COLIN EASTWOOD

'I turned up on the first day in a miniskirt. The queue to come and have a look at this funny, new, female young doctor wearing a miniskirt stretched all down the street.'

GILL WAKELY

'Occupational therapists have always been trained both in physical rehabilitation and mental health. Even in physical rehabilitation, the person you are dealing with has a mental side as well.'

MARY KEER

*'… there was a word in those days, called a "spastic".
And that's an awful word. But that's what you were considered.'*

ELSIE MCMAHON

*'People would take dietary histories to see what they'd
eaten and see if we could improve it. But basically,
the doctors didn't know what caused heart disease.'*

WENDY PARKER

*'Abortion was illegal. Women went to backstreet people
who would start them bleeding, and then they
would arrive bleeding on your doorstep.'*

SONYA BAKSI

*'[A patient's husband] turned to me one day:
"My wife said it was like having the baby on the
banks of the Ganges." I took it as a compliment.'*

NORMA MURDOCH

*'My mother came to take to thalidomide
because her father had just died.'*

GEOFF ADAMS-SPINK

*'So although it was the swinging sixties,
I don't think it reached Hope Hospital.'*

EILEEN HILL

*'That way we built up a two-bedded unit to learn a trade on.
We had to teach nurses. We had to teach ourselves.'*

DAVID MORRISON

JUNE HEWETT

Since before the NHS, hospitals had argued that child patients settled better with-out the emotional disruption caused by parental visits. But the distress experienced by many parents and children led to Sir Harry Platt, professor of orthopaedic surgery at the University of Manchester and president of the Royal College of Surgeons, being appointed to review the arrangements for the welfare of children in hospital. Published in 1959, his report recommended unlimited parental visiting and parent participation in care of the child. June was an early pioneer of this new involve-ment of parents in their child's care. As a schoolgirl, June spent time in the summer holidays working in a day nursery. At the age of 16, she began as a cadet nurse at St Martin's Hospital in Bath: 'Looking after babies, that was my forte.' Once she was 18, she joined the Preliminary Training School for nurses at the Royal United Hospital in Bath.

In September 1959 I became Sister on the baby unit at the Bristol Chil-dren's Hospital. That was the best time of my whole career. It was my own ward and I had students. I was the first one at the hospital to introduce free visiting. I asked parents to come in when their baby's feed was due so that they could feed their baby, which was important to keep the baby-mother bonding going. Visiting had been limited to morning and evening. I felt that the bond between the mother and baby was very important. I didn't ask anybody if I could do this, I'm afraid, I just did it off my own back. Nobody challenged me. I don't think the consultants or anybody even knew. I told matron eventually. She was alright about it. It was important that it wasn't just the nurse that was bonding with the baby. I would let the parents come in whatever time they wanted to. It might be ten o'clock at night, if that was the only time Dad could get in and wanted to feed. It was never challenged. The parents felt more at ease. They were encouraged to change their babies and do what they could for the baby whilst they were there. I may only have had three mothers in at a time, 'cause the feeds were at different times so I could spend time with the parents, which gave them confidence. If there were problems with the feeding, I could advise.

I had a system whereby all the babies in the ward were in a book and each baby had a first nurse, a second nurse and a third nurse. The nurses would choose which babies they wanted as their first. They only had about three or four. We only had 12 cubicles. If the first nurse was on duty, she would look after her babies. If she wasn't, then the second nurse would. It sounds complicated but it worked quite well. I had some rather difficult and sometimes peculiar babies in. I never had a baby that I didn't have a first nurse for. There was always somebody who loved that baby and wanted to care for it. Sometimes they needed a bit more help because it was a difficult baby, but that's what I was there for. I trained my staff nurses to do the same.

I had one baby in straight from the maternity hospital under the paediatrician. She had pyloric stenosis, which is unusual in girls. There's a muscle around the exit from the stomach into the small intestine called the pylorus muscle. And in pyloric stenosis this muscle thickens and, consequently, the children vomit after feeding. They have a very typical vomit. If you had a medical student who thought he knew it all, or even a new doctor, and you had a pyloric baby in, not treated, you would say, 'Go and feed that baby.' The baby would have a big projectile vomit all over him at the end of the feed!

This particular baby had an abnormality of the skull whereby the parietals had already fused with the occipital and temporal bones, and would hamper the growth of the brain. She came to me and was going to have surgery at Frenchay Hospital. This baby couldn't swallow. We had to tube feed her. She had to go three times for surgery. And this brings me on to the importance of paediatric training. First time she came back to me, she was absolutely bloated. The staff nurse was a male staff nurse from Frenchay. I said, 'What have you done to this baby?' He looked at me quite blank. 'What do you mean?' I said, 'Look at her, she's overhydrated.' But he didn't know anything about it. So I got the consultant up and she was absolutely furious. They had given this baby a subcutaneous infusion and overhydrated her. Then she had to go and have more surgery because her wound opened up. She came back to me that time dehydrated. They didn't have paediatric nurses on the surgical unit, you see, or the doctors didn't know much about paediatrics. The surgeon from Frenchay kept ringing up and asking how she was and I would tell him. 'Oh, I'll have to have her over again.' 'Look, the first time you sent her back to me, she was overhydrated, the second time she was dehydrated. This time, can she be a day case? We'll get an infusion up before she goes. I will send a staff nurse with her to stay with her and look after her so she comes back okay.' Sometimes you had to treat the surgeons like this because they didn't know much about paediatrics. So that's what I did. And she came back okay.

The father had been told so many times that she wouldn't survive, he didn't let Mother visit that child for six or eight months. He came in regularly, every day, but he would not let Mother come. He didn't want her to see her baby, who was going to die. When she was about six months old, she was still being tube fed. 'I'm going to try her on solids. Her pylorus must be alright now.' She took it quite well from the spoon. Only a little bit to start with. I thought, 'Oh, this is good.' I didn't say anything. The consultant came around just after this. 'How is baby getting on? I think it's time we tried her with some solids.' So I took a big breath, 'I've already done so.' 'How did she get on?' 'Quite well, really.' 'Oh, good.' And it was left at that. When she was 11 months old – Mum had been allowed to come by then, and we had taught Mum how to tube feed her, how to feed her with solids – she went home. She died a few months later, but at least Mum had a little bit of her.

June was persuaded to progress her career by becoming a nurse tutor in 1963, and she taught in Bristol until her retirement in the 1980s. 'My personal thought is that a degree is not necessary. I think we had a far better grounding in nursing, doing it the way we did, than these university students do. They come out of university knowing a certain amount of theory. But they haven't had any practical experience.'

COLIN EASTWOOD

Colin became one of the first male assistant matrons in the NHS, and a strong supporter of the Salmon Report, which introduced a new staff grading structure for senior nursing staff, including chief nursing officers. By the 1960s around 10 per cent of the nursing workforce was male. He had vivid memories of his mum dying from TB when he was four years old, and he too developed TB shortly after leaving school. Colin spent two months in Monsall Hospital, followed by six months at home with daily visits from district nurses to administer streptomycin by intramuscular injection. After recovering, Colin applied for nurse training.

Tuesday July 8, 1958, I was met by Miss Ashurst, who was one of the assistant matrons. 'I'll take you to the sewing room.' She was lovely and used to hum to herself walking along the corridor. We went off to G block and down the steps into the cellar where the sewing room was. Miss Ashurst was responsible for the sewing. Being six feet, three inches tall, they couldn't find trousers long enough for me to wear without them being half mast. I had to wear, for the first 12 months, at least, two or three pairs of trousers, which had at least eight inches sewn on the bottom of them. And that was my uniform. Male nurses had a dental jacket with buttons across the collar and down the side. Short-sleeved jackets, really. In those days, male nurses didn't even have the epaulettes. We just had the plain uniform and a little name badge.

There was three male nurses and 16 ladies. The first sentence of the first lecture we had in Preliminary Training School was: 'In hospital, it is necessary for all the nurses to learn a certain code of manner.' Full stop. That meant you would say 'Dr Smith' and not 'Colin Smith'. Or, 'Yes, matron', 'No, matron', and 'Yes, Miss Kelly', 'No, Miss Kelly'. Nowadays, you know, it's 'Hello Gladys, how are you getting on?' Discipline is good, really. When the consultants were about, we were hiding in case they asked you any questions. You would be in awe of consultants, really. I qualified in October 1961. So I was a staff nurse on neurosurgery for about nine months, followed by a staff nurse post in Edinburgh for nine months, doing neurosurgical training.

Colin returned to Crumpsall Hospital in 1963.

I was appointed as a junior charge nurse on neurosurgery: 13 female beds, and 13 male beds. There was a patient there who was unconscious for five years, and not a mark on the skin – not one bedsore. After doing that for about 18 months, I was getting a bit fed up with brain surgery and unconscious patients. 'Would matron allow me to do night duty covering the general wards to get some experience with medicine and surgery, orthopaedics, or what have you?' 'Yes, I'll give you 12 months experience.' When it was the acting superintendent's night off, I was left the admin bleep and I had the whole responsibility for the hospital.

About 11 o'clock one Sunday evening, my bleep went. A rather upset and distraught mother said, 'My daughter started holiday on Friday, and she's not come home. Can you tell me where she is?' 'Where was your daughter working? 'She was doing obstetrics.' I went to the ward and said to the Night Sister, 'Do you know anything about this young lady?' 'Well, she adopted a patient. And I think she's been taken home to wet the baby's head' – i.e., she'd gone to a party! I got the address of this patient. 'We'll take the bull by the horns and ring matron.' This was almost midnight. 'Matron, it's Eastwood speaking. I've got this problem.' 'Meet me at my car in half an hour.' She came down immaculate. Can you remember her apple blossom perfume? We didn't have sat navs in those days. But we found this house. You could hear music blaring out. Matron went up to the bell and a young man came to the bottom of the hall. 'Hello, come in.' 'No, thank you. Is Nurse Bloggs here?' Nurse Bloggs appeared at the bottom of the staircase. 'Nurse, are you aware that your parents are worried about you? I suggest that you ring them up immediately and let your mother know, at least, that you are safe and well, and when I speak to her in the morning, I'm going to tell them I've found you in a den of iniquity. Thank you, goodbye.' She drove her car back and by this time it would be towards two o'clock a.m. 'I'll see you in the morning, Mr Eastwood, at 7.45.'

In 1966 I was appointed the first ever male assistant matron at Crumpsall Hospital.

Each day brought different problems, different aspects – and, as administrators, you had to sort them out. There's not anything I didn't like about the job. I was quite proud wandering around the corridors and wards with

'Assistant Matron' on my lapel. One of the best things since sliced bread, to me, was the advent of the senior nursing staff structure, known as the Salmon Scheme. Prior to Salmon, you had a hospital matron who was responsible for all hospital nursing things. She had assistants, each with their own role. Salmon brought out a senior nursing staff structure, which was marvellous because assistant matrons were given responsibility for units. So you could have a nursing officer for surgical, a nursing officer for medicine, and so forth. That gave them the power and authority to sort their own staff. If they were short-staffed it was their fault, because they hadn't noticed that it hadn't been done properly. Nursing officers gave nursing a voice at unit level. Prior to Salmon, a Sister or charge nurse would say to the assistant matron, 'Could you give me some …?' She'd say, 'Oh, I think you'd better speak to matron about that.' With Salmon, matron would say, 'Well, you're the nursing officer, do the audit.' So the introduction of Salmon, in my eyes, was really a marvellous thing in nursing administration.

We went through a period of time where nurses didn't have a pay rise and so, in 1969, the Royal College of Nursing decided that nationwide there would be the Raise the Roof: Fair Pay for Nurses campaign. We demonstrated quietly with placards in the streets of Manchester and we got a 22 per cent pay rise after that. The Confederation of Health Service Employees had a branch for nursing administration and I joined in, although we broke all the rules there was. We crossed picket lines and things like that, because we were managers.

In the 1980s Colin retrained in nurse education and retired after 40 years' service. He was interviewed in 2017 by Gwen Crossley, who also trained in nursing at Crumpsall Hospital in the 1960s. Colin died in 2019.

GILL WAKELY

The contraceptive pill was developed in the US, and in December 1961, it was made available through the NHS. Before this date women had been able to obtain contraception through charitable family planning clinics, but the morals of the time restricted access to married women. In 1967 the Family Planning Act made contraception more readily available, partly in response to concerns that there was a rapidly growing population and the poorer families were at risk of struggling economically if they had more children than they could support. Gill was a strong advocate for women's rights to sexual freedom. She decided to be a doctor when she was very young, but her school thought it was more reasonable for her to be a nurse. After leaving school and working in a children's home, she got a job at Oxford working in a laboratory and was encouraged to apply for medicine.

I applied to medical school in 1959. One of the London hospitals didn't know why I'd applied to them because I didn't play rugby. I said, 'Well, I could if you like.' They didn't seem to like that. In fact, they looked very disapprovingly at me when I tried to be funny. 'What will you do if you get married and have a family?' 'I can't see what that's got to do with my training. I should just go on working. I mean, my mother always worked. So I can't see that there's any problem.' They weren't expecting me to be so assertive. I think they thought I should be terribly grateful for having an interview. I didn't get offered a place. They made it quite clear that they were looking for people who could play good rugby. [*laughs*] The following week, I had an interview at Bristol. 'I noticed you haven't put us down as the first choice. If we offer you a place, would you take it?' 'Are you offering me a place?' 'Yes, I think we could.' 'In that case, I'll take it.' I thought, a bird in the hand and all that.

There were 62 people on the course and 14 were women. So quite a lot more men – well, I thought they were boys. The quality of training was very mixed. A lot of it was still the 'see one, do one' approach. I did find it quite hard work. Partly because during my training, I got pregnant. I had six months off. I managed to find somebody to look after the baby. The dean was a little surprised when I turned up and said, 'Can I start again?' But they were very helpful and supportive. In those days, we worked in a group of students who you stayed with throughout your student training and rotated around the various specialities. I had to join a new group that were a year below. They put me in with a group of mature students, which was very helpful. They were all very ambitious and much more emotionally mature, so the standard within the actual firm was very good.

When I was a student, I started doing family planning training. I used to go to the local family planning clinic. In the 1960s you had to be married to go. You were allowed to attend the family planning clinic before your marriage night, provided you brought some sort of evidence that you were actually going to get married. Otherwise, the receptionist would not let you in. I was keen on family planning because I thought it was one of the freedoms of women to decide whether they were going to get pregnant or not. And women were getting much more sexually liberated then, and they were getting pregnant. I thought they needed some help with that. Also my personal experience of having had a cap failure made me keen. The availability of the Pill and intra-uterine devices from the early 1960s meant that there was much more to offer people than the rather unreliable rubber goods.

What do you remember about your first employment in six months' surgery and six months' medicine?

Not a lot, because you never seem to get any sleep. I was trying to do that and occasionally see my child. It went past in a blur. I was too busy getting on with it. From the physical point of view, it was difficult because it was so exhausting. On the other hand, we had spent the last year of our training doing locums, providing temporary assistance as house officers. Unlike now, when they're thrown in the deep end, I think we'd already practised a lot of the skills that were needed to do the job previously. During the training you could do an elective – a period of three months when you could choose to work abroad, do some research. One option was to do three months in general practice, which I thought might be quite interesting. It was also convenient from the point of view of not having to go anywhere else, which would have been a bit difficult for me with a small child. I did this elective with a GP practice in Bristol. I thought it was absolutely wonderful. I was very impressed with the work that they did, and that they knew so much about the people they were dealing with. Doing GP training at that time was quite unusual. One of my female friends did it, but I think she was the only one in our year who did. Most people just went into general practice with no experience whatsoever.

After house jobs I did this six months' locum in a single-handed GP practice in the red-light area of Plymouth. The patients were lovely. They taught me everything I knew. I turned up on the first day in a miniskirt. The queue to come and have a look at this funny, new, female young doctor wearing a miniskirt stretched all down the street. Most of them patients didn't have anything wrong with them, really. They just came to see this funny arrival. [*laughs*]

You managed a lot of things then at home that nowadays, you send somebody into a hospital. Things like, for instance, a heart attack or strokes. You wouldn't send anybody into hospital then. You'd manage them at home. Not very well, because there wasn't very much in the way of treatment. Of course, you did all your own calls at night, too. So you were on duty as a single-handed practitioner for 24 hours, seven days a week. It was quite hard work, but the patients were extremely considerate of you, because they knew that if they called at night, they'd be getting you personally out of bed. So you didn't get very many calls. They managed themselves, mostly. A lot of the older patients especially still had memories of having to pay if they went to the doctor, so they wouldn't have done that unless there was something seriously wrong with them.

Gill reflected on the difficulties of balancing children and work at that time. 'It would have been much more sensible if I'd have gone into public health straight away. But the career structure wasn't there. Public health and small children fit together much better than general practice and small children.'

MARY KEER

Mary wanted to train as an occupational therapist on leaving school, but had no financial support. Instead, she went to art school and, after having the first year paid for, she supported herself through teaching in the evenings.

I went to art school and did a three-year course in textiles at Camberwell School of Art in London. I then took a desk job with John Lewis, working in the textile production side. I got so bored with it. My friend said, 'Oh, for heaven's sake, Mary, what do you want to do?' 'I've always wanted to be an occupational therapist.' 'Go away and be one.'

The course was very broad and gave you a lot of opportunities. I worked in a big psychiatric hospital with 1,500 patients. I was frankly horrified by it. It was north of London, had a 20-foot brick wall completely surrounding it. Some of the patients had been there the whole of their life. I was told that some of them weren't mentally ill – they were born illegitimate, so they'd been put in an asylum.

I helped somebody design an altar cloth for the chapel. She was a very long-standing patient and could already weave beautifully. I set her up with this design and the hospital bought the silk that was necessary. I can remember going and buying special gold and tassels for sewing onto each corner. They asked me to go to the consecration of this piece of fabric. I turned up in the ward and she took me into her little side room on the ward. On the bed there were three handkerchiefs, a pair of gloves and a purse. We had to choose what she was going to use. That was all the variety she had. Broke my heart. But she looked so pleased and she had woven the cloth beautifully.

I got the job I really wanted, in physical rehabilitation at Gravesend and North Kent Hospital, in the late 1960s. It was a Nissen hut in the grounds of what was then a geriatric hospital, which had previously been the workhouse. I started there as a basic-grade occupational therapist and later on became the head of the department.

We had patients who were dockers and worked on the Thames. They needed to be really strong, especially in their upper limbs. We had the weights room with ropes and pulleys so we could assess whether they were able to do that sort of work. I had a bathroom and a kitchen where I could do assessments of how people could manage at home. I can remember assessing an old lady as to whether she could get in and out of the bath unaided. She insisted on keeping her hat on and sitting there in the bath, fully clothed. With a great deal of self-control, I didn't laugh. We also had a little corridor with a full-length mirror at the end. I had a nun as a patient. She was talking to herself in the mirror. Because all nuns look the same, she thought that was somebody else.

Many patients underestimated themselves. I can remember interviewing somebody: 'What's your job?' 'I'm only a housewife.' I said, 'Yes, and so for that, you do all the washing, the catering, the household chores and take the children to school and you're *only* a housewife?' You could see her blooming during this conversation as to how valuable she was. This was very helpful, because then people were much more positive about their treatment.

Clinics were held on Friday and we would go in with notes and give the doctor a report in clinic. We would usually do it in front of the patients. I found that quite useful because sometimes the doctor talked to the patient in terms that they didn't understand. When they came back to the department, they'd ask me, 'What did he mean, Mary?' I could explain it in words that they understood.

Occupational therapists have always been trained both in physical rehabilitation and mental health. Even in physical rehabilitation, the person you are dealing with has got a mental side as well. They need to have the opportunity for that to be healed, as well as whatever it is they're trying to improve in the way of function. The confidence is just as important as the stairlift, or long handle.

In the 1970s Mary moved to Wolverhampton to set up a School of Occupational Therapy from scratch at New Cross Hospital. The School later moved to Coventry Polytechnic, and when occupational therapy became a degree course in the 1980s, Mary led its design. She was interviewed in June 2020, aged 92, and died later that year.

ELSIE MCMAHON

Elsie was born in 1949 in Altrincham and shares her memories of growing up with a sight disability.

I'm registered partially sighted and I have been for all my life. I was born at six o'clock in the morning in my granny's front room. I weighed 10 and a half pounds. When I was born they thought I could have been blind because my eyes rolled around a lot, which they still do. My mum took me to hospital and it was discovered I was partially sighted. I am not an albino, but I have albinism. I haven't got pink eyes. My eyes are blue. But I can't cope in very bright light. And my sight is very poor. So I did struggle, and my mum did spend a lot of time with me at Manchester Eye Hospital. My sisters and my brother were both dark; there's nothing wrong with their sight. When I started school I couldn't cope. In those days there was no special needs or anything like that. I couldn't see the blackboard. The teachers found it very difficult to teach me ABC or anything like that. So the doctors put me under the care of Chester Blind Welfare. I had a lady that used to come and visit every month. They advised my mum and dad it would be beneficial for me to go away to a school in Fulwood, Preston, for partially sighted children. My dad didn't want me to go, but my mum said it would be better if I did. When I was eight, I did go to the home. It was difficult. I can remember feeling very homesick and I can remember the day they took me and I was deposited in this school with people I didn't know.

I settled down and we were very well cared for. When we woke up in the morning, I was taught how to make a bed, and it was a hospital-type bed. The food was plain but it was very good. We were taught how to cope. How to handle money. I don't look at money, I feel it. I still do that to this day. I never think about it. It's just something I've done all my life. Walking along, I don't look where I'm going, I follow a hedge or wherever. With my children, or friends, they give me an arm and I link with them. Without going to school I wouldn't have been able to lead the life I have led. I grew up in a very happy environment. We played netball, we played volleyball. It might have been a bit hit and miss – we didn't always catch the ball! [*laughs*] But there was no one to make fun of us. We laughed it off. Ninety-four children in the school, ranging from five to 16. We had a religious upbringing, but the Catholic children had their own.

We came from the north of England and the north-east – there was nobody from the south. We did country dancing. We used to have social evenings. We were taught to dance. All the old-time dances, the Veleta, the foxtrot. Around 1963 I remember when the twist came out, we had a proper three-piece band came to play. 'The headmaster will allow you to do one twist.' I hadn't got a clue what they were talking about. One of the teachers showed us how to do the twist. The headmaster frowned on it because he thought the dance was very suggestive and didn't consider it right for us to do. But we did it! When I left school I found it difficult because I missed all my friends. It wasn't like having friends around here. There wasn't the telephones and things like Facebook to keep in touch with each other.

You were considered a bit of a … there was a word in those days, called a 'spastic'. And that's an awful word. But that's what you were considered. You had something wrong with you, so you weren't quite right. I didn't feel like that – I just couldn't see. I can remember when I went to the eye hospital. Because I couldn't see in the bright lights, they prescribed glasses for me. I must have been one of the first people to have tinted glasses, and they were royal blue. I got my leg pulled something chronic at the normal school, before I went to Preston. The children were awful. I can remember standing in the playground and physically breaking them so I didn't have to wear them because the children were so nasty. They were nasty to you anyway, if you wore glasses. They used to call you 'speccy four eyes' and things like that, which hurt. Children are cruel to each other, aren't they? Nowadays, children accept children with glasses on – it's the norm. My children grew up thinking that everybody had a magnifying glass or glasses and hearing aid because I did.

I left at 16 but I found it very difficult to find work. Even though I've got a very good report, I had no qualifications. I got quite a few interviews. But as soon as they saw 'partially sighted', or looked at me, nobody would employ me. Every job I went for, I got turned away. I didn't give up because

I went to stay with my auntie one weekend. She used to go every week to this hairdresser's. I went with her this Saturday morning. The lady who owns the salon asked me about school and everything. 'Would you like to help out sweeping the hair up, or possibly learning to be a shampooist?' She couldn't pay me much. My auntie said, 'Why don't you go for it?' 'Well, I'll have to ask my mum and dad.' Which you did in those days. If you weren't 21, then you didn't make your own decisions, did you? My dad could take me to the train every morning and see me on the train on his way to work. The salon wasn't far from the train. It was a safe route for me to walk. I started sweeping the hair up, keeping the salon tidy, wiping the dryers down, shampooing, and the lady taught me to put rollers in. I did that until I got married in 1969 when I was 20. Then I had my first baby in 1970.

How many children have you had?

Six children. Being partially sighted has never stopped me. [*laughs*] My husband was wonderful. I don't think his family was quite happy. One of his sisters knew that my sight was poor. I think she thought he was taking on a bit of a burden. But he wasn't. I knew he wasn't. I knew what I could do and what I was capable of. I loved him and he loved me and we had a very happy marriage. We were married for 38 years when he passed away.

Elsie became ill with Covid-19 in March 2020 and shared her experience of being sedated in further interviews with the project.

WENDY PARKER

Wendy graduated in 1967 with a diploma in dietetics. She spent the first few years working in some of the London hospitals.

The wards in all the hospitals I worked at in the sixties and seventies tended to be the long Florence Nightingale wards. Thirty-odd beds in there on both sides, often with a table or cupboard in the middle with flowers on top. The nurses' station was at the end of the ward in a glass office, which was always full of cigarette smoke. The patients' notes were kept there, and you had to fight your way through the smoke to find the notes because the nurses were always smoking in there. The patients would be smoking in the day room as well. Men and women were never on the same ward. There would be a couple of individual rooms at the end of the ward near the nurses' station for very sick patients who were likely to die. It was very hierarchical on the wards. If we were sitting at the nurses' station having a handover about patients and a consultant walked in the wards, we had to stand up and stand to attention.

The patients might be diabetic. They might have kidney disease or liver disease. I would talk to them and organise their diet with them. We had a separate diet kitchen with diet cooks who were trained. The dietitians would work out the plan and then talk to the diet cook about it. The other part of the dietitian's work would be doing outpatient clinics.

One of the hospitals had a neuro unit, and we used to tube feed unconscious patients. We used to have lots of head injuries, because in those days people didn't wear crash helmets on motorbikes. I remember seeing so many young men who had come off their motorbikes and got badly brain-damaged. Crash helmets were a wonderful thing when they came in. To tube feed we used to put a Ryles nasogastric tube up the nose and down into the stomach. The Ryles tubes were huge. It must have been most uncomfortable. As time went on, we got the fine-bore tubes which were much easier to put up a patient's nose and get them to swallow it to go into their stomach. We dietitians had to work out how to feed these unconscious patients. It would be Complan, raw eggs, milk, a teaspoon of Marmite, protein powder and a couple of other things. These feeds would be made up in the diet kitchen and put in wax cartons on the bottom of the food trolleys. So you've got this milk-based feed going into a sick patient after sitting on the bottom of a warm trolley. It was not the best thing.

On one of the wards, staff asked some of the relatives for a whip round. They got some food blenders, which were just coming in the 1960s/1970s. They put ordinary dinners in this blender and would then stick it down the tube. They were a law unto themselves. I tried to get them to stop, but the consultant wanted it done that way. When you're unconscious and injured, you need lots of extra protein and extra calories because the body is in a catabolic state. Just sticking a pulverised dinner down was not the best thing. I'm telling you things that make me shudder now and would make any dietitian today shudder. But we did the best that we knew at the time.

My second job was at King's College Hospital, where Dr RD Lawrence was 'the' chap for diabetes. It tended to be what we called 'type one' diabetes. There was no great mention of type two diabetes, because there was very little obesity. That's the thing that jumps out at me when I look back: I would do a general outpatient clinic, and there'd be people with coeliac disease or kidney disease, and there might be one overweight patient.

At King's College Hospital, I worked in the liver unit with Professor Roger Williams. I had the first ever liver transplant patient in this country. He had to have this very special diet. It was very high in calories because of the trauma of the operation. He's one of the patients who has stuck in my mind. I also worked in the renal unit, which was very new as well. Dialysis machines were just coming in. I remember the meetings when the doctors had to decide who could have a dialysis machine and who couldn't, depending on age and whether people had children. They had to decide, in a way, between life and death.

When I spoke to a consultant in 1967/68 about all these patients who had heart attacks, I remember him saying, 'We don't know what causes heart attacks. We're beginning to think it's not just one thing that causes a heart attack. We're beginning to think it's lots of different factors.' Patients would come in and if they were overweight – there weren't that many – we'd put them on a weight-reducing diet. People would take dietary histories to see what they'd eaten and see if we could improve it. But basically, the doctors didn't know what caused heart disease. Now, of course, we do know, so the incidence of heart disease has dropped.

It's a different profession to how it was in the 1960s. I think the National Health Service has improved in leaps and bounds. The way of working and the professionalism is so much better today than it was 50 years ago.

Wendy had two children in the early 1970s at a time when women were still expected to leave work and become a housewife and mother. But the shortage of dietitians led to her being asked to come back to work. She fought to get childcare from the hospital crèche, as she wasn't a nurse or a doctor. 'I battled away and, eventually, matron gave in. That meant that the children of cleaners, porters, whoever could go in the crèche because I broke the mould.'

SONYA BAKSI

After qualifying in medicine Sonya took a post in New End Hospital, Hampstead, caring for women who'd had illegal abortions. 'The sixties to the mid seventies was a really good time to work. They called it the 'swinging sixties' and you've got The Beatles and everything was so much lighter after the post-war years.'

This is 1963/1964. I finished 100 illegal abortions in the six months. Abortion was illegal. Women went to backstreet people who would start them bleeding, and then they would arrive bleeding on your doorstep. My consultant was Catholic, and she wouldn't work with them. I had to use the registrar [junior trainee] and sometimes I was on my own. And it was terrifying. I remember a Finnish or Swedish au pair girl. The anaesthetist saying to me, 'Sonya, I've already given six pints of blood, you've got to stop her bleeding.' You don't forget these things. She survived. I remember another woman who wouldn't talk to me. But she talked to the other women on the ward. Not only had somebody started her abortion off, they'd stolen her handbag and dumped her on the doorstep of our hospital. The women on the ward had a whip round to get the money to send her back home again.

In 1964 I joined the Abortion Law Reform Association, which estimated 100,000 illegal abortions a year. The law was reformed in 1967. We didn't have the Pill. It was either the Dutch cap, or the coil or sheath, for years. Afterwards, I did family planning clinics myself as part of my work in the maternity and child welfare services. I fitted umpteen Dutch caps. The women that I saw really upset me. I was determined to do health education in schools – which I did for a long time – and educate people so that we could do prevention.

My first job was in Camden Town, where I was the medical officer for two homes for unmarried mothers and their babies. One of them was Catholic, and the girls in 1966 were coming from Ireland, even as they come today. The other was Church of England. The girls told me how the matron would make them take the potato peelings out of the dustbin because they hadn't taken enough potato off the peel and scrape it off again. They would tell me how they had to go down on their hands and knees and polish the fender. Women that were nine months pregnant. Absolutely disgusting. I did the antenatal checks on them and I saw them at six weeks to give them a postnatal check. I also examined the baby to make sure the baby was fit for adoption. And I was callous. Those girls had been breastfeeding those babies for six weeks. Until I had my own pregnancy of my own child, I did that in a clinical and not a human way.

My clinic was Camden Town and my families were Greek Cypriots. A lot of the population of Cyprus had come to live in London because of their war. They all lived on my patch because we had two Greek Orthodox churches. I had a Greek nurse allocated to work with me, but she was from mainland Greece and she looked down on the Cypriots. We had to try and teach them about contraception and help them with immunisation. It was really hard work. We also had a lot of Irish, a lot of West Indians. They faced poverty, overcrowding, disgusting accommodation, language barriers, cultural barriers, everything. A lot of the multiple-occupation Victorian houses had sinks in the corner. How can you give a woman a Dutch cap when she's got to wash it, insert it and wash her hands afterwards, if she hasn't got the privacy of a bathroom? And the husbands. One woman told me the husband kept her Dutch cap locked in a cupboard and only gave it to her when he wanted sex, because he thought she might use it with somebody else. Another one told me her husband punched holes in it because he thought she'd be having an affair with other men.

The Abortion Act 1967 enabled women to terminate a pregnancy if there were health risks to the mother or her unborn child. But the decision had to be authorised by two doctors, one of whom had to be a gynaecologist/obstetrician. Doctors were allowed to opt out of the process if they were anti-abortion. Sonya continued her career working in community health, advocating for health education in schools. Seconded to the Department of Health to contribute her expertise to the development of the Children Act 1989 in that year, Sonya undertook the first inspection of mothers' and babies' health in prisons. Women were being treated with appalling cruelty and forced to do punitive, hard work. Sonya cried when reporting her findings to the Department of Health: 'The table of civil servants and medical officers went silent. Totally. I've never silenced them as much as I did at that time.' She succeeded in stopping these inhumane practices.

NORMA MURDOCH

Norma trained in nursing at the Victoria Hospital in Glasgow and, after qualifying, became a staff nurse on the orthopaedic ward. She and two of the other nurses got married to their husbands in the autumn of 1960.

We changed history because we got married and we were the first married staff nurses. In the Victoria, once you were married, you could work as a 'white coat', working on the wards, but you couldn't work as a Sister or anything. It was very weird and wonderful. I used to feel quite embarrassed because white coat nurses were so senior, but weren't allowed to be in charge of the ward. When we got married it caused quite a furore. Everybody was incredulous that all of a sudden they were going to have married staff. It's incredible when you think about it – it sounds ridiculous.

Norma moved into midwifery.

I loved mider [midwifery]. But I loved nursing, you see. It didn't matter where I was. I liked it all. I was a 'green lady'. The Glasgow Corporation had district nurses and they had midwives, and we all wore these green uniforms. The hat was like a cowboy hat. I had often been offered half price on the bus because they thought it was a school hat. Oh, it was fun! My husband was at sea and he was away for two or three months at a time. So it worked very well. And we lived in Clarkston then. My district was from Muirend right down Victoria Road. There were three of us who did one big district, and we shared. In those days women could choose to have their babies at home. Some of the GPs didn't like patients to have home confinements.

Nowadays, mothers are in and out the day that their babies are born, but they don't get the care that we gave them. We spoiled our patients. As soon as they registered with us, we went to visit and we took all their particulars. Sometimes we knew them for seven months before the baby was born and you would visit them once a month until the baby was two months. We went in and chatted and got to know them. You just kept an eye on things.

It was more social. We had a book for each of them. You would measure the tummies, take their blood pressure. We did all these things routinely.

What was it like, attending home births?

Oh, some of the stories I could tell you, you couldn't print it! But I loved it, I really did. What I liked about it was that when you went out to the house, hopefully they weren't just ready quite to deliver. You'd do an internal examination to see if the baby was on its way. There was a big box that every patient got. It had all sorts of dressing and pads. There was paper that was always waterproof. Some of these folk wouldn't have anything, so you were prepared for any eventuality. We had special white gowns that we wore. You'd get dressed and covered up when the babies were being born. Oh, happy days.

I had been sent out to this house in Gorbals, just to check this lady. It was her eighth or ninth baby. Everybody knew her. I went in and the first thing that I noticed was the smell of frying. The husband was cooking a great big frying pan of sausages for lunch. I can see all these sausage links. They had a big radiogram in the corner and there was a lot of paper on top of it and then this cooking area, one of these portable heaters on top of that. I'll never forget it. Mum was in bed, one of the beds in the wall – 'hole in the wall' beds were a feature of Glasgow tenements.

At the time there was a lot of Pakistani people coming in. They took over the [Glasgow] Corporation, they were driving all the buses. They had joss sticks burning and the smell just about knocked you out, it was so powerful. 'Could you possibly put that out?' 'Oh, of course.' The mums couldn't speak any English. It was lovely. You were welcomed with open arms. The women weren't used to having their babies in bed. They would squat. I said to the husband, 'Could you try and persuade your wife to have the baby in bed?' She did and everything went beautifully. The husband could speak English. He turned to me one day: 'My wife said it was like having the baby on the banks of the Ganges.' I took it as a compliment. She had already a couple of children, but she'd had them in Pakistan.

There were no mobile phones. For goodness sake, they didn't even have phones in the house. They would have to go and phone from outside, from a telephone box. I had a telephone at the side of my bed, and you were called in the middle of the night. I would phone the Corporation and they sent out a car. By the time I was dressed and had all my bits and pieces organised, there was a beautiful dark green Corporation taxi waiting at my door to take me, with the gas and air machine, to the patient.

I loved every bit of my job; I was very happy with wherever I worked. It's great to have all these things to talk about. I could talk the hind legs off a donkey, all the different stories!

Norma retired in the mid 1990s. 'The very idea of the NHS not existing doesn't bear thinking about,' she reflects.

GEOFF ADAMS-SPINK

Developed in the 1950s as a sedative or tranquiliser, thalidomide had become a popular treatment for pregnant women suffering from morning sickness. Just before the contraceptive pill was made available in December 1961, distributors of the thalidomide drug withdrew it from the UK market because it caused a range of disabilities as babies grew in the womb. Geoff was born in Leicester in 1962 and was one of the 10,000 or so babies affected worldwide.

My mother came to take to thalidomide because her father had just died. She had three young children and her mother to look after. Because of the grief – mother, father and daughter were very close – she'd spent several nights without sleep, and got to the end of her tether. The GP had prescribed thalidomide for her mother, who was equally grief-stricken and disturbed and unable to sleep. It was the new sedative that everybody was taking. So my mother took one pill, thinking, 'All I need is a good night's sleep.' And what you see before you is the consequence of that one pill.

I was born without a right eye. Instead of there being an empty socket, there was a something there that was like an eye, but wasn't an eye. When I was three, I was admitted to one of the big hospitals in Leicester, and that was removed. For me that was quite traumatic. My parents weren't allowed to stay with me. It was probably the first time they'd ever left me anywhere and I was frightened to death.

What memories do you have of that?

I was on a children's ward. It was incredibly noisy. There was always somebody crying. Feeling disorientated. Dreadful food – awful. I mean, I'm a lover of shepherd's pie, for God's sake, but even my three-year-old, not-very-discerning self knew that this was way below par. The other thing was it was the first time I'd encountered anybody who was Black. There was a very big, very smiley Black nurse on the ward. I was scared to death of her because I'd never encountered a Black person. In my village, you never saw a Black person at all. So, wow, that was a shock. I had another follow-up operation when I was five. Again, my mum and dad weren't allowed to be with me. They insisted that I was put on an adult ward because I found that children's ward too cacophonous. These old guys who were on my ward made a huge fuss of me and that was quite nice.

From the age of five, I was at special schools. Being born with impairments caused by thalidomide profoundly affected the way I grew up. It was 60 miles away and my parents were only allowed to see me once every three weeks. For the first four weeks, they weren't allowed to visit at all because there was a so-called 'settling-in period'. For a little kid who was five? I think that was quite tough. Look, I'll tell you how my mind and body rejected being away from home. Every morning, I defecated on the floor. And even now I don't know why I did that. The staff were horrified. And they obviously asked my mum and dad, 'What's going on?' Because if you had a dog that did that, you'd wonder, wouldn't you?

The other children had varying degrees of physical and/or learning disabilities. I was more mobile than most – there were an awful lot of wheelchair users. I was one of the lucky ones because I had a mum and a dad who took me home for the school holidays. A fair number of those kids had been in the position of the thalidomide children who were born and the doctors told their parents, 'Leave this one here and go home.' They had left that one there. They were in that place 365 days of the year. One or two developed relationships with local families who were eventually allowed to foster and adopt them. I felt lucky. I'd grown up with a mum and a dad and siblings, and it was a shock to me that anybody wouldn't have that because that was my only experience.

We were spoon-fed religion, but it was a very benign environment. All the staff were there for the right reasons. A lot of the kids at my first school had various surgeries. You had to be very careful, once somebody was in a plaster cast, not to bump them or jog them. Also to make sure that the door doesn't slam when you leave the room because that shock people feel goes right to the scar. It made me be very sensitive to people's extra needs when they were recovering at an early age. You take the average little kid who goes to the primary school. How many of their friends have their legs from toe to hip in a plaster cast?

There was a huge drive when we were thalidomide kids to normalise us. I'm showing you my left hand and on this left hand, I've got two fingers that are fused. That finger on the outside there doesn't have any bone or anything in it. The doctor said, 'Oh, we could just separate those.' My mum said, 'Why?' 'Well, it would look better.' 'That's not a good enough reason. Would it help him?' 'Not really.' 'In that case, no. I withhold my consent.' Although she wasn't able to counter the prevailing tide of 'your child has to go to a special school', when it came to things like this, she was able to say, 'No, you're not doing that to my son.' For those kids who didn't have parents, there was nobody for them to say, 'No, you're not separating those two fingers.' It would have just happened. That's a bit sad, really. There was too much lopping off of bits. I had a little friend called Wendy – still in touch with her now. She's a fellow trustee at the Thalidomide Society. She and I were best friends at school. I always call her my first girlfriend. She had little feet on the end of her little legs – she used to walk on the sides of her feet. We'd hold hands and cross the playground. Then she was taken into hospital and those feet were lopped off. Why? So that she could wear prosthetics. Now I always tell her how upset I was when that happened. But she always counters and says, 'But I'm still using my prosthetics.' So, in the end, it was for the greater good and I think the right decision was made. But my six-year-old self is still processing the fact that her little tiny feet were cut off for no good reason.

I was only there for three years, because the staff very quickly realised that, although I might have a couple of bits missing, my brain was fully functional. I was sent to Exhall Grange [School] when I was eight, and I remained there until after I finished my O levels. It was a very different sort of environment. It was halfway to being a prison camp. It had 300 kids: 100 girls and 200 boys. It was a very tough environment. Academically, it pushed kids really hard. The headmaster, George Marshall, was ahead of his time in two aspects. Firstly, in respect of saying that every child must maximise the use of their residual vision. No white canes, no guide dogs, no Braille. Large print? Yes. Magnifying glasses? Yes. You were given what they called low-vision aids and the teachers wrote on the board, very big. Also, he was way ahead of his time in thinking that kids who have various degrees of partial sight needed to get on in the world. That they needed to get certificates and qualifications. We were encouraged to work hard, so there was a huge amount of competition to be top of your class. The exam board allowed all of us 12 or 15 minutes per hour extra. There was an accommodation made for time, but that was about it.

My sister, when I spoke to her about my birth in adulthood, described it as like a nuclear bomb going off in the family. It was a disruptive event, shall we say. My mother and father had to make a lot of adjustments very quickly without any support or guidance. They just had to do their best. A lot of the thalidomide families were in that same situation: it was a shock. It was literally a shock. The NHS and the secretary of state for health at the time, Mr Enoch Powell, weren't geared up to support the families because they didn't know what the bloody hell was going on. Some thalidomide children were left at hospital and were put in the care of the state. At the time, doctors thought they were being kind. But these were people's lives. My dad had been involved in the Thalidomide Society in the early days of setting up. They had to make huge sacrifices to fund their own legal costs. They fought very hard on my behalf.

When I think back to medical advice then and now, it's chalk and cheese. For a start, I think doctors were seen as gods, and ordinary people didn't challenge the advice of a doctor. For me, thalidomide was one of those episodes where the deference given to people wearing white coats was suddenly undermined because these children were produced as a result of medication administered by these all-knowing, all-seeing, all-powerful doctors. It started a slightly more sceptical, I think, more healthy relationship with the medical profession, which was to say, 'Yes, I hear what you say, but I will go home and consider your advice. I'll maybe go and talk to some other people. Then I will come to my own conclusion because you're not always right.' If I throw that right forward to the whole anti-vaxxer debate, I understand how people feel when their GP says, 'It's safe. It's totally safe, don't worry.' If you want to look at the roots of what's behind the anti-vaccine movement, look at thalidomide, because that was what started to chip away at that polished, almost untouchable sense of medical men – and it was usually men – always being right.

I still think there's an awful lot more that needs to be done for families with disabled kids. I notice that people still have to fight like bloody hell to get kids the medical treatment or education. But my goodness, at least now the norm is that kids stay with their families.

Geoff gained a first class honours degree in Politics and French and then had a choice of a 'fast-track' Foreign Office post or a traineeship with BBC News. He opted for the BBC and became a writer, presenter and broadcaster. Working with the Thalidomide Trust, Geoff was instrumental in getting a new financial settlement from Diageo PLC, successor to the UK distributor of thalidomide, to support the health needs of thalidomide survivors as they age.

EILEEN HILL

Eileen grew up in Swinton, in Salford, and wanted to be a nurse from a very early age.

I can remember being with my friend at the entrance to the hospital. It was May 1966. We were very excited. It was Sunday. 'I'm going to start on this training on Monday.' We walked towards the nurses' home and there were cherry blossoms out. We were met by Home Sister. She took us to our rooms, and on our beds was our uniforms that we thought were absolutely wonderful! Blue dresses with starched white collars. We had to learn to put the hats on. And the best of all was the cloaks that had a red lining. We all put them on with the aprons and paraded up and down the corridor. A lot of us knew each other because we'd been cadet nurses at the hospital. On Monday morning we waited outside the School of Nursing for the senior tutor. She was very tall and imposing. I remember she smoked cigars. She was a fountain of knowledge. She was always very kind and nice. We absolutely adored her. Outside was a statue of Florence Nightingale, and we all thought, 'Oh, we get to be nurses.'

It was very strict. If you're on a ward with your best friend, she wasn't allowed to call you by your first name. I was Nurse Crumpton. My friend was Nurse Allcroft. There were only about 20 of us. I think there was one male. A lot of nurses in those days came from places like Jamaica. A lot of Irish nurses came across. So there was a mixture of cultures, which was new to me. We learned a lot about Irish girls. At the time, Irish music became quite popular. A lot of them were quite religious, so they did tend to stick together. We had a girl from Jamaica; she was lovely. We did have nursing nuns with long, white robes. One of them taught me to dance, because they'd not always been nuns. We got on quite well with different cultures. Found them very interesting. There was an Indian girl, but she had problems with the language so she didn't stay. She used to do a lot of Indian dancing for us. It was the sixties, so times were changing. We used to go out to a lot of clubs and things. So although it was the swinging sixties, I don't think it reached Hope Hospital [now Salford Royal Hospital]. We lived in the nurses' home. No men could go in.

We rebelled against the food they served us. The *Daily Mail* came. We had placards and banners. We sat down in the grounds and it was on the television. We demanded better food, because the problem was when we used to do split shifts. We'd work in the morning, have some time off in the afternoon, go back till eight o'clock when the night staff came on. Then we'd go over to the nurses' home for our meals. Sometimes you go across and there'd be no food left. We were paying for that. And the food wasn't very nice. So we had this rebellion. We didn't tell matron. She was absolutely livid with us. But we managed to get something done. A new restaurant was built for all staff, and the meals were much nicer. It meant that all the staff from the hospital could eat there, from doctors down to everyone, and I think eventually some of the relatives came in.

Eileen married at the end of her training and had a baby.

Were you well supported in trying to combine a career and a family?

Not really, no. I went back when my child was six weeks. When I worked nights my husband looked after the baby. But in the days, I had to get up and feed her and try and get a little bit of sleep. It was too much, really. I did go live with my mother, who helped a little bit. But it was very hard work. That would be the winter of '69. There was a flu epidemic and there was very little staff on the ward. I can remember being on the orthopaedic ward where you had quite a lot of young men who've been in motorbike accidents, for instance, in plaster. On my own there with 30 beds. That's when you ran. You couldn't walk because it was so very busy. Today, it's all very specialised, but then, you were a general nurse so you're expected to be able to go on all the wards. The hospital didn't have intensive care. Sometimes you'd be allocated to go and 'special' a patient who was very poorly. That was one-to-one nursing and you even had to 'special 'somebody on these very noisy respirators.

There weren't many things I didn't enjoy. I always remember having to clean somebody's false teeth. It was very busy in the sluice, where the bedpan washer was. I emptied the cleaning agent down the bedpan washer and the teeth fell in. I had to put my hands in and get them out and disinfect them. That was awful! [*laughs*]

Eileen trained as one of the first nurse prescribers in the 1990s. Now retired, she volunteers at Salford Royal Hospital in the 'meet and greet' service for patients. 'You see the doctors and nurses there. They have a coffee, and I do look back and think how different it was to when I worked there. I don't think the nurses would ever have had coffee with the doctors then.'

DAVID MORRISON

The 1960s saw rapid development of new medical technologies that benefited the most severely ill patients, including babies and children. David was one of the pioneers of intensive care units. After qualifying in medicine, he'd spent several years in the Royal Army Medical Corps before taking up a post at Crumpsall Hospital in Manchester.

I became known as a gadget man who was good with machinery. When the first defibrillator [a device that sends a pulse to the heart to restore a normal heart beat] was bought, and the physicians didn't understand how to use it, somebody said, 'Dave's a gadget man, take it down to him.' I took it apart and read the manual. We had a porter who had a coronary that night and they hadn't a bed for him. I put him in one of my beds and stuck him on this machine. The next morning I was standing with the senior medical registrar, talking about this machine, and the trace suddenly went flat. We really didn't know what to do. Bill said, 'Try pacing', because there was a pacemaker on it. I held the electrodes up in my fingers on the patient's chest while Bill switched it on. The patient started to jerk, and so did I, because I hadn't any rubber gloves on. The heart started again. We were so inspired by this that we set up a cardiac arrest team. That took a bit of doing in a major hospital – 2,000 beds – because we had to go round all the wards and standardise the trolleys so they'd all have the right equipment. And teach all the kids how to do mouth-to-mouth and cardiac massage. It was totally new in those days.

At that point, around 1965, we decided we'd have to have some form of intensive care unit. We were trying to do this on ordinary wards with ordinary nurses, and it was obviously impossible. I went to the medical superintendent, 'Look, we need to build some sort of a unit.' 'Well, if you can find a room, you can have it, but the place is full.' [*laughs*] So we found a room. He said, 'You can't have any money.' [*laughs*] So we stole all the equipment from other departments. [*laughs*] I'll never forget the dental surgeon coming in one day to see a patient and he'd got his foot on a brand-new piece of equipment. He said, 'Do you know, I've been waiting 10 years to get one of these and some bastard's pinched it.' [*laughs*] I said, 'The world is becoming a very dishonest place.' We had a tin of white paint, and everything we stole we used to paint white over-night and then paint ICU in large black letters on it, and it was ours. It was great fun. That way we built up a two-bedded unit to learn a trade on. We had to teach nurses. We had to teach ourselves. We didn't know what we were doing.

Was there much way of finding out the current state of ICU medicine at the time?

The only way was to go to conferences and talk to other guys. I used to pay my way to a lot of foreign conferences, because that's where you really learn. The Germans would give a paper that was fact, fact, fact. The British would give a paper that was waffle, waffle, waffle.

Did you ever sleep?

No, no. I started on my own and was given four nurses eventually. One of the nurses was one of the most experienced Ward Sisters in the hospital, who'd run a 30-bedded ward. She was useless because she couldn't adjust to dealing with one or two patients. When everybody went to sleep, she'd bath them, wake them up. 'Oh, these people are being rested,' we'd say. The best kids' nurses were the young. They were all extroverts. They became our family.

One of our nurses who had trained at another hospital came and worked for us. She was on one weekend, on her own in the unit. The anaes-thetist brought up a guy from theatre who needed long-term ventilation. He'd never used our type of ventilator before, so she had to explain how it worked and demonstrate this to him. Then the RMO [resident medical offi-cer] arrived wanting a blood-gas test. This needed an arterial blood sample and the RMO missed the radial artery. She said, 'Oh, give it here.' Took the syringe off him, stuck it in the femoral artery and took a sample. Then they tried to get one of the technicians from the path lab to work the blood gas results. Both were off. The nurse said to this guy, 'Look after the shop for a minute and I'll be back.' She dashed up to the path [pathology] lab and did the blood gases and came back with the results. Nobody had believed that nurses could do this sort of thing. I taught them all sorts of things that nurses weren't supposed to know. We formed probably one of the best teams ever.

We built the ICU up to eight beds, then they gave us a new unit. We decided to add a coronary unit. A bloke from the regional board came round and said it was not the policy of the regional board to mix coronaries with intensive care patients. I said, 'You tell that bugger there to go away and die somewhere else.' I got a new coronary unit. Then we added a dialysis unit because they were trying to transplant in Manchester.

All the other units were using junior staff to do the work – and this was wrong. If a bloke's really ill, he needs the guy with 20 years' experience. It's a job for senior people because you're going to have some very difficult decisions, a lot of ethical decisions, and you've got to have the clout to do it. You've got to be senior enough to put your foot down and say, 'This is what's going to happen.'

There were five hospitals in the Manchester group. Everybody said they wanted an ICU. That was obviously impossible. We couldn't afford it. The only answer was to find a way of getting people to the unit safely and swiftly, so I built an ambulance and we used to go and fetch the patients. We'd got a Volvo estate car. We turned the front passenger seat the wrong way round, so that the stretcher went into the doctor's lap, sitting in a reverse seat, and he could intubate. The cutaway back seat had the nurse in it and on the back of the driver's seat was a fixed case with all the drugs, syringes and needles in it. Behind the nurse was the defibrillator, ECG, etc. The only thing we couldn't do sitting down was cardiac massage, so we bought a pump and I worked out that we could alter the design so it would sit in a gantry and be swung over the patient. Every fifth pump it blew as a ventilator, so it was another pair of hands.

I looked at my intensive care quite differently to most people, and in a way started a new subject. It set out a way of thinking. And that's what I'm proud of. It didn't entirely catch on. A lot of the people who are in intensive care nowadays are anaesthetists who know all about ventilating people, but sod all about what you do in kidney failure. It was a great life. I had a great time. Whether I achieved anything is a very different matter. But I tried.

David retired in 1989 and returned to his north-east roots, building his own house in Northumberland. He died in December 2022.

At the end of the 1960s

In 1961 the NHS had become the UK's largest employer, with a workforce of more than 600,000. The easing of post-war austerity meant that there was more leeway for investment in the NHS, and the 1962 Hospital Plan for England and Wales included 90 new district general hospitals and more than 130 redevelopment programmes. The Plan was significant because, for the first time, it took a population-based approach to healthcare, setting out the range of services and norms for bed capacity and staffing. Technological advances like cardiac pacemakers and new drugs like beta-blockers meant that more complex diseases and conditions could be treated – and hospitals evolved to create new spaces of care, including intensive care units, as David Morrison recounted.

The more liberal attitudes of the 1960s played out across the NHS, and women gained ground in regard to equality in the workplace and access to contraception. Nursing norms began to flex to accommodate women like Norma Murdoch and Eileen Hill, who wanted to return to work after marriage and then combine work and family life. Nurses also became more vocal about their grievances around low pay and poor conditions, and went on strike. Women gained better control over their sexuality through the contraceptive pill and the reduction in stigma around unmarried sex. The Abortion Act 1967 gave women new rights to terminate a pregnancy – although this often remained difficult in practice because of resistance from some doctors.

But the decade also witnessed the tragedy of thalidomide that affected more than 10,000 families across the world and raised new questions about the ethical responsibilities of scientists and doctors. It brought more scrutiny to medical processes and marked a watershed in the testing and regulation of medicines. The Committee on Safety of Medicines was set up in 1964 to regulate the use of new drugs, and the Yellow Card Scheme was introduced for the reporting of adverse reactions to drugs. Nevertheless, the more liberal attitudes of the 1960s did not change the experiences of people with disabilities like Geoff Adams-Spink and Elsie McMahon, who were still excluded from mainstream schools and sent away from their families for education.

The NHS's anniversary in July 1968 was marked by a conference, chaired by Kenneth Robinson, Labour minister of health.[13] It reflected on the NHS's remarkable achievements through technological advances and the huge increase in new drugs. It also raised questions about the need to rethink aspects of the service, particularly the need to better coordinate services across the three parts of the system – hospitals, primary care and public health services. 'Forward into the 1970s!' was the closing remark from Robinson. It was to be a turbulent decade in which the NHS underwent its first structural reorganisation.

Chapter 4: 1970s

'When the list came for specialisms, all the white girls were given obstetrics and all the Black girls were given geriatrics.'

CAROL BAXTER

'Bloody Sunday was the first major disaster in Northern Ireland and a lot of the patients had gunshot wounds in their legs, and parts of their body.'

URSULA CLIFFORD

'I said [to Barbara Castle] … "the arguments they use for the 1974 NHS Reorganisation are very compelling and we have to put the patients first."'

DAVID OWEN

'We always had a Ward Sister or senior nurse on the ward round. They actually ran the show.'

GEORGE BENTLEY

'I mean, they wouldn't have me in a golf club then because I was the wrong colour.'

RAJ MENON

'I went to the student health centre … "I'm pregnant."
"Okay, what size shoes do you take?"'
KATHRYN BRAITHWAITE

'I asked very pointed questions about patient involvement
and I really made myself a bloody nuisance.'
EDWINA CURRIE JONES

'…predominantly young Black patients were brought to the
hospital in severe, painful crisis due to sickle cell.'
ELIZABETH ANIONWU

'So an engineer and an electrician – we did 99 per cent of the work.'
PETER MOORE

'I can remember … having conversations of a polite but strained nature
with some of the staff who didn't really believe in patient power.'
DIANA

'It broke your heart if you looked at any of the children in depth,
to see all the things that had gone wrong with them.'
MASUD HOGHUGHI

'When you have a sickle cell crisis, you have a lot of serious pain.'
BASIL BRAMBLE

'It doesn't matter whether the patient's conscious or unconscious …
We treat them as if they can hear us and they can feel us touch them.'
PATRICIA MACARTNEY

'He manipulated her feet … while her bones were still more supple … I was
crying outside the door and she was crying the other side of the door.'
MARION and CERI WATERS

CAROL BAXTER

The NHS continued to recruit staff from overseas during the 1970s. Whereas, in 1948, people coming to Britain from former colonies were granted citizenship, the Immigration Act 1971 withdrew the right of entry for prospective nurses from these places. In the same year, the Royal College of Nursing, with very little evidence, made claims to the Briggs Committee on Nursing about educational levels of overseas nurses. Carol was born in the seaport town of Port Maria in Jamaica. As she got older she began to look for opportunities to widen her horizons. 'It was the sixties. I was coming of age and it was the Black Power movement. People are becoming very globally conscious of the Vietnam War. I began to understand the world in a bigger way. I thought, "It's probably a good idea to try and link all my interests together in global health, and perhaps train in the UK."'

I happened to be sitting on a bus and picked up a *Mirror* newspaper from a Jamaican woman who'd brought the newspaper back from England. It had the Profumo affair splashed all over it. I read the juicy gossip and turned the pages to see snippets about the NHS. I began to understand the concept of the National Health Service. 'It sounds like an amazing idea.', I'm thinking. I started studying as a scientist at the University of West Indies in Jamaica, knowing I was biding my time. I saw the advertisement to study nursing in England in *The Gleaner*, which is our local Jamaican paper. I was selected with a group of other young women to come to study in the UK.

I found myself in London on a train to Manchester before New Year's Eve 1970, all organised by the Jamaica High Commission. I was put in a taxi to Hope Hospital [now Salford Royal Hospital] where I was met by the nursing home Sister. That was the start of the nursing journey. It was cold. I was fascinated with the smoke coming from the chimneys. I'm thinking, 'Where are the leaves on the trees?' The next night there was a New Year's Eve party in the nurses' home. I had a whale of a time listening to the music people were singing: 'She'll be coming around the mountain when she comes,' which is the first time I'd heard that song. In all honesty my first few days here surpassed my expectations in terms of that sense of wonder, that sense of difference, that sense of excitement.

When we went on the wards, that's when I began to really realise some of the inequalities that I saw. When the list came for specialisms, all the white girls were given obstetrics and all the Black girls were given geriatrics. That seemed, to me, a signal that something's wrong. I asked the tutor about it innocently: 'Did I remember you saying that if you ask early, you would get your specialism? And I was the first to ask.' She denied it. That opened my eyes up to some of the wrongdoings that went on, along with all the good stuff that happened. It began to spark consciousness in me to try and see if some of those things could be changed, or addressed, or at least flagged. There was total agreement with the other Black nurses that that was unfair. We talked about it an awful lot. I was the one who tended to represent and turn up and challenge, because that's who I was.

I didn't get any support from white nurses at all – even down to when a patient would be rude to you because of your colour. It was not a big issue for me, because usually, they're geriatric and old. Old patients are confused. They would say, 'Take your filthy Black hands off me.' You'd look to your nurse friend, but they would say they didn't see it, didn't hear it, or denied it. Or they would say, 'Oh, come on, grow up, and don't be so sensitive.' It meant that because the white nurses didn't see it or didn't want to see it, it took longer for it to be addressed. It was never addressed in the hospital setting in my time.

When the nursing exam results came out, all the girls who did well got a book inscribed, except for the coloured girls going back to their own countries, who were told that they would get a cheque for £5. I thought, 'Well, that's not fair. I was top of the class in medicine. I'd like a book inscribed.' I challenged them. 'I don't want your £5, thank you.' They would have been taken aback by someone refusing what they thought was a gift. It wasn't a gift for me. It was an insult. I wrote a letter to the matron. I didn't take the cheque. I had just applied to become a health visitor. I thought, 'Well, I've done it now, and nobody's going to give me a reference. I've been arguing with the nurse tutors for three, four years; I've been asking too many questions.'

When I went for the interview, they said, 'Yours is the best reference we've ever had from any student coming to study public health nursing,' and that's stayed with me. It helped me to understand that sometimes being authentic and being who you are, and speaking out, may not be popular at the time, but somebody will stop and listen, and then give you that respect. I think this is what I did. I mean, the other side of it could be, 'If we don't give her the reference, we might still have her here with us for another few years, and it's the best way of getting rid of her.' But I'd like to give them the benefit of the doubt in that.

The mindset at the time was, we were foreigners coming into their country – but they were very dependent on us. We did a good job, and we cared for people very well and we were a saviour to the NHS. We came when there was nobody else here to deliver care, and these people knew that.

At the time, The Race Relations Acts 1965 banned racial discrimination in public places, but did not cover employment organisations. Carol continued to play a pioneering role around raising awareness of racism and discrimination, and later moved into research and academia.

URSULA CLIFFORD

Ursula worked through the devastation of the Troubles in Northern Ireland that began in the 1970s and were to last until the Good Friday Agreement in 1998. 'I hope you become as good a nurse as your aunt,' Ursula was told by matron at her interview. 'My aunt was a district midwife. That sowed the seed for me to decide I wanted to be a nurse.'

I was one of the most junior people at the opening of Altnagelvin Area Hospital in Derry on 1 February 1960. It was the first hospital opened after the war, and was on the National Health Service. We had newspapers and magazines and radios at that time – no television – coming to the hospital and talking to us and asking our opinion. And it was very exciting.

What was the most challenging of your experiences?

The beginning of the Troubles in Northern Ireland, because the operating theatres played a big part in the immediate care, which meant we were first responders. It started all off on Bloody Sunday – a massacre on 30 January 1972, when British soldiers shot 26 unarmed civilians during a protest march in the Bogside area of Derry. Everybody was confused and didn't know what we were doing. Running around with lists of patients. We didn't know where they would be operated on.

Bloody Sunday was the first major disaster in Northern Ireland and a lot of the patients had gunshot wounds in their legs, and parts of their body. I remember distinctly, one of the surgeons coming to the orthopaedic surgeon, and telling him to 'lay it open'. Now a gunshot going through soft tissue in the leg, for instance, you have an entry wound and an exit wound. He came in and he said, 'Lay it all open.' The surgeon muttered to me, 'Oh, that was done in the Spanish Civil War.' So, in a sense, we were still using treatments from as far back as the Spanish Civil War. When it came to saving legs that were blown up and things like that, they developed methods of screws and plates. Same in the facial injuries. We developed these methods of screws and plates and bolts that saved their legs and you didn't have to amputate them, which they would have had to do even up to the Second World War. Even all the gunshot powder up around their face and how to scrub it off. The patient then eventually got new skin and looked perfectly normal. The treatment of burns was another thing that we got more efficient at as well: how to dress them and prevent infection.

I became, eventually, the manager of critical care, managing operating theatres, casualty department and ICU. I was in charge whenever we had a tragedy. Everybody was so competent. Everybody knew what they were doing. We very quickly were able to put the patients through the system. To me, looking back, that was the evolvement of critical care and first responding. We became so proficient because of having to deal with injuries that were previously not known to us. We developed treatments for them, especially the facial maxillary people dealing with bombs on the face, and rubber bullets and things like that. How we dealt with it … taught the world. That was my highlight before I retired.

'I had a wonderful career,' reflects Ursula, now in her eighties. She delights in the fact that her daughter now works in the NHS and gives her a day-to-day account of 'what's going on in the place'.

DAVID OWEN

The NHS underwent the first reorganisation of its structures in 1974. It was intended to improve coordination of health and social services by aligning health and local authority boundaries. A new three-tier structure of regional, area and district health authorities was introduced, and public health was brought out of local authorities into the NHS. Local authorities retained responsibility for environmental health, communicable diseases, housing, clean air, pollution, food safety and pest control. David unexpectedly found himself at the centre of the 1974 changes. After qualifying in medicine in 1962, he had worked on neurological research until 1966, when he was elected as Labour MP in his home town of Plymouth. He served on the board of Charing Cross Hospital while they were in the midst of planning a new hospital. 'It was the best investment that the health service made in me. When I later became minister of health, I had some idea how the damn thing ran.'

1974 – I remember it well. I'd just been appointed parliamentary under-secretary for health by Harold Wilson, Labour prime minister. 'Who's my boss?' 'Barbara Castle.' 'But Barbara Castle is secretary of state for health and social security. She can't run the health service.' 'No, you'll be doing it.' 'Harold, an undersecretary? The BMA [British Medical Association] will eat me up for breakfast. They won't ever agree to talk to me. They'll endlessly say Barbara has to.' 'Well, I've run out of numbers of ministers of state and I have to legislate to increase the number – but I promise you I will increase and make you a minister.

I went to Barbara. She lifted up the phone in front of me – she knew Harold pretty well, and she was a remarkable woman. She was Labour's equivalent to Margaret Thatcher: ideological, attractive, used her feminine wiles. Very difficult to argue out of a position, but if you're still standing after 10 minutes, usually she would listen and would change her views. She rings up Harold: 'David is right, I never thought of it, but the BMA … Are you promising me, Harold, you'll make him a minister? 'Yes.' So he kept his word.

We went straight into a meeting. I hadn't even formally been appointed. The chief civil servant came in. 'My colleagues and I have come to talk to you about the fact that Sir Keith Joseph's legislation for the 1974 NHS reorganisation has all gone through Parliament, but the appointed day is in three weeks' time. Now, we will argue against you changing that and postponing it, but I want to say right at the start, if you do decide to do that, we will loyally serve you and carry it out.' Barbara said, 'Fine, go ahead, explain your views.' They gave their views and she turns to me. 'David, what do you think?' Bloody hell. We knew each other and we'd been on the National Executive Committee on the Health Service and things, so I admired her even then. I said, 'Well, it isn't easy to say, Barbara, because you and I were on the committee that made the recommendation for the general election manifesto that we're going to give this reorganisation up, but the arguments they use are very compelling and we have to put the patients first, so I think we have to bite on the bullet and accept it.' To my great surprise, she said, 'I agree with you.' So we accepted it. That's to her great credit and it's to the credit of the civil service, the way they conduct themselves.

That reorganisation had many problems and it was a difficult issue for us for a while, but we've weaved our way through it. We made more of the Community Health Councils [CHCs], and I do regret their passing. By the way they evolved, they were beginning to have a very good consumer voice in the health service and they were also listened to by quite a lot of the health service. That reorganisation had merits and considerable demerits, but one of its merits was that hospitals had catchment areas – and by creating areas and districts, it stopped going down the route whereby hospitals would be detached from their catchment areas.

What do you think is the most significant achievement during your period as health minister?

I had two great advantages. Barbara Castle was secretary of state for health and social security and she was very keen to try and get an all-party agreement on basic pensions, which she did really, in many ways, achieve. So she was ready to delegate quite a lot to me and there were two big things at that time: abortion and cigarettes. Barbara smoked like a chimney and she's now written about the fact that she had an abortion when she was younger. She had supported abortion law reform in 1965, and her constituency was a very big Catholic population and she lost quite a lot of votes. I think she got worried about that.

It was an extraordinary Labour government 1966 to 1970. We didn't have any money, we were having endless financial crises, but we had this new input of young Labour MPs and we did abortion law reform. David Steel was responsible for that, on a Private Member's bill. Homosexual law reform, divorce law reform – we put all these things through. In '74, we were facing a very difficult situation around abortion law reform because there was an argument about 24 or 28 weeks as the time limit for termination. The previous government had set up a commission, and they made a sensible minor change in the number of weeks. Pressure was up for us to legislate. Now the problem about that is, in those days, we didn't have a majority in the House of Commons. Any bill that was going to deal with this recommendation would open up the whole Abortion Act – so it was very dangerous. So I dealt with that. We kicked it out of touch.

The second thing was a much more pressing problem. There were endless stories in the *Evening Standard* – 'London's the abortion capital of the world', and the opening up of private abortion clinics. The 1967 Abortion Act didn't introduce licencing. I said, 'We will introduce a licencing system inside the Department of Health.' The legal advice was: you will be acting *ultra vires* – beyond the power of law. You will be taken to court. 'Well, I'm prepared to be taken to court. If they sue me, I'll say I've overridden the advice because it was a state of emergency that abortion clinics, which were totally unsanitary and not with any proper basic standards, were endangering the lives of women.' I looked at the bill and thought it was within my powers to introduce licencing schemes, so I did. I did wonder whether I would be in court arguing that I'd acted beyond my powers, but there was never a beep and it went through.

David left the Labour Party in 1981 to form the Social Democratic Party, leading it until its demise in 1990. He was appointed a Life Peer in 1992 and sits in the House of Lords as an independent social democrat.

GEORGE BENTLEY

George grew up in Sheffield, which, in the late 1930s, was a major steel town and mining area. His father managed a steel mill and his mother was a seamstress. His mother had an ambition for him to become a doctor. George liked that the local GP had 'the best car in town'.

I inclined towards surgery right from the beginning. I loved the drama of the operating theatre – I suppose a feeling of power and being able to control something and to do something. The other thing is the feedback you get from the patients. For most surgeons that is a drug, you know.

George specialised in orthopaedics, working during an exciting time of the introduction of internal fixation for fractures.

Internal fixation is a routine treatment for most fractures now. If you had a fractured femur, the standard treatment would be going to bed for 12 weeks with traction with a pin through the femur, waiting for it to heal and doing exercises every day. The orthopaedic wards used to be full. Now it's a nail down the femur and you're out in a couple of days. It's amazing. So exciting.

Surgical training was very busy but very exciting. It was a wonderful team effort. Each one of those people – consultant, senior registrar, lecturer – would take it upon themselves to teach you those things. Over six months you could learn so much. You didn't see much of your wife or family. It was all work. We didn't mind that. It was what we were there for. People backed you up when you were up for a job. You would have to go for an interview, and it was open. The great thing about the surgical scene is that it has been pretty well egalitarian. I moved 10 times during my training so, on average, we moved every two years until I became a consultant. We talked about it at length and my wife said, 'I really want to be with the children.' We were always short on money, but my wife never ever interfered with my training.

George was appointed professor of orthopaedic and accident surgery and consultant orthopaedic and spinal surgeon in Liverpool in 1976, and in 1982 moved to the Royal National Orthopaedic Hospital in London.

Each ward had a Sister who ruled with a rod of iron. At that time you couldn't be married and be a nurse. They were tremendous people. The women had given up an awful lot to dedicate themselves to their profession. We learned an awful lot from nurses. When you first started, if you didn't get on with a Ward Sister, boy, you are in big trouble. But they became your friends as you got more senior. They ran the nursing side. We ran the medical side. If we had a problem, we used to combine meetings and discuss it.

To talk about the emergence of consensual therapy later on is nonsense. It was going on already. At Royal National Orthopaedic Hospital Stanmore I had Sister Hart for about 20 years. If I had a problem, I would go and see her and say, 'What do you think, Sister?' Everything about the patient's care in bed was their province. We'd never interfered with that. Occasionally, we'd say, 'This wound's bleeding, or a dressing needs changing.' But never, ever would we interfere with any of the other things. These nurses became supremely expert at dealing with people. Whether they had enough pillows, whether they'd opened their bowels, whether the skin was getting sore. 'Are you comfortable? Do you need anything else before you go to sleep?' The level of care and dedication was very, very impressive.

One of the crises in the health service has been the lack of good relationships between doctors and nurses. There has been a serious breakdown. It really came around the mid seventies. What was happening was a complicated thing. I hope I can say this to you without seeming to be reactionary. I'm actually being factual. Society was changing, women wanted independence. There was a big fuss about it and they restructured nursing with the Salmon Report in 1967. When I started, the senior nurses were people who had more or less decided they weren't going to get married ever. So they dedicated themselves but, boy, they were expert. The senior nurses ran the ward and taught junior nurses, and it went down the line. None of that was interfered with by the doctors. A lot of those nurses, particularly in Sheffield, were not necessarily very well educated. But they were compassionate, caring people. That's absolutely critical if you're going to be a nurse. When they introduced the idea of degrees that tended to recruit more people who were interested in personal ambition and progression, and who were usually better educated; the problem was that there was a period when the only way you get more salary was by going into nursing administration – and I think that was bad. All of that led to a tension between the doctors and nurses, and we've never really resolved it, I don't think. For me personally, the relationship between doctors and nurses was never a problem. As you get more senior, it's less of a problem, because they'll take it from the chief. But there were a lot of strains in the system. Nowadays, the juniors have a rough time with the nursing profession.

I'm proud of the career I've had. I've been very lucky. The people really influencing your life are the people you work for. I've had some wonderful experiences and I've got a huge respect for the people in the service.

Now in his eighties, George continues to be involved in research and writing on orthopaedics and musculoskeletal science.

RAJ MENON

By the 1970s many overseas doctors, particularly from South Asian countries, worked for the NHS. But the racial discrimination of the times led to the 1975 Merrison Report, which raised questions about the clinical competence and language skills of overseas doctors and led to a complete reappraisal of the professional registration of overseas doctors in the NHS. During this period a group of doctors set up the Overseas Doctors' Association 'to protect and promote the interests of overseas doctors in the UK'. Raj Menon's family originated from Kerala, India, but became first-generation immigrants in Singapore, where Raj was born in 1948.

My father was Indian origin. My mother was Indian origin. I was very fortunate the government of India gave me a scholarship to train in medicine. I qualified from Andhra Medical College in Visakhapatnam, which is now a city in the state of Andhra Pradesh in South India. But in 1970, just as I went into a clinical year, the government of Singapore decided to de-recognise all Indian degrees. It was mostly a racial attack on the Indian population, because a large number of Indians were doctors and lawyers. A predominantly Chinese government felt that was not right. The only way to bring them down was to de-recognise Indian degrees, and then to give an aptitude test – only for Indians.

So I knew that I couldn't go back to Singapore. I applied for a clinical attachment in Leeds, St James's University Hospital. I took a charter flight with money I borrowed from my eldest brother. I borrowed £40 from my second brother. It was the first time I wore a suit. 'I will return this money to you.' (By March '75, I settled all the debts.) I landed in Gatwick Airport at 2 a.m. I didn't know anyone. But there was someone there from the British Council. 'Look, I need to get to Leeds.' He provided the transfer from Gatwick Airport to a British Council place in London, and he got me a taxi first thing in the morning, as soon as the day was light, and I got a train from King's Cross Station to Leeds. I arrived in Leeds on 16 August 1974. I booked a room in the YMCA in Leeds in Chapel Allerton. My bag was full of medical books, very few clothes. I asked the warden how to get to

St James's Hospital. I took a bus as instructed. She told me to get down at a public house called Dock Green. And I didn't know what a public house was! I took the reverse journey to come back and I thought, 'I must remember how to do that.'

Within two weeks a consultant called me and said, 'Look, you can apply for jobs. And you can give my name as reference.' Some of my white colleagues took me to Leeds Infirmary, to personnel department, and introduced me. 'This is Raj, he's free to do locum jobs.' I stayed there until January 1975 and came back to St James's to do my medical pre-registration jobs.

My first stint in general practice was a rural practice in Todmorden. It was quite tough, being called out middle of the night. For the first month or so, my trainer would come out with me. The demands patients made, I thought, were unfair. Patients used to call you out in the middle of the night. And you had to go. My parents never had the money to call the doctor out. But I couldn't say all that. I just kept it to myself. But I did tell my trainer: 'You know, you are lucky here. I grew up in Singapore, where my parents didn't have much money. We had to grit our teeth and go and see a doctor the following morning.'

The first call on my own at night was a sheep farmer. I went in my jeans and my turtleneck sweater. I knocked on the door at 11 p.m. in a godforsaken place in Todmorden up in the hills. It was February, March, extremely cold. 'I am Doctor Menon.' He said, 'Doctor?' He slammed the door shut and he rung my trainer. 'There's a chap outside in a pair of jeans and sweater.' Unbeknown to me, my trainer went out on call at night in a full suit. I'm used to the hospital, where I was on call. During daytime I had a tie and a white coat, but at night I was wearing jeans. He opened the door and said, 'Come on in, then,' and he was quite rude.

A lot of my patients when I first joined the practice had been in the [First World] War. I used to tell them of my father's experiences as a Japanese prisoner of war in Singapore. My father never spoke to me about what he went through. But suddenly there was a connection between us. 'Doc, we didn't tell our children either,' one patient told me.

In the days when I was a trainee, you had a morning surgery and evening surgery, and afternoons, the GPs are free. Some of the partners used to play golf or do whatever. I never went anywhere. I mean, they wouldn't have me in a golf club then because I was the wrong colour. They euphemistically call it 'blackballing'. So if you are an Asian, one black ball is the equivalent to 10 white balls or whatever. So there was no chance of me playing golf.

But I developed smear clinics, antenatal clinics, baby clinics in the afternoon, which wasn't existent in my practice when I took over. My senior partner said, 'Okay, well, I'm going to retire, so you can do.' Monday afternoons, we had baby clinic, Tuesday afternoon, an antenatal clinic. All the afternoons were filled up as I went along, and by the time I retired, we had them every morning, afternoon and evening. The surgery was always full of people.

By the time Raj retired, the practice cared for 6,500 patients and had four full-time partners. 'I've had a difficult, at times painful, journey, but when I look back, I'm happy.'

KATHRYN BRAITHWAITE

The National Childbirth Trust was set up in 1956 by Prunella Briance, who had suffered two traumatic childbirths. It began lobbying to reduce medical intervention in childbirth in the late 1960s, and through the 1970s, became prominent in middle-class mothers' experiences of birth. Kathryn had her babies at a time when the National Childbirth Trust was a strong influence on mothers and childbirth.

I must have been about 17, going to get contraception from a GP. That was very traumatic. I was still at school. The GP was a friend of my parents. I knew that there were places that you could go. I think it was called Marie Stopes. But that was in London, and I was in Ruislip. And that's a hassle. Even though I went to school in Hammersmith, it would have been a pain to go and find one. If you lived in the suburbs, it was just your GP. He gave me what I wanted. I think it was the Pill in those days. When I've looked back on it, with hindsight, it just seems not great. I think these days, young people have much better access to the things that they need. You had to have a lot of self-confidence to obtain contraception, which luckily, I had. There was a stigma.

When I was at university, I got married at the end of my second year. And I got pregnant quite quickly. I went to the student health centre. This is now 1974. 'I'm pregnant.' 'Okay, what size shoes do you take?' 'Six and a half.' 'That's fine, okay.' 'I want to have the baby at home. Because I'm not ill, I'm just going to have a baby.' It was that era. Barefoot and pregnant, Laura Ashley dresses. The shoe size was relevant because of the pelvis size. They told me that if I'd had smaller feet, they wouldn't have let me have the baby at home.

I had a lovely midwife called Sister Rainbow, and she gave me most of my antenatal care. I went to see the professor when I was studying for my finals. 'How's it going?' 'It's really difficult because I keep looking at the Mothercare catalogue.' You learn a lot from the Mothercare catalogue about babies if you know nothing. The day I went up to get my degree, he shook my hand. 'Obviously, you weren't looking at the Mothercare catalogue all the time.' I'd got a 2:1 and done okay. But yeah, it was difficult.

It was the days of the National Childbirth Trust. Birth is not an illness. You learn about all the stages. You learn your nursery rhyme for tapping on your leg. You're going to do it naturally. You don't have drugs. You're under a lot of pressure, actually, to be that person. I read about the first stage of labour, the second stage of labour and the transition. When Sister Rainbow said, 'I think it's time to push,' I remember saying, 'But I haven't been through transition yet,' because I was looking at it in an academic way. I had my second child at home as well. Same midwife, Sister Rainbow. Another home birth.

I look back and think, 'Gosh, that was mad.' When I think about childbirth now, about when my grandchildren were born, it's all such a big deal. It's not just that you don't have any drugs to help. It's just that you're in a room with a midwife. There's no doctor nearby.

Soon after the birth of her second baby, Kathryn and her family went to live in South Korea, 'leaving the joys of the NHS behind. Most of our early experiences with a baby and a toddler were done on the other side of the world, where things were much harder.'

EDWINA CURRIE JONES

Edwina was born in Liverpool and remembers being taken to child health clinics in the 1950s, where cod liver oil and orange juice was handed out.

The NHS is one of the reasons that I chose to live in this country. All my family come from Eastern Europe. They're all Eastern European, Jewish immigrants, Ashkenazi immigrants – and they started coming to the UK in the 1890s. They got as far as Liverpool and got stuck! Growing up in Liverpool, there had always been a strong interest in public health before the NHS came into play. We had one of the first medical officers of health in the country, and health was very much part of the education service and the child health service. My dad didn't believe in doctors and medicine. He thought they were all quacks because he'd had TB when he was a child and the doctors had not been able to help. He refused to have me vaccinated against smallpox, so he had to go to court. What really annoyed my mum was not so much that he didn't want me vaccinated, but that he couldn't remember the baby's name. [*laughs*] When I was about 13 years old, my dad refused permission for the BCG [Bacillus Calmette–Guérin] vaccination [for tuberculosis]. So I waited. On my sixteenth birthday, 1962, I went to the school nurse and I had everything done.

After winning a scholarship to Oxford, Edwina visited New York to stay with her aunt.

One of the things that pulled me back was the health service. It rapidly became apparent that I am an asthmatic and would not get the care that I needed in the United States. I couldn't afford private care and I wouldn't get insured. The basic principle of the NHS was that it was everybody's insurer. It came home to me very forcibly when I had an abscess on a tooth and my insurance in America didn't cover dental care. I ended up losing a front tooth. I'm 18 years old, and I got a denture … It was a long time before I could afford to do anything about that. I found myself thinking, 'There's something fundamentally different about being British.' If go home, and I go to my college course, I have a duty to put something back. I don't know how, but I will. The NHS has always been very much part of what makes me British, I think.

By 1974 Edwina was married and expecting her first child, and the family moved to Birmingham, where she rapidly became involved in politics.

Off we went to Birmingham, and we found we had really landed on our feet. The only thing I really insisted on was that we live inside Birmingham, not outside. Debbie was born just after the October general election of 1974. Our local candidate was Mr Cadbury. And so we had the meetings in our house. I made chocolate cake. The baby was passed around and cooed over. Then the 1975 council elections came up and we had a vacancy in our ward, so I was a shoe-in. I remember saying to them, 'Well, I'd be happy to have a go, but I'm going to need some help.' 'What kind of help?' 'Babysitters.' Every hand went up. By 1975 I was on Birmingham City Council. The great thing about Birmingham was it was a nonconformist city with a very strong tradition of local government. The Birmingham way of doing things chimed with me. If you're going to spend public money, you have a strong responsibility to ensure it's spent well. That may sometimes mean spending more, not less. You have a strong responsibility to explain to people how their money is being spent, and why.

I volunteered to go on the central Birmingham Health Authority Board as a council representative, often taking the baby with me. I got myself on the maternity subcommittee because Debbie was born at the maternity hospital, and I was not happy with some aspects of the professor's care there. I asked very pointed questions about patient involvement and I really made myself a bloody nuisance on this committee. We were able to do a number of things that helped women. For example, the main slots in the car park, right next to the door, were all the consultants, so we banished them and we made those spaces for patients. We got the buses to divert to go through the car park, so pregnant women could get off the bus and go straight in for antenatal clinics. So attendance at antenatal clinics went up.

Edwina's challenging of medical authority and paternalistic attitudes reflected the rise in patient and community activism during the 1970s. The 1974 NHS reorganisation introduced Community Health Councils (CHCs), which were the first mechanism for patients and the public to have their voices heard. Edwina stood for Parliament in 1983 and served in Margaret Thatcher's government between 1986 and 1988. She was involved with campaigns on heart disease, and women's cancer screening and health promotion, as well as the government's first AIDS campaign. She is now well known as a writer and broadcaster.

ELIZABETH ANIONWU

Elizabeth was inspired to become a nurse after receiving sensitive and compassionate treatment for her severe eczema from a nun: 'I really thought she was the most wonderful woman in the world.' During the 1970s attention began to focus on the health needs of some of the UK's new ethnically diverse communities. Sickle cell anaemia is a rare inherited blood disease which, in the UK, affects people of African and Caribbean origin. There is no cure for the condition, and care focuses on patient education and screening. NHS staff of African Caribbean heritage like Elizabeth were crucial pioneers in advocating for appropriate services.

I went on a health visiting course and I got involved in local Black community activities in West London. We're talking now early seventies, and we had a significant arrival of families from East Africa because of Idi Amin's expulsions, for example. I practised as a health visitor for three years in Brent. I loved it.

In the mid to late 1970s, I was working as community nurse tutor in Brent, based at the Central Middlesex Hospital. My role involved service development and training for all community nursing staff, district nurses, health visitors and school nurses. I really loved that work but, as I was doing that work, I got more and more aware of sickle cell. We'd had a couple of families on my caseload who had young children with the illness and who were just distraught. They felt they were getting reasonable care by the paediatrician, but they just didn't understand the illness. They were petrified their children were going to die very young. People didn't know about the illness. They felt very isolated – and these were families of Caribbean origin.

One of the main reasons I became formally involved was because I saw a newly arrived haematologist called Dr Misha Brozovic. We're now talking 1975/76. She gave two lunchtime talks on sickle cell. I asked a lot of questions and, at the end of the second talk, Dr Brozovic ran after me. We got talking and we realised we had a lot of areas in common, particularly about wanting to improve the services. She also had a much broader view of medicine, such as the importance of family-centred community. She understood the race dimensions as well, which is very unusual. Maybe because she was an immigrant herself?

We got together and I started to visit the patients on the wards first, and to see the picture from the patient's point of view. Meeting the doctor and working with her informed me to help other Black nurses and set up a support group for sickle. So that's how it all happened. We were asking, 'Where are the gaps? How can we address them? Who do we need to talk to? Is it in education? Is it in housing? Is it in health? Let's bring all these people together to try and solve the problems that the families are facing.'

You know, a child has been told at school they can't go to the toilet, or drink water. This child has sickle cell anaemia, so they do go to the toilet more frequently, they do need to drink water more frequently. They're not playing up when they say they can't play out in the cold weather because they're going to get sick or into crisis. When we come to housing, every which way, problems were being added to the family's life, simply because whatever agency it was never had heard of the circumstance. So it was very much problem-solving and giving a voice to the families, because they've never really been asked their opinions or what the problems were.

I would say two areas caused problems within the NHS. One was that predominantly young Black patients were brought to the hospital in severe, painful crisis due to sickle cell. We're talking severe, requiring diamorphine. In the old days it was pethidine. So put all this together – a condition that, in those days, many people didn't know about – young, apparently healthy-looking individuals demanding pethidine or diamorphine now. These are drug addicts, they must be drug addicts – and they're making a fuss, they're shouting, their family get angry because they felt that their relatives weren't being treated respectfully and speedily.

There were deaths of patients with sickle cell disease. I remember when I started setting up the Brent sickle cell service in 1977 onwards. There'd be three or four deaths a year, and these deaths were young people. I mean, the tears we have wept over these painful deaths. Sometimes it's unexpected deaths, young deaths, due to chest syndrome, and the sudden deterioration and intensive care, and the family is desperate for information and you hear, you know, 'He's 23, he's died.' It's just horrendous, it's horrendous. I sort of unwittingly walked into a sort of advocacy role, because ... I knew where the tensions were, and I knew there were reasons for tensions. There was a lot of anger at times and there was a lot of fear, not only from the patient, but also from the staff. Because some of the staff saw patients with sickle cell as difficult patients. They were getting angry, Black, and they were loud, because the patients themselves had a good awareness of signals – they had to be.

Let's say you're 17, and every time you go to the accident and emergency – and we're talking about a high prevalence area in London – why don't the nurses know about it? Why don't doctors know about this condition? I became a specialist in sickle cell disease, and the first nurse to run a sickle thalassaemia inflammation information screening and genetic counselling. Brent was the only such service for five or six years and then, in the mid eighties, Manchester, Islington and other places developed similar services. So the specialist services started to be developed and then the NHS started to take on board sickle cell. You have the Sickle Cell Society now. Things are still not okay, but they're a heck of a lot better than they were. There are still inequalities in the provision of care at the time of need, which still need to be addressed.

Later in her career Elizabeth became professor and dean of the nursing school at the University of West London, and in 1998 she set up the Mary Seacole Centre for Nursing Practice at Thames Valley University to address issues of racism in nursing. She was made a Dame in 2017 and awarded the Order of Merit in 2022. She has written in depth about her experiences of coming from a mixed-heritage family and a lifetime's contribution to the NHS in her 2016 autobiography, Mixed Blessings from a Cambridge Union.

PETER MOORE

Peter joined the Royal Mineral Water Hospital in Bath, in 1974. The hospital dated from 1742 and was known locally as 'the Min'. It was famous for its use of Bath's geothermal springs in medical treatments and has long specialised in rheumatology and chronic fatigue.

I've only ever had three jobs in my life: the Air Force, the Navy (at Corsham), and the health service.

I saw a job vacancy for an electrician. Those days, I was up at Corsham working on the naval radio equipment. I applied for it. My boss, who was based at the Royal United Hospital [RUH], came in and says the job was mine. It was 1974 – a year of the floods of Lynton and Lynmouth. If you look at the records, there was a tremendous flooding down in Devon and Somerset. My colleague went on holiday on Saturday and I started work in the Mineral on the Monday. I was thrown in the deep end and learnt a lot, which was good looking back.

I was very fortunate inasmuch that, my boss being in the Royal, anything I needed was provided. There was a good understanding between myself and the management from the Royal. Plus the fact I had an engineer who was permanently there with me. So an engineer and an electrician – we did 99 per cent of the work. Any carpentry, or plumbing or anything that wasn't within our bones, they will bring somebody over from the RUH to help us out. It was good. I not only stayed in the Mineral, I worked all the north side of the river. I used to look after the fire station, the ambulance station, and some doctors' surgeries, doing all the electrical maintenance. My colleague would do his engineering side of it. Also a 300-bed nurses' home. That was an ex-hotel. It was taken over by the Admiralty during the Second World War and the health service bought it back as a nursing home.

We would get in there for an eight o'clock start and do all the maintenance, which was allocated for certain pieces of equipment to be checked. We had a swimming pool in the Mineral to keep up. That's one complete day's work.

First thing, we'd make sure the pool attendant was aware and we would drain the pool. After 12 o'clock, it'd be empty. The porters had to come up and scrub the pool. It's not a 25- or 50-metre one, don't get that idea. It was just a proper treatment pool with steps and hoists to put patients in and bring them out. We would then start filling about two o'clock. That never, ever finished until at least half past six because we had a pump down in the pump room at the Roman Baths. It pumped up the water, up into our tanks in the roof at the Mineral. They were huge iron tanks. The water would come in 118, 120 degrees, and it had to be cooled down. Then we had to do all the filtration of the equipment and temperature controlling. If it was too hot, you're scalded. If it's too cold, nobody'd jump in. Simple as that.

Another day, I could be working purely and simply on different jobs that cropped up within the hospital bounds itself. We had outside buildings as well, on the site. We had the accommodation for the staff for the Mineral. The nursing officer or the matron, she was over in one of the houses. She kept an eye on it, and all the trained staff will be in the other house. It was like doing general repairs and simple things like light bulbs and repairing switches. Even had to do washing machines and that, so the variety was there. I had such a variety. It was a wonderful life.

Did you ever have to go in down to the pumps?

Yeah. Very much. In the Mineral, our workshop was down in the gunwales, as we used to call it, where the boilers and everything were. In our workshop we had a manhole cover. We used to have to go down it three or four times a month. Sometimes it was a lot more. When you went down that manhole, the bottom was a channel approximately about a metre high. And in the middle of that channel was a pipe, which was where all mineral water came up from the Roman Baths through a pipe which ran down the road.

We had a very ancient, very unusual three-piston pump, which used to make a most peculiar noise, but it pumped our water up. That's why it took us from two o'clock in the afternoon to half past six at night to get it all the way up to the swimming pool. It used to be a lead pipe until 1976.

In 1976 there was a bug, an amoeba, found in the water. Somebody died. Everybody was trying to say where it came from and what happened. We used to have to go into these large tanks up in the roof, and clean them out, trying to get rid of this bug. So there was a lot of work involved then. Once again, it's a little bit of history that I know and am a bit proud of.

The Min moved in 2019 and is now known as the Royal National Hospital for Rheumatic Diseases (RNHRD).

DIANA

Diana was born in Yorkshire in the early 1940s. She had her tonsils out in hospital aged five, and still remembers the distress she felt when a nurse took her doll away to show to another child: 'I can remember as a young child thinking this was unreasonable.'

I graduated from Newcastle University in 1964 with a degree in social science. I found out about medical social work. In those days social workers were called 'lady almoners' because they were largely dealing with money. They changed their name to 'medical social workers' in 1964. One of my friends said, 'That's because we aren't ladies anymore.' Then I got a place on the postgraduate course in Cardiff for the one-year training, which is where I met my husband, who's also a retired social worker. I decided that I would do hospital social work. It was a very interesting position in which to be as a social worker. You were not like some of the lower echelons of the hierarchy, but you weren't a doctor either.

Diana worked for almost three years in London.

I remember there was a senior gynaecological consultant and he used to hold a tea in the Ward Sister's office every Tuesday afternoon. At this tea was himself, his registrars – who all seemed to be men – the house officer, the Ward Sister and me, as the social worker to the unit. The real example of a hierarchy was one day when there were no sandwiches. He looked around to me and said, 'Maybe you could go make some sandwiches?' It took great courage to say, 'I'm sorry, but I really don't think that's my role.' The result of that was that the Ward Sister went off and made them.

It was a very interesting time in healthcare. There were very new things coming about and one of the things that was very relevant to me was the passing of the Abortion Act in 1967, which made abortion legal, with two signatories. I started to get asked for social assessments on people requesting abortion, which was quite a dilemma really because my belief was that this should be available to people who wanted it. I also knew if I just said, 'Oh, yes, this person's circumstances are really severe,' for all of them, then they weren't going to do them all.

I wasn't making a decision, but I was laying out information, and I think that was really quite difficult. People who'd been raped or assaulted, there'd be no question about it. They'd get an abortion. Or somebody who was having an extramarital baby would get an abortion to stop the husband knowing. But more straightforward cases or single girls who felt they couldn't cope – they would tend to get refused unless there was something particular.

Diana worked until she had her first child in 1970.

In those days women just gave up work. You didn't have maternity leave. It never occurred to most of us to go back to work. When my son was born, it had only just become standard practice that fathers were allowed in the labour ward. I was generally quite nicely treated when I was in the hospital. Some of the regimes in 1970 were still sort of thirties and forties, you know, feeding your baby every four hours. They weren't really very good at encouraging breastfeeding, which I was very keen on, and a regime like that didn't help either. That's where I found the help from the National Childbirth Trust [NCT]. I became active in it and coordinated the postnatal support group and discovered that there were people not so lucky as me with a straightforward delivery. Those mothers had quite difficult times because of restrictions on things like when you could go and see your baby and visit the premature baby unit. I can remember going with an NCT teacher to the hospital and having conversations of a polite but strained nature with some of the staff who didn't really believe in patient power at all. It was just the beginnings of the interface between patients and the hospital.

When I was involved with the NCT, the hospital ran a milk bank for premature babies, because breast milk was better than formula and not all mothers can do it. The NCT organised the rota of drivers, who would be people with slightly older children, and breastfeeding mothers. It's funny really, when you think of it – the little bottles into which the mothers expressed the milk were just in the cold box, you know, like a sandwich box, not even a freezer box. We took them to the milk room at the hospital where they were, I suppose, pasteurised or sterilised in some way, and sent up to the ward. It was quite a satisfying thing because they were so glad of it. They didn't have enough breast milk and they knew it was the best thing for little babies.

My daughter was born in 1974. Once you've got a child, you start to be more involved with the health service for vaccinations and things like that, or when they're actually ill. I can remember in our GP surgery, sometimes you'd have to wait for hours because there were no appointments. You'd have to wait for hours with a yelling child on your knee. The worst and most terrible experience was my daughter having meningitis at the age of 15 months. We'd no idea what it was. I just knew this was a child that was very seriously ill. I looked at my *Dr Spock*, which was the baby and child-care manual that everybody used in the seventies, and it mentioned polio. I thought, 'Well, this can't be polio.' The GP came. 'She has an ear infection.' I've never forgotten that because he was wrong. Her life was saved, as we had a GP living next door. I would never have consulted her but my little girl was so ill. Immediately, she felt all around her neck and said, 'All the meninges are swollen. Call your doctor back and I'll stay with your little boy.'

Diana's daughter was admitted to hospital.

When she was better I got involved with the National Association for the Welfare of Children in Hospital, which advocated for parental involvement. I discovered that my hospital was by no means as bad as other hospitals up and down the country that still had rigid visiting hours. But mothers were not expected to stay overnight and there were no facilities. They already thought I was quite eccentric because I was there the whole day, until my husband came back in the evening to do his stint. When they had a ward round all the mothers were supposed to vanish. The Ward Sister said, 'Oh, you can stay there, if you sit nice and quiet.' I remember the consultant coming round and going through the history with the Ward Sister. He looked to me, 'Ah, the mother's here. We could ask her.' This is now 1975 and we're still moving on fairly slowly.

Diana joined the Community Health Council in 1978.

That was fascinating going to visit hospitals and taking up complaints, which were sometimes well received. I'm very aware all this sounds very critical. I'm 100 per cent supportive of the NHS but, like any institution, it can have entrenched people and attitudes.

Now retired, Diana is a user of NHS services. She says her experiences have been good on the whole. 'I'm delighted to see how young and enthusiastic most of the staff seem to be.'

MASUD HOGHUGHI

Masud was born in 1938 in Tehran, Iran. 'I was the invisible member of the family, so I became a bookish kind of boy.' As a young boy around 1955, Masud was sent to finish his education in England. 'My father had the belief, I think, sometimes almost literally, that it was the British who would determine the shape of clouds, and whether there was a wind or whether there was a drought.' Masud began studying at the London School of Economics, but his plans were cut short when his father became bankrupt.

In 1960 I started a degree in Hull. I had a wonderful teacher. I took my last year as speciality in clinical psychology. I had three months in De la Pole Hospital, a mental hospital outside York. I was as green as the hills. The hospital did not have a psychologist. I was put in the admission ward. On a beautiful sunny day, the window was open and a patient went to jump out. I went for him with a rugby tackle. I was out of action for 10 days with a bad back and have continued to suffer from a bad back the rest of my life. But as things go, this was mild. Sometimes patients attack viciously and badly hurt people. I wasn't hurt, in part because I wasn't afraid. I was lean, I was strong; I knew how to look after myself.

In 1970 Masud gained his doctorate and moved to Aycliffe Classifying School in County Durham, which provided residential care to young offenders who had been committed by the courts to an approved school. Attitudes towards children were changing and, rather than punitive approaches, the Children and Young Persons Act of 1969 emphasised the need for care and protection of juvenile offenders.

When I joined Aycliffe as the senior psychologist, the director showed me the four canes that he kept in the corner of his room in an empty cardboard tube. I said, 'I'm afraid I can't work here if that happens. If you have a problem with a child, I am the senior psychologist – hand them to me, and I will deal with that.' He was a big man. This was a direct challenge. But I was green and I was idealistic and I just couldn't bear the thought. These are children, for God's sake. I said, 'I will walk out, I will resign, I will just have nothing to do with the place.' By the time I was appointed director, much to his enormous credit, that had completely disappeared.

This was the largest collection of children who nobody else could deal with. It was open. There were unlocked wards apart from three wards out of 12 which were locked. Simultaneously, the law changed and what had been a responsibility of the Home Office became responsibility of the Department of Health. Because the Home Office had made an almighty mess of the whole thing. Times were changing, people's views were changing. Children were beginning to be talked about as children – not delinquents, not approved-school boys, or approved-school girls. There was a shift in perspective and perception. The change of the law was part and parcel of that. That little children had no business to be part of the penal side of the Home Office. They were children. I was both instrumental in, but also dramatically the beneficiary of, a change in the times. If I can take any responsibility at all, and I don't, it is that I brought in the concept of *children* to deal with young people who did terrible things. I eventually changed Aycliffe's name from Aycliffe Classifying School to Aycliffe Centre for Children. That was what we were about. We were for children. We were not for delinquents. You don't classify people. That was an old-fashioned, deeply disgraceful way of looking at children. I got my managers to change the name of the place to the Centre for Children. And overnight, the staff started looking at themselves as something different. I say to them, 'You're looking after children, please remember that.'

Treatment is for human beings. We treated these children because they had more problems than I had had Sunday dinners. It broke your heart if you looked at any of the children in depth, to see all the things that had gone wrong with them. All the things that had been done to them. You don't really expect, dealing with 100 boys, to find that something like 60 per cent of them have been buggered. I steeped myself in the notions of abuse of children. This is long before it became fashionable. All of it goes back to this power differential that is between children and other people. It applies to other people, it applies to prisoners, it applies to patients. But you have to be profoundly aware of your own status in relation to the people you're dealing with. I could afford to do that because I came from a background which had given me the status that I didn't have to worry about, you know. We had servants, I was from that background. When I translated that to Britain, that was not the case. We were riven with social class differences, with stigmatisation, with pointing fingers at people, putting great big labels on them.

It was a cumulative, iterative exercise and I was continuously going back on what I've learned and examining it. I began to see that the naming of these people as 'sick people', or as 'patients', obliterates the sometimes very dramatic individuality of these people. Although for some reasons you have to treat them as patients – you have to give them medicine as patients – but most of the rest of the time, you are dealing as one human being with another human being. If you look them in the eye, and if you relax and show no fear, you are okay.

Once at Aycliffe, a number of staff had been bloodied by a child who was under conditions of security because he had killed somebody. I then had to take charge. I would go into the unit. And it's happened more than once. All the staff have kind of amassed, because they're not sure where to go. The child is a 16-year-old boy, very, very powerful, very angry, very distressed. Nobody wants to be the first person to overpower the child because of the consequences of getting it wrong: tackling the child, breaking a limb or something of that sort. So they ring the boss. I call out from the top of the corridor, 'It is me, I'm coming along.' I stand at the door and here's this kid with a great big piece of skirting board. He had yanked it off the wall. I go in and look him in the eye and I say, 'Johnny, it's just me. Sunshine, you are safe.' I very often call them 'Sunshine'. 'Am I alright if I sit on the corner of your bed?' He looks at me. And he looks at what was in his hand. I have no defence. I can't conceivably be aggressive. I go and sit on the corner of the bed. Watching him with the corner of my eye. Eventually, he's sobbing, sitting beside me. 'Johnny, Sunshine, you know I will have to have you charged because of what you've done to Mr So-and-so. But I will look after you. I will try and make sure that you come back.' I went to his defence and I had him back. He eventually was transferred to our longer-term secure-treatment facility, and that was all right.

I was involved in the development of assessments which addressed the unique features of those children, the things that you could use as a kind of key to do something with the child. Above all, the parents. The work that you have to do with the parents who were the embodiment of profound disadvantage, of brutality, of all the wars that our society has to offer. Most of us couldn't really operate if we knew all the things that happened in our society. We've got to kind of shut our eyes. There are things that I will not read because I can't deal with it. There's nothing I could do. But I could do something about those children: feed them properly, give them nice clothes, talk *with* them, not to them or at them. And demanding that all my 300-and-odd staff do the same thing. Not giving one millimetre space for anything abusive towards those children. You want to be respected. You treat the child with respect. And that works. It takes time to get established, but that works because the children become acquainted with the notion of being respected. And they don't want to lose it.

One of my absolute hallmarks was that no drugs were used in the management of children, period. The only person who would approve it was me. These children had been medicated up to the gunwales. But they'd still managed to run riots all over the place. So what we did was we took them off the medication within a set period. 'Sunshine, nobody's going to give you an injection. Nobody's going to give you a tablet, unless you've got a headache and we'll give you a headache tablet. But you're a human being. You're one of us. We treat you the way we treat ourselves.' And it works.

I think what you remember are your failures rather than your successes. Your successes are all the children you discharged. You put back in school. You put the family together, after a fashion, and you send the child back. Let me give you one example. I have been up into Bristol. I am on the platform waiting for the train to come. And a tall man comes up to me. 'Hello, doctor. What are you doing here?' 'Do I know you?' He says, 'Have I grown that much?' I say, 'What was your name?' He told me, and I said, 'Hello, Sunshine, how are you?' He would have given me a cuddle if it had been appropriate. It's a nothing, but he actually recognised me. He approached me. And he did it with a smile. It was recognition of 'At least I haven't hurt him.' That's something to be profoundly grateful for.

Masud finally retired in 2015 and offers his reflections on the NHS in the final chapter.

BASIL BRAMBLE

Basil was born in London in 1958 and was very poorly as a child, needing transfusions in hospital for a blood disorder. It wasn't until Basil was in his teens that his parents found out they both carried the sickle cell gene. Basil had inherited the gene from both parents and was born with sickle cell anaemia. 'Blood transfusions make you feel better, but it was tough. It was really sore.', he says.

Sickle cell anaemia is a blood disorder. The blood cells are like half-moon, or banana, shape. A normal blood cell is round. That's why sickle cells don't go through the bloodstream as well as a normal cell. They clog and stick, and that causes the crisis. Blood cells carry oxygen round the body. If the sickle cells stick together, this means there's no oxygen. It's called a 'crisis', where you just can't breathe. You have to be hospitalised with strong painkillers and oxygen. If the haemoglobin is low, then you need a lot of fluid. Sickle cell sufferers have to drink quite a lot, although we're advised to keep off alcohol if you can. I drink quite a lot of water.

My parents didn't know too much about it, you know in the sixties and early seventies. I remember them coming back from hospital, I think when my youngest brother, who's 10 years younger than me, was born. I remember Mum saying, 'So that's it.' They worked out that they was both carriers and there was a chance of one out of three children having full-blown sickle cell like I did. After that we found out that my middle brother and my youngest brother carried the trait.

I spent quite a lot of time in hospital. Primary school was hard because I missed a lot of education. When I was about 14/15, my dad sat me down and said, 'It might be a bit tough for you out there son, back and forth from hospital.' I thought life was going to be challenging. I worried I'd never get a job, but I got my first job about 16, straight after leaving school. I feel blessed that I got that job.

It was in a photography studio. This guy was one of the most famous theatrical photographers of the time: Michael Barrington-Martin. I was assistant photographer, printer and messenger. Bruce Forsyth, Faith Brown and Dana (winner of the 1998 Eurovision Song Contest) were in the studio. I used to do the printing and take the photos to the London Palladium and all over. It was a lot more challenging in 1974 with photos than digital is nowadays. When you're in the darkroom developing, you do five at a time. It was challenging to get them all the same quality.

I was hospitalised for 10 days about six months after working there, then had to convalesce. My employers were really good. I suppose being truthful at the start really helped. I went into my first job and said, 'I suffer from a blood disorder.' It was never an issue. Other sickle cell sufferers have said I've been lucky because they haven't kept a job. I don't know anyone who's reached my age and had four jobs and managed to work that long. My last job was with Morgan Stanley, an investment bank. They gave me so much support. I feel blessed. I think the Lord must look down on me and says, 'Just be truthful.' I've worked for 40 years.

When you have a sickle cell crisis you have a lot of serious pain. I personally know whether I'm going to end up in hospital or not. I'll have a lot of pain, drink a lot of hot drinks, take a lot of painkillers. You do know when it's time to call the ambulance. You take painkillers, but when your joints are still hurting and you're struggling walking, you know it's 999 time. You're usually on all fours when the ambulance arrives. On the floor, collapsed, gasping for breath, screaming with pain. My pain is like four heavyweight boxers – Mike Tyson, Muhammad Ali, Lennox Lewis, Larry Holmes – and they've got six-inch nails and a mallet each and they're pounding on all parts of your body. That's what a crisis feels like. It's absolutely horrible. It doesn't matter how big or strong you are. You'll always just be in tears, crying your eyes out on the floor. Can't wait till the ambulance gets there. Certain sickle cell people I know have had a crisis and have gone before the ambulance arrived.

After undergoing an eye operation, Basil began to volunteer at Moorfields Eye Hospital in London and received a Stars Award for 20 years of volunteering in 2018.

PATRICIA MACARTNEY

Patricia trained as a nurse at Crumpsall Hospital in North Manchester and in 1969 took the opportunity to do a three month new specialist course in Intensive Care at Whiston Hospital in Merseyside as a Sister, where she worked with David Morrison (p.121).

Whiston Hospital in Merseyside was one of the few with the new two-bedded prototype unit. That was experimental. Nobody really knew what they were doing. We had patients that would have been written off. We got all sorts – a mix of surgical, medical trauma. Before those two beds had been established, those patients would have just come back to their appropriate ward. They wouldn't have been ventilated, so they would have been left – and died naturally. I learned more about interpreting ECGs, interpreting blood results, and then to contact the relevant medical staff, to add or change IVs, change ventilator settings. It was still very early days. 'We could try this,' or 'We could try that,' the medical staff would say. It was a lot of the medical staff sitting by a patient trying things.

Putting patients on ventilators, we used a paralysing agent along with a sedative. But when you disconnected the ventilator to do suction on them, that meant patients couldn't breathe or move. You were working on a one-to-one basis, so we were encouraged to bond with the patients. I was talking to a patient, 'Can I ask you a question about when you were on your ventilator? Did you ever feel panicky? Were you scared?' He said, 'It depended on who was looking after me. Some people you felt safe with and some not.'

We got the purpose-built intensive care unit, and that was developed by trial and error of the two-bedded unit. David Morrison, director of ICU, had a lot to do with the design of it. Where the beds went and having beds with access all the way around, with no trailing wires. On the central station, where you could see all the patients, we had two cubicles. One of them we tended to use for dialysis or barrier nursing. The other would be used for patients on ventilators. The patients weren't all on ventilators. Some of them were conscious, which made life difficult for the patients after they moved to a normal ward. The patient had a nurse close to them for 24 hours a day. Then they went on a ward and some had big issues about not feeling safe, or not having somebody there always.

The worst moment in Patricia's career came when three children and a baby had been in a house fire. They were rescued by firefighters and brought to the nearest Casualty. Patricia left the ICU to go and help.

The mother had left four children in the house alone with an electric fire. The three-year-old survived and the baby was okay. The five- and seven-year-old were on the same trolley, feet to feet. They were suffering from smoke inhalation and had arrested. We didn't have equipment for children. It was trying to find tubes and getting them intubated. We worked so, so hard on them and they both died. The atmosphere was just awful. The firemen were in tears. I was in shock and the doctor was in shock. I did what I could and then I had to go back to ICU. Luckily, the charge nurse that was on recognised I needed to talk it through. I remember smashing a couple of plates. He gave me them and said, 'Yeah, you need to do that.' I couldn't cry. I think there was so many emotions and I know the firefighters felt the same. There was so much anger with the mother leaving them. I know you're not there to judge, but you can't help when you see.

It doesn't matter whether the patient's conscious or unconscious, you do not go up to them and start any procedure without talking to them first and explaining what you're going to do. It's not our job to decide whether they can hear us or not. We treat them as if they can hear us and they can feel us touch them. You do not go up to a bed without talking, even if it's to take the blood pressure.

One particularly good student told Patricia she wouldn't want to work in the ICU because too many patients died. Patricia responded, 'But for all the ones that die, the successes are worth it.'

MARION and CERI WATERS

Marion and Ceri, from South Wales, gave a joint interview about the experience of Ceri's being born with a foot disability in 1974. Ceri was Marion's fourth child and she gave birth to her at St Joseph's Hospital, where much of the care was given by nuns.

Marion: I had a normal birth but Ceri was taken away before I even had a look at her. I just thought it was the routine. After about 20 minutes I asked, 'When's my baby being brought back? 'Oh, she won't be long.' They took me back to my room and brought me in a cup of tea. I said, 'I haven't seen my baby, where's my baby?' 'Oh, she won't be long'. Actually, it was about an hour. I think probably they were getting other people to look at her. My husband was in London, at the zoo, with the other three children.

The midwife was the one who came and said, 'She's the most beautiful baby I've ever seen delivered, but there is a problem.' Ceri was in a wheeled cot. The midwife said, 'She's got a problem with her feet.' She turned the blanket back and showed me, and Ceri had talipes in both her feet. It's what we used to call 'club foot'. Her feet, one was worse than the other, but they were both very inverted. My sister knocked the door and walked in with my 10-year-old daughter, and obviously I was upset, and my daughter went across to her cot, looked at her feet and said, 'They can put that right, Mum.'

Ceri: 'Bilateral', they call it. The doctor showed me my first X-rays when I was about 13. The one foot, the heel bone was up where the ridge of your foot would be, and the toe was almost wrapped and touching the leg. He said to me it was one of the worst visual deformity cases he'd ever seen – and he was a talipes specialist. He used to say that to me quite regularly, that he was so proud of what he'd done and what he'd accomplished.

Marion: My GP said he'll get a paediatric orthopaedic consultant to come out in nine days. He said if we're wanting the specialist to see her before then, we were going to have to pay. 'No, I'm not waiting nine days, I want him to see her straight away, as soon as he can.' He came and I had to pay him, but that was by the by. He saw her when she was two days old. He examined her and said, 'I can do something for her. I can promise you that I will get her feet flat to the floor, but I can't promise you she'll walk.'

He was NHS, but on this occasion I had to pay £20, as he did private work as well. He did not have a very good bedside manner, but he was a miracle worker. He said, 'I will plaster her up myself now,' when she was two days old. He took her into a special room with one of the nurses. I waited outside and I could hear her screaming, because it was very painful obviously. He manipulated her feet, and I think if he hadn't done it there and then, while her bones were still more supple, I firmly believe she wouldn't be as she is today. I was crying outside the door and she was crying the other side of the door.

I had my first appointment when she was 10 days old down at the Gwent hospital. His bill had arrived the day before. I'm sat outside waiting to see him when he walks along the corridor. He said to me, 'Oh, Mrs Waters, have you had my bill?' I was so embarrassed in front of all the other people. I said, 'Yes, it arrived yesterday.' I'd got on the telephone and I said to my husband, get your chequebook, write it and come to the hospital with the cheque. I said, 'I'm not going through that again.' But he was wonderful with her. In fact, he would bring all his students to see her.

Ceri: I think at one point some students came over from China, Japan, somewhere in the Far East. He asked me if it would be okay if they could come and see me – I must have been about 11, 12 maybe. He had a name for me; he never called me Ceri. He used to call me something like his 'princess'. He showed them the X-rays and then showed me standing, because I literally was like his proudest piece of work.

Marion: For the first couple of months of her life, the treatment was changing her plasters, realigning her feet and plastering them into position, which would happen once every fortnight. Then he wanted to get the first operation, which I think was an Achilles tendon operation. My other children had just had chickenpox and I had to take her to St Lawrence Hospital in Chepstow for the operation, which was a plastic surgery hospital. I took her in in the morning and I was changing her napkin, waiting for them to come and admit her, and I saw the first blister on her bottom. I said to my husband, 'I think she's got chickenpox.' In came this young intern. I said,

'I don't think she'll be able to have the op, she's got chickenpox.' He said, 'Oh no, no, no, it's a water blister.' I said, 'No, this is my fourth child. I've never had a water blister on one of them, but I have had three with chickenpox.' He said, 'Well, we'll keep her in isolation, but I'm sure it's a water blister, Mother.' So I was staying the night. Six o'clock the next morning, I was down to give her her first feed and to change her and she was plastered. In he walked. I'll never forget his face. He said, 'Oh my God, you were right, Mother. It's chickenpox, you'll have to take her out immediately.'

In spite of everything she was going through, she was always happy. But we'd walk into the plaster room and she'd see the nurses and she'd start to cry. Well, this Christmas it was skeleton staff. The nurses didn't have their hats on for some reason. Anyway, she didn't cry. I was very puzzled by this. I said, 'Would you mind putting your hats on?' They put their hats on and she immediately started to cry. So when I came back the Sister in charge of the plaster room said, 'Nurses, when Ceri Waters comes in here, hats off.' And every time we went in, the shout would go up, 'Ceri Waters is coming, hats off.'

Ceri moved to wearing boots when she was 14 months old.

Marion: The soles of the boots are metal and they're joined by a metal bar. They're very soft leather to lace around, across her foot, and they had to be adjusted and her feet turned. But she'd walked. She actually stood, balanced, on those, although they've got nuts on the bottom.

Her brother, who was coming up for seven, would stand her. For hours he would stand her there and say, 'You can do it, come on, Ceri, you can do it,' and she would come to him swinging her hips on these boots. She even had to sleep in these boots, and she couldn't turn. You try sleeping and not turning. So we had a frame, and every time she moved, you were out trying to put her comfortable. But, as I said, she was such a happy child in spite of all of that. She very rarely cried. When she eventually went into shoes, her shoes were specially made by the Remploy factory in Aberdare. Remploy had factories that employed people with a disability. They would deliver them to the Gwent hospital and come down and fit them for her. If I had any problems, I just rang them up and said, 'Look, she's worn it down, or she's done this, whatever.' I could go to the factory with her and they adjusted them.

Ceri learned to walk when she was about 18 months.

I can remember going to the Gwent and they took her out of her frame and they put the boots on her. I had to pass her to a nurse because I was so upset. I saw her and she was standing in these boots, and I said, 'Can you take her a minute, I have to go outside.' All the nurses were amazed at how much she'd come on and how she was trying to walk.

Nothing's phased her. Nothing's stopped her. She's played tennis, she's done disco dancing. Football. She was in her university football team.

Ceri: I learned to ski when I was 38. It was incredible, because learning to ski, the snowplough position was my natural feet position. It was the only thing that came easily! The only thing that I cannot and I've never been able to do is stand up on ice skates.

Marion became tearful in the interview remembering her first sight of Ceri in the cot. Now a mother herself, Ceri reflected that it was only once she'd had her own children that she understood exactly what her mother would have been through.

At the end of the 1970s

The 1970s was a decade of turbulence inside and outside the NHS. It began with industrial unrest and conflict, as successive governments sought to increase efficiency and innovation across industry. Trade union membership grew. The National Union of Public Employees (NUPE) and Confederation of Health Service Employees (COHSE) recruited white-collar workers from the NHS, local government and schools. A global oil crisis affected Britain badly, and by 1976 the Labour government was forced to apply to the International Monetary Fund (IMF) for a loan. The terms of the loan enforced deep cuts in public expenditure, which put enormous pressure on public spending. The government sought to control inflation by holding down pay levels. But this led to a drop in real wages and put many of the lowest-paid workers in the NHS into poverty, resulting in the first major collective action across the service. Selective strike action took place across the UK through the early months of 1979. Eventually, a pay increase of around 9 per cent was accepted.

Amid this discontent, the NHS underwent its first structural reorganisation in 1974 with the plans developed by management consultants. From the beginning of the NHS, there had been problems in successfully coordinating responsibilities for services between hospitals, general practitioners and local authorities. Aneurin Bevan, of course, had had to create the NHS from existing systems, and the intransigence of opponents led to a system split three ways. Proposals for the NHS reorganisation had been developed in a Conservative government with Sir Keith Joseph as secretary of state. But the 1974 general election brought a Labour government into power and as David Owen recounted, the new government had to make a swift decision as to whether or not the reorganisation would be implemented. (Similar reorganisations took place in Scotland, Wales and Northern Ireland). A three-tier structure of regional, area and district health authorities was introduced, but it rapidly became clear that the new structures were too complicated and impeded effective decision-making. The significance of the 1974 reorganisation in the longer history of the NHS was not the structural changes themselves, but rather that it marked the beginning of a continuing pattern of using reorganisations to effect change – despite evidence that they rarely achieve the intended improvements.

One positive benefit was the introduction of Community Health Councils (CHCs). For the first time in the NHS, patients and the public had a mechanism through which they could have their voices heard. They were also given powers around hospital closures. It reflected the rise in patient and community activism that was beginning to challenge medical authority and paternalistic attitudes, as exemplified by Edwina Currie Jones's work in Birmingham.

Through the 1970s the NHS remained very popular, and comparisons with other health systems showed the NHS continued to be highly efficient. The decade ended with the 1979 general election bringing the Conservatives into power, led by Margaret Thatcher, with a pledge to reduce the level of public spending across Britain. The NHS was on the brink of a decade that would bring irrevocable changes to the service.

Chapter 5:
1980s

'That van went around Liverpool … until we got 10,000 [breast cancer] screenings and sent the findings to the NHS.'

ETHEL ARMSTRONG

'It was topside, used to come in from Argentina … It was a national scheme.'

DERRICK STEVENS

'I think the NHS is a glory and a saving grace … I've had the most amazing treatment through my life.'

JONATHAN BLAKE

'Right from my teenage years, it's been about having control over my life as a woman and helping other women have control over their lives.'

LINDA PEPPER

"I can't guarantee that, even if you end your hunger strike here and now, you'll survive."

PAT SHEEHAN

'Almost the first thing I did when I came to London was to shoot off to Houston, Texas, to learn how to do a new procedure.'

AVERIL MANSFIELD

'When I came in, there were about 800 patients in the hospital. When I left, that was probably down to 200 … that was an achievement.'

DAVID ROTHBERG

'We had a different [general practice] model. We wanted to really overturn what was going on. I think we thought we could change the world.'

TOM HELLER and JACK CZAUDERNA

'It was so novel to prescribe morphine in what looked like relatively high doses to get on top of people's pain.'

ILLORA FINLAY

'Nursing has played an amazing path in allowing me to lead a very open life as a gay man since the age of 19.'

ROBERT DOWNES

'The Patients Association was representing the interests of patients. In those early days, it was a fairly new concept.'

LINDA LAMONT

'They introduced a thing called "general management". Until this point, doctors were gods.'

LIONEL JOYCE

ETHEL ARMSTRONG

Breast cancer screening was piloted in Liverpool in the 1980s. Ethel and her husband Harry (see page 38) had moved to Southport at the end of the 1970s, as Harry's job required him to be close to the Liverpool Docks. Ethel thought, 'Well, that's it, I've done enough now, I don't want to do anything else.' Then she spotted an advert.

I answered this one. It just said, 'somebody with experience'. They were looking for somebody who was up for a challenge. Professor Whitehouse sent me a letter: 'I know it's a bit unusual, but would you meet me at Little-woods in Crosby?'

Littlewoods had been set up by John Moores in 1932 as a football pools company but expanded into the mail-order business. By the 1980s it was the largest private company in Europe, with shops and catalogue retail.

I met him outside this huge garage with all Littlewoods vehicles for cata-logue deliveries. Littlewoods had got the pools, they'd got catalogues, they'd got a mail-order company – and everything went through that one big unit with these huge wagons.

I thought, 'I don't know what we're doing here.' I was looking at all these big, lovely, shiny wagons. Professor Whitehouse said, 'I'm meeting the Little-woods people here because they've got an old chest X-ray van.' Standing in the corner was this van. It looked like a reject from the wars. When I looked inside, it was just an empty shell with a cab on the front. 'What are we going to do with this?' 'Well, you've done some radiotherapy.' 'Yes.' He said, 'What would you really have liked?' 'Oh,' I said, 'many times I thought, I wish I could have seen this woman a lot quicker than I'm getting her. I wish there'd been some means of seeing what was going on, because she's got a history, a family history of breast cancer that would knock you sideways.' But there was no facility for picking up these people because there's no screening programme for them.

Professor Whitehouse said, 'The NHS will not entertain mobile breast screening because it means nationally, from Scotland to Wales and in

England, it's going to cost a fortune. Not for the staff, but for the equipment and the units. We want to prove to them that actually we can pick up early breast cancers and give these women a better chance.' With breast cancer, there's a start and a finish. We don't know how the disease will progress, but if you can get somebody a few months earlier, with less invasive treatment and surgery and a good outcome, it's a chance worth taking.

I was in the era where the only safe way was to remove not only the breast itself, but the big pectoral muscle. Women used to come to me for follow-up chest X-rays to see if there was any spread to the other lung. All you could see were white ribs with blue skin over the top. That was the only way a surgeon could be sure that he hadn't left any breast tissue back there. We still had the problem of – it's not the primary cancer that gives you the problem, it's the spread from that to the lymph nodes. If we can get somebody with a history of a grandmother, a mother, two aunties and a cousin all with breast disease, they can have earlier treatment.

I spoke to every organisation I could think of in Liverpool. Littlewoods came in. Then Vernons, another pools company. Then the Ocean Trading Company, the shipping companies, all their female staff. Up came the police, 'Will you do our ladies?' 'We can't do them for free, but if you will donate £10 per lady, we will move the van on site and we will do them there and then, take half an hour from your day.' That's how it worked. We had a very small grant from the University of Liverpool to pay the staff salaries. We were never paid by the NHS.

I trundled that old van, with one more radiographer and two experienced breast clinic nurses that wanted some part-time work to fill in with their kids. Every bit of water had to be carried to the van. It was cabled up with a big 30 amp. There was no dry photography done. It was all your old-fashioned developer, rinser, fixer, wash tanks. We did a full clinical service in there, full blood testing and full mammography, and processed on site. That van went around Liverpool from 1978 until we got 10,000 screenings and sent the findings to the NHS. We started it, then other groups – Scotland, Manchester, Nottingham, Guildford, Guy's, and Bart's – followed. Those were the seven pioneer groups that literally did the full clinical history of a patient. Full examination by the qualified nursing staff and then full mammography.

We did that from 1978 to the mid eighties, when it was then adopted as a national breast screening service.

In 1988 the NHS introduced breast and cervical cancer screening programmes. Ethel retired in 1990 after 42 years of service, but within days she was taken by friends to a meeting of the NHS Retirement Fellowship. 'Nobody said, "What did you do?" I had this lovely feeling that it wouldn't have mattered whether I'd peeled potatoes in the kitchen, or whether I'd folded sheets in the laundry. From day one, I was hooked.' We will catch up with Ethel when she's at the centre of the NHS seventieth anniversary celebrations in the 2010s.

DERRICK STEVENS

Derrick was born in a Cotswold village in 1959. 'Living in a Cotswold village sounds very idyllic, but as a child it's quite boring.', he recalled. He remembers the school dentist turning up 'in a caravan, motor-home type of thing'. It would park in front of the school and the children would be called up, examined and treated if required.

I left home at the age of 16 and went to work and lived in hotels and went to college one day a week. I was trained as a chef. You worked split shifts. Go in, do lunch. Have some free time in the afternoon, then go back and cook dinner. That was all very well as a single young man. I met my wife, who was a nurse and she was doing shifts. I was a chef in a hotel doing shifts. We ended up not seeing each other. So I applied for a vacancy as an assistant head chef at the Lister Hospital in Stevenage and I got the job. The reason I went for that job was because of straight shifts. Start at 7.30 in the morning, finish at 3 in the afternoon. We worked five days out of seven, including weekends. You did an early shift or a late shift. Latest finish six at night and earliest start seven in the morning. My wife was happy. We had a better social life.

When I first started at Lister Hospital as assistant head chef, my responsibility would be to cook the food and to supervise the section that I was allocated to. You have somebody that specialises in desserts, someone that specialises in main meals, in vegetables, and so on. Each section had an assistant head chef. Every three months, we'd change sections. If I was in the vegetable section, then peeling the potatoes – in those days, we used to peel potatoes, and chop all the vegetables. Everything in those days was cooked fresh. We used to cook everything fresh on the day. It was a busy environment, but it was always fun working there. There was lots of us working. If I was in the vegetable section, let's say, and I'd be supervising, I'd have a couple of cooks and a couple of assistant cooks also allocated to that section. About five of us allocated just to the vegetable section. Labour was very intensive.

In the larder section, for preparation we used to dice all our meat ourselves. We used to get this meat coming in which was called 'intervention beef'. It was very good, actually. It was topside, used to come in from Argentina. A whole topside of beef would come in. The whole topside of beef would come in in these boxes. And we'd have to break it down, cut it into joints and roll it, or dice it. We even minced it as well. Because it was so cheap. It was a national scheme. We used to have national butter come through. All these things we used to get nationally, that used to come cheap to the NHS, has gone now.

We used to have different diets like low fat, high protein, low protein, diabetics, what was then classed as a 'reducing diet'. These were the days before the word 'obesity' was used. We'd have the liquidised diets, puréed diets and all that. Certainly, allergies were not as prominent as they are now. There seems to be a lot more people that have allergies than certainly they did back in the eighties when I first started working in the NHS.

The therapeutic diet aspect changed drastically. When I first started, we had separate menus for all the different diets and each different diet had a menu card. When I left the NHS, which was in 2018, we had incorporated therapeutic diets into the standard menu. Patients were given the choice to select from the main menu through dietary coding rather than having a bespoke menu for their requirements. There was always the chance that people would choose the wrong options, but we had a safety net. They used to have a sticker that they put on the menu card to indicate what dietary requirements they were on. If they had chosen that wrong dietary require- ment, then we used to pick that up within the administration office. It changed the emphasis on responsibility to the catering department, away from the nursing staff. The nursing staff in the old times would have given out the bespoke menu to the different patients. Whereas with the system when I left, it was really down to the catering staff to keep an eye on making sure that the right selection has been chosen.

Derrick witnessed enormous changes in food preparation over the course of his career.

My last employment was at Dorset County Hospital in Dorchester. My position had changed. I was in a management position, not just covering catering, but multiple departments. The food preparation had changed in the sense that a lot of stuff used to come in pre-prepared. All our meat used to come in ready diced and ready minced. That was a labour that was taken away. All our vegetables come in ready-prepared, so our potatoes were ready-peeled and cut. So they just went straight into the pot and was cooked without any preparation at all.

How did you attempt to maintain a good standard of incoming foods?

Towards the end of my career, it was about lots of local sustainability and buying local-produced products. At Dorset County Hospital I used milk which came from a small farm just on the Jurassic Coast. That farm produced the milk, along with four other farms along the coast. We used to get that direct to us, straight from the farm. We used to benchmark it. When we benchmarked it against the national suppliers, we're about a penny a pint cheaper. So it was local, food miles were reduced and from a budget perspective, it was better as well. Also, the fat content of the milk was higher, so it was more nutritious for the patients and building up the patients. One of the other ones I used was a local ice cream producer in Corfe. I also used a local specialist producer of gluten-free products just outside Sherborne.

Derrick shared his recent experience of having a heart procedure.

It wasn't the nicest environment. It was attached to a day unit, classed as a minor procedure. On a half trolley, half bed. You sleep there overnight with a curtain around you.

I was dropped at the door; no visitors were allowed. My son picked me up the next morning. I don't want to sound dramatic about it. I'm familiar with hospitals, so I'm not apprehensive or frightened of hospitals, but lots of people are. Now, heart procedures are seen as minor. You worry as a patient. Will I survive it? General anaesthetic. Having something inserted into the centre of your heart. Healthcare professionals become a bit blasé and don't consider the apprehension and worry the patients go through. I was only there overnight, so it was a sandwich. It wasn't the best sandwich. I wouldn't have been happy sending it as a caterer. As a caterer I always liked to make them on site and send them up on a plate rather than in a box.

Derrick retired in 2018 and reflected on the increased stress and pressure on staff compared to when he joined in the 1980s. 'Everything is a bit more cut-throat. It's about meeting targets – not always to the advantage of the patients.'

JONATHAN BLAKE

The AIDS epidemic was one of the NHS's major challenges of the 1980s. The fear and stigma around homosexuality, HIV and AIDS among healthcare staff and the wider public compounded the awful treatment some sufferers experienced. Patient advocacy came to the fore, and sufferers and supporters got involved in every aspect of research into AIDS treatments. It built on the ongoing gay rights movement and challenged historical views about sexuality and stigma. Jonathan was born in Birmingham in 1949 and was one of the first people diagnosed with HIV/AIDS. This led him into activism and advocacy.

I think the NHS is a glory and a saving grace. For me, it's always been there. It became even more important because in October 1982, I was diagnosed with HIV – or it was then called HTLV-III [human T-cell lymphotropic virus type III]. So very early on in the saga of London and this country's HIV epidemic. I've had the most amazing treatment through my life. I'm still here.

My father sold furniture. We were a nice Jewish middle-class family in Birmingham. We were sent away to boarding school, which was horrendous. Actually, it wasn't horrendous, because I already knew by the age of six or seven that I was homosexual – or I was 'other'. Being in boarding school, you were surrounded by boys; it was heaven! That might get edited out. As a teenager it was difficult because when I was born homosexuality was illegal. I knew that it was considered dirty. I remember sitting around at a family meal, and a relation talking about these horrendous 'homosexual perverts' that lived on the King's Road. He thought that they should all be annihilated. By this time I was at drama school, and used to go to the King's Road to a couple of bars there. I used to think, 'You don't know shit. You're sitting here at the table telling us all that, and you haven't got a clue that I'm homosexual, have you?' When you know that something that essentially gets you excited is against the law, that you are a criminal before you've even had a chance to explore, that is quite a heavy burden to deal with.

From 1967 to 1970 Jonathan studied at Rose Bruford, a drama college in Sidcup, Kent. The Sexual Offences Act 1967 legalised homosexual acts in England and Wales on the condition that they were consensual, in private and between two men who were both over 21.

Every weekend I would go up to London and explore the gay scene. It was vibrant because, in July 1967, the law was partially decriminalised, which was of no use to me because I was still 17. In July of 1970, I hit 21. I woke up on that morning and my parents and two brothers were there. I announced at breakfast that I was homosexual. Because now I was no longer breaking the law. I knew that I couldn't have told them before because they were law-abiding citizens, and they'd have given me to the police. You see, this was in my head. My younger brother knew already, because we were at school and close, and so that wasn't a problem.

Can you describe the sexual health clinic?

You were considered a modern-day leper if you'd got gonorrhoea, syphilis. You really were 'unclean'. Not a fit member of society, whether male or female. People were still only getting their heads around the fact that homo-sexuality could be tolerated. That was the attitude of the general public, and it fed into medical staff. There were always issues particularly around gay men, and venereal disease. If it wasn't for Afro-Caribbean women, the NHS would very probably have collapsed. They were the mainstay of the nursing staff. And whilst they were great, they had a lot of difficulty around homosexual men. They had sincere Christian beliefs, and homosexuality was beyond the pale. It was difficult. It's not like, as a white man, that it was racially motivated. It absolutely wasn't. It was religiously motivated. It was a difficulty and it was a barrier. I remember having to go and have syphilis injections. One of the things when they jab this big needle in, pushing the penicillin in, is they slap you. She gave me a whacking thump and I said, 'What did you do that for?' 'We need to make sure that it's in.' I think that it was more I was getting punished. I was being spanked.

Were you aware of HIV?

Not really. I mean, I had lived in New York. I'd got connections with people in America. An American friend of mine in 1981 was getting married in San Francisco and wanted her gay friends to come over as ushers. I had an ex-partner who was living in San Francisco, so I went to stay with him. I was getting a whole lot of information that, ordinarily, people wouldn't know. It wasn't on the streets of this country. But I was beginning to get a sense that something was going on. That there seemed to be this weird, strange, horrible disease that was affecting young gay men. I was a young gay man. It was awful the information that one was getting – that you die a horrible death.

I received a diagnosis in October 1982, which was very early on. I was diagnosed at the Middlesex Hospital in London and my hospital number was 'London 1'. So I was the first person at the Middlesex diagnosed with HTLV-III. What had happened was that I increasingly was aware I'd become ill. Every lymph node was up in my body. I was in a lot of pain. I was walking like a gorilla. I couldn't put my arms by my side. I couldn't put my legs together because the glands in the groin were up. It was just awful. I remember going to my GP – wonderful GPs, backbone of the NHS. I was living in the East End at that point. As I walked in, she looked at me and said, 'Shake my hand.' I put my hand out for her to shake. As she shook it, her free arm felt the lymph nodes at the crack of my elbow. I went, 'Ouch, what did you do that for?' She said, 'Well, that's the sailors' handshake. Whenever the sailors got into port, they would shake hands, whether it was a woman or a man. And if that little lymph node, in the crux of the elbow was up, that was a sign of syphilis and they wouldn't go with them. Have you had a syphilis test recently?' I said, 'Oh, no, I've had syphilis, but not recently.' 'I suggest you go and have one'. That's why I went to the Middlesex – to investigate syphilis.

I arrived there. Because the glands were all so enlarged, they wanted to do a biopsy. I was taken in. In those days, if you are homosexual, you were put in side wards. We're not there to contaminate the rest of the population. There was one other man who was in my side ward. You got a sense that he was not long for this world. I'm lying in my bed, feeling awful because of the pain from these enlarged glands. They've done the biopsy. We were waiting for results. I suddenly realised that I knew this man. I had met him in 1976 when I had been out on tour in Norwich, and we'd had this relationship for a week. Here, in 1982, is the same man.

I didn't put two and two together. But they come back and tell me that I have this virus that is called HTLV-III. That it is an incurable, terminal virus. There is nothing that they can do for me. There is no medication. I've got between three and six months to live. I was 33.

I couldn't believe it. My life was over before it had even begun. I was feeling very isolated at that point. I felt I'm a modern-day leper. I had got this killer virus that was coursing around my veins. I didn't want to pass it on to anyone. If I was going to go to a bar or pub, I couldn't meet people, because I didn't want to explain. Who's going to want to have sex with me, or meet me or give me love? It was really, really wretched. In the December of that year, I decided that I was going to commit suicide. But when push came to shove, I was brought up a nice Jewish boy. That you clear up your own mess; I basically couldn't do it. So nice Jewish boy, you get on and you live. That's easier said than done, since my self-esteem is on the floor and I feel like a modern-day leper. It's horrendous.

I remember going to The Landmark and I was saying, 'God, I desperately need a new HIV doctor because where I'm at in Chelsea they want to put me on X and I don't want the medication. I don't know what to do.' Someone says, 'Oh, I've got this fabulous doctor at King's College Hospital.' So I make an appointment. He said, 'Let's see if you tolerate this,' – it was a really inexpensive antibiotic. If you could tolerate it, it kept PCP [pneumocystis pneumonia], at bay, which was one of the killers. I kept getting herpes and shingles. I'd had about three attacks of shingles. He said, 'We'll put you on Acyclovir prophylactically as a preventative measure. Because Acyclovir is what is used to lessen the effects of shingles. We'll use that prophylactically, so you take it every day.' Basically, that was it. I would see him every two weeks, and they would see my CD4 count [count of white blood cells that fight infection]. I'm back at work and that was fine. But it was hard.

Jonathan remembers the policies of the time.

There was a certain amount of bravery on the part of Norman Fowler, who was the health minister at that time. We're talking now '87. He was extraordinary that he told Margaret Thatcher that there was HIV within the heterosexual population of Edinburgh. What he didn't tell her was there was HIV in the heterosexual intravenous drug users of Edinburgh, because she would very probably have said, 'Let them die.' The point was that he was economic with the truth, but it galvanised things. Suddenly, she threw huge amounts of money at HIV in terms of research, to getting drugs, to see what could be done. Money was brought in for drop-in centres. I mean, just extraordinary. There was a lots of positive from a negative. But having done that, they then absolutely cut it dead by bringing in Section 28. It just was a nonsense.

Clause 28, or Section 28, of the Local Government Act 1988 prohibited the 'promotion of homosexuality' by local authorities.

Clause 28 was a very nasty piece of legislation that was brought in by the Conservative government under Margaret Thatcher. There could be no discussion of homosexuality in terms of sex education, or in family units to be taught in schools. It had this really dreadful effect, as a good percentage of the population were completely scrubbed out. Their sexuality was totally negated, not acknowledged, would not be allowed to be acknowledged. So it led to huge amounts of ignorance. What was just so appalling about it was that it came at the time of the HIV epidemic, which the government had acknowledged with a very nasty piece of advertising, that played on fear: the 'Don't Die of Ignorance' campaign.

Jonathan is now one of the oldest survivors of HIV/AIDS and continues to advocate for LGBTQ+ rights issues.

LINDA PEPPER

Linda was born in 1948 in Doncaster, South Yorkshire.

My dad was in antiques. My mother was a chorus girl with the Windmill Theatre in London. She was a professional dancer. My dad would say he 'rescued' her from that kind of life. It was that sort of era that, if you were on the stage, it was a bit dubious. I was 10 when my mum got diagnosed with MS [multiple sclerosis]. It took years to diagnose her. I was very well aware of the whispers in the shops. My mum was 'a drunk' because of the way she walked. It was horrible hearing the whispers when you queued up in the grocer. I wanted to shout to everybody, 'My mother's got MS – lay off!'

I left school at 16, then became a secretary with British Rail in Doncaster. With a big greasy boss, who kept saying, 'Come and sit here, Linda, while I dictate.' I kept saying 'No, I'm sure if that was right, they'd have told us that at college.' Then I went to America. I looked after the children of Richard Rodgers, of Rodgers and Hammerstein [musical theatre writing duo]. I went from Doncaster to a rather glitzy life in Manhattan – Central Park with Frank Sinatra for dinner. I grew up so quickly.

In the early 1970s Linda returned to the UK.

I thought I need to have a career. Social work turned me down. Probation turned me down. They didn't value all these life experiences I'd had. The only thing would take me was psychiatric nursing. I trained in a long-stay hospital in Bristol. Some of the patients had been there for 30 years because they'd had an illegitimate child. I found it interesting. But I think nobody should be allowed to do psychiatric nursing at 18, because you need to have life experience. Some of the younger nurses really struggled because they hadn't got that.

A lot of the family therapy stuff I was doing related to issues in people's childhood. That's what made me go into child psychiatry. I was on a children's hospital on the Wirral. It was all psychosomatic disorders with kids.

They were known as the 'pissers and shitters'. A lot of kids would be middle-class families. The parents or mother would take them to the GP, 'There's something wrong with this child.' And I'd end up with them. I thought, 'There's gonna be a lot of kids from disturbed families – and nobody realises this problem till they come before the courts.' I moved then into assessment of children in local authorities.

This led to Linda doing a PhD and becoming deeply involved with campaigning for women's health services in Liverpool during the 1980s, including establishing a new hospital for women.

Politically, I wanted to be empowering women to take responsibility for their own health and to fight the system. In Liverpool I led a lot of demonstrations. With a megaphone. We had anti-abortion issues in Liverpool. Consultants saying, 'These women who want abortions should have their vaginas filled with concrete.' I'd hire a cement mixer for a demo. We ran something called LASS – Liverpool Abortion Support Services – for the women coming over from Northern Ireland for terminations. Nobody back home knew where they were going. They'd go to some horrible, grotty B&B the night before. We set up stuff with groups in Northern Ireland. We had a rota and we'd meet the women off the boat. We'd take them to our home for the night and give them a really nice night and we'd take them the next morning for the termination. We did that on a big rota. I was part of the National Abortion Campaign, which became the Women's Reproductive Rights Campaign. We changed the name because a lot of Black women were saying, 'We have no problem getting abortions. We would quite like not to have an abortion, but we're coerced into it, and it's a wider issue.'

Hospital consultants were also blasé about the waiting lists: 'So what, there's only 400 women on the waiting list for gynae ops? What's 400?' I got 400 women in lines of 100, all dressed in white, to take over the centre of Liverpool on a Saturday. Me with a megaphone to show this is what 400 women looks like. So, yes, I'm an activist. We got some of the actors from the soap *Brookside*, which is set in Liverpool, to be there and hordes of people came. It was a time of much more interesting ways of demonstrating then than now – that got the media attention. We campaigned to get services that women should have, including the Women's Hospital, and because of those politics I wanted to work then in communities.

Lynda re-evaluated her approach to activism.

In Liverpool I'd been chair of a Community Health Council, and I'd stopped going on the street with my megaphone and decided to work through formal structures. I thought, 'If I'm really going to change the NHS, then I can't always be out on the street with a megaphone.' There must be ways of getting involved formally that are part of the system. So Community Health Councils seemed a way of helping patients have a voice through a formal structure.

Right from my teenage years, it's been about having control over my life as a woman and helping other women have control over their lives. Knowing how to demand respect. I had abnormal cervical smears and I had to go for an appointment. Nobody could tell me why. The doctor comes up. He doesn't greet me or anything. I'm lying, you know, the way you are – with your legs in stirrups, with your fanny on show for the guy sweeping the floor. The doctor puts the notes in one hand and he shoves his other hand up me. He says to the nurse, 'Why am I seeing this patient?' I am now responsible for assessing the communication skills of doctors in obstetrics and gynaecology. That's why I do it, because it's really important that doctors respect and understand the effect they might not mean to have on women.

Linda continues to advocate for patient and public involvement in the NHS and became the patient editor for the British Medical Journal's Sexual *and* Reproductive Health *quarterly in 2018.*

PAT SHEEHAN

Pat was the seventeenth Republican inmate at Long Kesh Detention Centre, later known as 'HM Prison Maze', to join the 1981 hunger strike, a culmination of the five-year protests during the Troubles, which were aimed at gaining political status for Provisional IRA and Irish National Liberation Army prisoners. He began fasting on 10 August – after nine prisoners had already died – and ended when the hunger strike was officially called off on 3 October. He survived 55 days without food.

My real contact with the health service came when I was in prison. When I was 19 years of age, I was convicted for a bombing attack that had been carried out by the IRA.

Just before the hunger strike began, when Bobby Sands began his hunger strike, I had a visit, probably February 1981, with my mother and father, and my sister Louise, who was a year older than me. At the end of the visit, my sister and my mother had walked on, but my father held back a bit. He says, 'I want you to take your name off the list of volunteers for the hunger strike. Louise has been diagnosed with leukaemia, and has been given five or six years to live.' You can imagine. It was the first time there was any bad news like that in our immediate family. I was absolutely devastated. She was just a year and a half older than me. She would have been coming 24 and I'd be 22, going on 23 in May. I went back to my cell and thought about it and decided that I would carry on with the hunger strike if I was chosen to replace any of the ones who had died.

When you go on hunger strike, you have to have a particular mindset. The view you have going on a hunger strike is that you have a job to do, you have one job to do. That's it.

I had already mentally prepared myself for what was going to happen, what I had to do. Some people will say, well, it was cruel and selfish on my parents. Cruel, it may well have been. But going on hunger strike to the death is like the antithesis of selfishness, you know.

I began hunger strike on the 10 August 1981 up until Saturday 3 October, which is 55 days.

On hunger strike we were examined by a doctor every day. Our weight was taken, blood pressure, all that sort of stuff, our urine was tested. We were drinking just water. And took a small amount of salt each day. Like your finger tip and dip it in the salt. It has never been made clear to me why we were advised to take some salt. Someone told us that if you didn't have the salt, you could have hallucinations, or whatever. We were also examined on a weekly basis by a consultant from one of the big hospitals in Belfast.

On hunger strike, we were treated quite well. We remained in the prison H blocks for a large part of the hunger strike. Most people were moved, around 20 days, to the prison hospital. I was there for nearly 35 days. That was only because the main prison doctor was on leave. I asked the guy who was standing in, 'When can I expect the move to the prison hospital?' He said, 'Well, are you in a hurry to get moved'? I said, 'No.' He says, 'Well, I'm happy to leave you here as long as you're happy.' So fair enough, so I got to spend longer in the block than any of the other hunger strikers. Most of the doctors were very professional.

On the Wednesday before the hunger strike ended, I was examined by Professor Grant from the [Belfast] City Hospital. I was totally jaundiced. Seven and a half stone, almost totally blind, very, very weak. The blindness was caused by deprivation of I think one of the B vitamins. It affects the muscle that controls the eyes and allows the eyes to focus. One of the doctors explained that it's a bit like sea sickness. If your eyes can't focus, that creates nausea. You begin vomiting up the water and eventually you're just throwing up green bile. The doctor asked me to lie flat on the bed. He pressed his fingers on the right ribcage on the right-hand side here. I nearly went through the ceiling with the pain. He wasn't trying to hurt me. He said, 'Your liver is badly enlarged and is beginning to shut down. I can't guarantee that, even if you end your hunger strike here and now, you'll survive.'

Our officer in command of the IRA prisoners had come to the hospital to see me. He said they were making arrangements to bring the hunger strike to an end the following day. Would I be okay until the Saturday? I explained to him what the consultant had said. I said, 'Well, I'm not coming off hunger strike. I'll come off it when it ends, and that's it.' And I had this crazy notion, that night, that if I was able to keep myself awake, I would, by sheer willpower, keep myself alive. As it turns out, I got the best night's sleep of the whole hunger strike.

I was the longest of all the lads on hunger strike. In theory, I would have been the next to die. We gathered in my room in the prison hospital the next day. At 3 p.m. I called in the chief medical officer and told him that I was terminating my hunger strike. That signalled the end of that hunger strike that had begun on the 1 March, in which 10 people had died. I was then moved to Musgrave Park Hospital in Belfast. There was a secure wing in it, and I was placed in a ward with three other prisoners who had also survived the hunger strike.

Before I left the prison, they gave me two vitamin injections. One was a multivitamin. And the other vitamin specifically for the eyes. I suppose within an hour, my eyesight had returned almost to normal and the nausea had disappeared. At Musgrave Park Hospital, they came in with what looked like a glass of milk. They told me it was half milk and half water. If I could keep it down, I could have as much as I wanted. If I couldn't, they'd have to put me on a drip. So I tasted the watered-down milk. It was the sweetest, most beautiful thing you could ever imagine. It was nectar from the gods. I was in Musgrave Park for four weeks after that. It was nurses and doctors from the hospital who were dealing with us. It was a normal hospital setting, apart from the fact that our ward was locked.

Of the four of us who were in the ward, I had probably been the most seriously ill. And yet I was forced to go back to the prison. One of the other lads had no appetite whatsoever. He was in the hospital for maybe three or four months after the hunger strike. I was lucky and I've survived without any ill effects that I'm aware of since then.

I'm an Irish Republican and we don't believe that Britain should have any influence at all over Ireland. We believe that Ireland should be a united, independent republic. However, that's not to say that nothing good ever came from Britain. The one thing that all of us would be thankful for is the National Health Service. There's no family, irrespective of political allegiance, that hasn't been affected in some way by ill health, cancer and other diseases, and people who have been involved in accidents. And it's always a great comfort to people that there's a health service there that can take care of their needs. It has its problems, make no mistake about that. But by and large, it's been something that's been good for the people of this part of Ireland.

Pat was released from prison in 1998 as part of the Good Friday Agreement. He is now a member of the Legislative Assembly of Northern Ireland.

AVERIL MANSFIELD

*Averil was born in 1937 in Blackpool. Paying for healthcare before the NHS was diffi-
cult, and her parents kept a pot on the mantelpiece, into which some of her father's weekly
wages were put. Her mother feared that Averil's ambitions to enter medicine were 'above
our station'. 'Nobody had been to university from my family, so it was a new venture.'
Averil was to become the NHS's first female professor of surgery.*

Medicine interested me as a child. Surgery was the bit of medicine that
grabbed me. I read lots of books about the history of medicine and how
people started to do something for the first time. I thought, 'That's for me,
it's what I want to do.' I applied to Liverpool and Manchester Medical
Schools. I set off in my hat, coat, shoes and gloves – all matching. They both
offered me a place, which was quite surprising because there were not as
many women in medical school in 1955 as there are now. I chose Liverpool
because I liked the atmosphere and the relaxed and humorous way that
people went about their lives.

*After finishing medical school, students worked for 12 months as house officers before
receiving full registration from the General Medical Council. Averil did her house jobs at
Broadgreen Hospital in Liverpool.*

It was a good, big general hospital, run by Dr Finlay, who was the physi-
cian superintendent, with a hospital secretary and a matron. Dr Finlay was
so lovely with the young doctors, supporting and guiding us, and giving us
responsibility when responsibility was due. I can remember saying to my
boss in the first week, 'Is there any time off in this job?' He said, 'Oh, I
suppose you could go into Liverpool on a Wednesday evening, provided
you're back in time to do the night round.' Those were his exact words. You
got two weeks' holiday during your six months. It was a terrific atmosphere.
It didn't matter that we were on all the time. Yes, you got tired. I can remember my registrar – an Australian to whom I owe a great deal and who knew
I wanted to be a surgeon – was assessing not just my skills, but my stamina.

Was I able to get up the morning after I'd been on call all night? Able to get up and get on with the job. Yes, you did need stamina, and I was blessed with plenty of that. I don't think anybody grumbled about the hours we worked. We knew that was the year you had to get through. If I look back on it, it was one of the best years of my professional life because everything was new and exciting.

I knew I wanted to be a general surgeon. I was pretty cagey about admitting it in my year, because there were quite a few of the men who wanted to be surgeons and I thought they're going to say, 'No, no, don't be silly.' I never varied in my desire to become a surgeon, but I didn't shout it from the rooftops. At that time there were one or two scattered women surgeons in the north of England. There was a paediatric female surgeon, Miss Forshaw. She'd taught me when I was an undergraduate. She was quite something to be reckoned with, a very strong-minded lady and a really good surgeon. She had spawned one other female trainee, who was a little bit older than me. There was a lady surgeon around Wigan. I think there was somebody in Manchester. So female surgeons were very sparse. It really didn't bother me because I didn't see that that mattered very much. I thought, 'This is what I want to do, this is my future, and there's really no reason why I shouldn't.' And of course, Liverpool's a great place for supporting the underdog. If you're mad enough to want to be a surgeon, they'll give you a hand. It's very much the Liverpool way.

I loved operating from day one. My first proper internal operation was an appendectomy, and I was guided by this lovely Australian registrar who was teaching me how to operate. He took me through it, and it all went well. I remember ringing my parents up from my room, 'You'll never guess what I've just done.' That was very nice. Because I managed the first one well, the registrar then gave me other operations, always assisting me, always making sure it was within my scope. By the time I'd been a house officer for six months, I'd done 20 appendectomies. Some of my young trainees would give their eye teeth to have done 20 appendectomies ever, let alone in their first six months. Unbelievably different.

By '72 I was a consultant. I was very lucky. It was unbelievable how quickly I rose through the ranks to a consultant. People always assumed that because I was female it would take a lot longer; and it didn't. If I was the best person for a job, I got it. I'm certain there was no impediment from the fact that I was female. I got my second application to be a consultant. The first one I applied for was in London, and I was relieved not to get it because I looked in the estate agents' windows and thought, 'I can't possibly come and live here.' The second job that I applied for was in the teaching hospital in Liverpool, and I got it. So it was very fair.

I'd done so much surgery that by the time I became a consultant, it wasn't that big a deal. It was different and you had a different responsibility, and you had your own trainees to look after. But in terms of being overwhelmed by the work – no, it was what you had trained to do and you were ready for it. So that was good.

Averil's passion for vascular surgery began when she was a house officer at Broadgreen Hospital. Her consultant had visited the US to learn about the new speciality of vascular surgery and wanted to develop it in the UK.

One Sunday morning we all gathered to operate on an aortic aneurysm. I'd never seen one before. I don't think many people had seen one before, because aortic aneurysms were things that you really couldn't operate on. I was captivated. It was the most amazing day. I'm almost certain it was the consultant's first operation of this kind. I thought, 'This is something I really want to do.' And that's really where it all started.

When I became a consultant in 1972, I declared at the interview that I would want to develop vascular surgery in my job while remaining a general surgeon. It was fascinating because people were not used to vascular surgery. They were rather frightened of it. They assumed it was going to be very difficult and unpleasant, and mostly got quite a nice surprise when they discovered it actually did work. So I did more and more. While I was in Liverpool, I retained my general surgery and did everything: breasts, bowels, gallbladders – you name it. But when I moved to St Mary's Hospital in Paddington in the early 1980s, the professor of surgery had a little chat with me and suggested that it would be a good idea if I dropped the general surgery and just did vascular surgery. My predecessor at St Mary's was a man called Felix Eastcott, who had done the very first operation in the world on the carotid artery to prevent stroke. He was developing vascular surgery as a speciality, so it was easy to follow on from there and build it up. Almost the first thing I did when I came to London was to shoot off to Houston, Texas, for 10 days to learn how to do a new procedure for an extensive aneurysm operation. I'd done one of these while I was in Liverpool, and that was probably a first in this country. I became the expert because I'd done one. And I knew I wasn't the expert. It was just beginner's luck that this had gone straightforwardly. So I made it my business to go and learn how to do it properly, from someone who was an expert. So we then settled down and did these more complicated vascular procedures.

What was your sense at that time of the risks of new procedures?

That very first procedure that I did in Liverpool, I'd never done one before. But I was absolutely straight with the patient. I said, 'Look, you could go to Houston, Texas, where they know how to do these things properly. I've tried to send you to London, but nobody there seems to want to do it. I've never done one before. I don't know whether it can be done. All I can say is that you've got a problem that will take your life, probably quite soon, and this gives us a chance. But it's no more than that.' I think he fully understood what he was letting himself in for, and was absolutely straight about wanting me to do it. And fortunately, it all went well. But you're right, it could just as easily have gone the other way. I probably never would have done another one had he died; but he didn't, so that was good.

Somebody has to do it the first time. I think that's very dominantly a surgical problem: the fact that there has to be a first patient. I don't think we can get round that. Felix Eastcott, my predecessor, who did this first operation to try to prevent stroke – that patient could have ended up with a big stroke; happily, they didn't and happily they remained well for many years to follow it. But it is a risk.

Most of my discussions about things that were relatively new were not so much with surgeons as with anaesthetists, because it was often as big a problem for an anaesthetist to take on something new and different as it was for the surgeon. They may not know how the patient would behave in these circumstances, particularly with things like an extensive aneurysm, which is what I was embarking on up at St Mary's. The anaesthetist was vital to the development of that. Anaesthetists are your closest mates, there's no question about that. You have to get on with them. When I moved to London, I acquired the anaesthetist who had worked for my predecessor. That was the first time I'd ever worked with somebody who clearly was a little unsure about the idea of a female surgeon. He was quite old-fashioned in his approach. We became very good mates and we worked together extremely well. But those first few weeks it was, 'We'll be doing such and such, won't we, Averil?' 'No, we won't. That's how my predecessor might have done it, but I do it this way.' So there were a few months of learning how to get on with each other, but we did in the end, and it was a very good relationship.

When I first started in the 1960s, you didn't tell people they had cancer, let alone what you were going to do to them. It was really completely different. For me it became more and more time-consuming explaining things to patients – particularly as, towards the end of my surgical career for some of the operations that I did, there would be two alternatives. A big open-heart operation, or a minimally invasive procedure like keyhole surgery. Both would be possible. Both would have their pros and cons. You'd spend half an hour with a patient, describing the pros and cons. You do have to be sure they fully understand what's going on, and they're not doctors, they're not familiar with the territory, so it does take time.

I was always very much of the opinion that you needed to talk to patients about what you were going to do to them. But not in the detail that I ended up having to talk to patients by the time I retired in the 2000s. I mean, it was in a completely different league. And things like the complications that can ensue after a procedure – you almost worry that it's become easier to say that every possible complication in the world can happen to you. You've got to include them all, because that's the only way to safeguard yourself. That can't be right; it must be terrifying for patients to have to listen to all that.

I can remember one patient who – I'd put the two possibilities for his aortic aneurysm to him. He said, 'Right, I'll go away and think about it.' 'Good. That's fine.' He spent the next two weeks on the internet, and he came back and said, 'Bloody well make my mind up for me.' He'd no idea what was right. So I said, 'Well, that's fine, then. I'll do this.' It's hard sometimes on patients to give them that choice. A lot of the time, there isn't that much choice, it's just you have to tell them a bit about what might go wrong, but they still have to have it done. I think they're more used to hearing about things that could go wrong now, aren't they? I guess the man in the street knows a bit more about what goes on in a hospital than they used to. It's an amazing feeling when you can restore somebody to normal working life.

I have managed to have a family life, and a happy outside-of-surgery life. Very happy. But it did need tolerance, on behalf of the people that you are living with, of your lifestyle. There were times when I would feel guilty that I was putting a completely unknown stranger ahead of my family because that stranger had got into surgical difficulties when I should have been at home cooking supper, or whatever it was. That is a difficult dilemma. People are not nearly so concerned now because they accept that they're either on, or they're off. If they're not on, they're at home, and that's it. Finished. Done. I didn't really have that distinction in my life, because I knew that at any time I could be called. I just coped with that, put up with it and got on with it. And regarded that as life. Maybe people don't want to do that anymore. They want to feel that there is a secure time away from work. I think that's perhaps the upshot of it, really, the central issue is that you want to be certain that you can be away from your work for a period of time. As I got towards the end of my career, we had slightly more time off. That did help. It meant you could have a glass of wine without fearing that you might have to be dragged in to do something. But it wasn't all that onerous, and more than compensated for by the pleasures of doing the job.

In 1999 Averil was awarded a CBE for services to surgery and women in medicine. She retired in 2003 and reflects on her experience of the NHS as a patient in Chapter 10.

DAVID ROTHBERG

David Rothberg was born Salford in 1950.

I did an MSc in probability and statistics at Manchester University. In 1972 I saw an opportunity in the NHS working in a pilot scheme. Three units across the country were collecting information to be used to improve the efficiency of the NHS. I applied to Oldham unit and got the job. There was the NHS graduate training scheme. That was the best way at that time to get into the NHS and to progress. But I didn't know anything about that, so I joined directly.

NHS trainees had a training programme drafted out. I didn't have anything, so it was a matter of doing it yourself and signing up for the Institute of Health Services Management qualification. I also later signed up for the Institute of Personnel Management, which is a broader, non-NHS qualification in human resources and personnel management. One good thing at the time was there were lots of training opportunities. The NHS ran its own courses on management training, or specific subjects that were relevant at the time. I went on lots of management training. As I became more senior, the decision-making became, if you like, a bit more political. I know some of my wife's relatives probably had a view that I was closing hospitals and things like that, and didn't like it.

I did my first post for a year, but I didn't enjoy it. I was more interested in the mainstream, day-to-day side of the NHS. I moved over into other junior posts. My impression was the NHS was pretty badly managed. There wasn't good coordination between doctors, professionals, administrators. Everybody was running their own show. GPs were totally separate from the hospital side. It was very much separate empires and was a bit of a hodgepodge. Resources were being wasted. No one was looking at the whole situation in the hospital and saying, 'Well, it may be better to spend some money here rather than there.' The money was coming from different places. So the people providing the money were accounting for what they were doing, but they were separate funding streams.

In 1983 the Thatcher government launched the NHS Management Inquiry, led by Roy Griffiths, director and deputy chairman of Sainsbury's supermarket. Griffiths recommended the appointment of general managers and advocated for doctors to become involved in management. The aim of general management was to improve efficiency by establishing chains of responsibility and accountability.

When the Griffiths Report on NHS management was implemented, I was based in Epping, managing hospitals in that area outside North-East London: Epping Hospital, Waltham Abbey, Ongar War Memorial Hospital, and Great West Hatch and Little West Hatch Hospitals in Chigwell. The Griffiths Report was a massive change. That was the first real change where they tried to give one person, a general manager, responsibility for all the resources. The NHS brought in people from outside and encouraged people from the army and the RAF to come in. The RAF and the army were very hierarchical, whereas the NHS is about teamworking. You have to get the doctors working with the nurses and all the different professionals. There's a lot of professionals in the NHS and a lot of egos in the NHS, so that's the big challenge. I don't think the people brought in from the outside fully appreciated what was involved. They were used to issuing an order and the order being carried out. That wouldn't work in the culture of the NHS.

I moved to manage the mental health services for Bromley Health Authority. I was in charge of the old psychiatric hospital and it was my responsibility to develop new services in Bromley and, at the same time, manage the consequent closure of the psychiatric hospital, which was called Cane Hill Hospital. There were lots of challenges because we needed a lot of money from the region to buy properties and to run new services while services were running down – the transition. I personally put a lot of work into that, into making the case and so on. I've fronted lots of meetings where people have not been happy because their local hospital was under threat. When I was running mental health services for Bromley, people liked the old mental hospitals. Their relatives were relatively well looked-after in the main and any change from that, people were, 'Well, I'm not sure that my relative could manage in the community.' They'd want guarantees that there'd be the proper levels of support. I mean, when you've got economies of scale in the mental hospital, everybody's under control. You've got everybody there. When you start to resettle people in the community, then you lose those economies of scale, and you need more people looking after the same small groups of people in community homes. So that was obviously quite stressful.

A lot of the work that was done, I did personally. Working out what we needed to do in the transition so we could resettle people from the hospital to the community. I didn't assess individual patients, but I decided they would go in that home, based on the aggregated information I had. I knew we had so many people of this particular type who could live together. So I did an aggregated-level model. I worked that out and tied in the finances. We set in motion the whole change. When I came in, there were about 800 patients in the hospital. When I left, that was probably down to 200. Some had died, some had been relocated to other NHS facilities and some were going to be resettled. And the financial plan to back up that was all in place. Obviously, that was an achievement.

The hospital was very much part of the local community. The local community felt like they own the hospital. I thought that was something strange at first, because I hadn't worked in an environment where there was that attitude, that sense of ownership. Once I got used to that, I enjoyed it – and we lived in the community as well.

David retired in the 1990s. 'I've been a good client for the NHS in recent years. I have a pacemaker in my chest. I've also got severe sleep apnoea. I use a CPAP [continuous positive airway pressure machine, which keeps your airway open] machine at night and I wear a mask, which puts air in. So I've got my money's worth out of the NHS. Apart from working in it for 24 years!'

TOM HELLER and JACK CZAUDERNA

Primary care changed significantly during the 1980s, including the upgrading of old premises and the building of new health centres which could accommodate a growing number of health professionals working in primary care. GPs treated an increasing number of patients suffering from depression and other mental health issues, and became more involved in health promotion. After qualifying in medicine in London, Tom worked in Nepal, including time spent at the Kunde Hospital at the foot of Mount Everest. He worked in development studies in East Anglia on his return, and moved to Sheffield to train in general practice. Jack met his life partner, Maureen O'Leary, while training in medicine in Bristol. Maureen specialised in psychiatry, Jack in general practice. In 1979 they decided to move north, and Jack became a GP trainee in Tom's practice.

Tom: All I needed to do was to come to Sheffield and do a year in general practice as a trainee and a few weeks in obstetrics and gynae. There was no medical school in Norwich at that time and it wasn't quite satisfying politically. I also had a young family and I thought, 'It's probably better to be in a bigger place.'

I went for a whole year with a really excellent, lovely doctor, single-handed. A guy of Indian origin. The daily schedule was come in about 9.20, chat with him, have a cup of tea and rich tea biscuits and then start surgery at 9.30. Finish about 10.45. There may or may not be a visit. Then you're free until five o'clock in the evening. It fitted my lifestyle with having a young family. It was brilliant. Also, I could carry on with working on sociological studies.

I was a trainee and then went almost immediately into being one of the trainers for the Vocational Training Scheme. There were three of us who shared the organisation, and we were pretty innovative. I ran one of the groups of trainees, and I ran it with a psychotherapist. The sessions were partly about medical knowledge and what you need to do clinically. But a lot was to do with support and how they were getting on. These groups were quite influential in setting the tone for general practice in Sheffield over the next decade at least.

There was a job coming up as a single-handed practitioner in Darnall, a really interesting, lovely area. Very much connected with industrial service. People who live there might have been coal miners, working in the steelworks, traditionally. As people bettered themselves, indigenous people, a lot of immigrants who again worked in the steelworks, bus operatives and people like that came to the area. A GP couple retired, so it became a single-handed practice. I took it over. They had built a little offshoot so that people didn't have to come into the house. Part of the deal in those days with single-handed practices, you had to buy the house as well. So we bought the house but didn't move in. We converted the whole thing into the surgery. For the first time, people were allowed into the house itself. They were standing there looking at these high ceilings and big green settees. That was their waiting room. We built new consulting rooms and things like that as well.

I was still pretty politicised. We decided to run it as a collective. So people who came along, like the practice nurse who was a political friend, the cleaner, the doctor, we all got an hourly rate by seeing what the takings were over a year and dividing it by however many we were. We had big clinical meetings but also a practice meeting. Deciding what to do as a practice. Trying to be democratic. If there was money to spend, we would decide between us all how to spend it. We took on a trainee, and it was a radical time. Sheffield attracted doctors that wanted to work in this way. We called ourselves TCP – Towards Coordinated Practice. We were the first practice to show people their own notes. We employed a psychotherapist.

Jack: There were exciting things going on in primary care in Sheffield. In the early eighties Sheffield was called 'The Socialist Republic of South Yorkshire'. The buses were really cheap to get around in the days of David Blunkett and Clive Betts – these people became MPs later on. The infrastructure was there. There were some very young, idealistic, full-of-energy doctors who wanted to work in a primary care setting as GPs. Half a dozen of us used to meet and think about how we were going to do this. General practice in the 1980s still tended to be single-handed practitioners in their own buildings. We had a different model. We wanted to really overturn what was going on. I think we thought we could change the world.

Jack became a GP trainee in Tom's practice.

It had one receptionist who was allowed to answer the telephone. A tiny waiting room with a one-room surgery attached to the house where the GP's mother had lived. The records used to be kept above the desk. Tom and a whole load of other people, including me, set out to change things. I finished my GP training in 1981. There was a requirement by the GMC [General Medical Council] to be GP-trained – you had to do three years post-qualification to be a GP, but before that, you could just go straight into practice.

The practice had a general medical services contract. So we're independent contractors, like all other GPs, but we set up the practice internally, as an equal pay, collective practice. In other words, everybody who worked there got the same amount of pay per hour. This was revolutionary and I'm still proud of what we did, although it was completely off the wall, in a way. So from receptionists to the doctors, we got paid the same hourly rates. We thought it was important in challenging the power relationships that health workers had between themselves, and also attempting to look at the way that we treated the relationships we had with patients as well.

We were among some of the first practices that had counsellors looking at people's mental health. These are standard things now, but at that time, in the early eighties, it was very radical. We had interpreters because we started to get a lot more people from Pakistan, Bangladesh, Yemeni people, Somali people over the years. We had to adapt our practice to look after people whose first language was not English.

The Sheffield steel strike in 1983 really motivated a whole group of people to set up what became the Sheffield occupational health project. These were not professional people. We were all activists, I think. Some of us had professional qualifications and some didn't. But we worked in working men's clubs, talked to the steelworkers, miners, of course – there was the miners' strike. The health service would pay 70 per cent of the wages, the salaries, of people GPs employed, that was part of just standard contract at the time. GPs would have to find 30 per cent of people's wages and salaries for reception staff, for practice nurses, the interpreter, and we employed some of the occupational health workers, which were funded via the council.

The occupational health workers would sit in the waiting room talking to people about their work and how that impacted on their health. Doing things like hearing tests for steelworkers who've been in noisy environments, asbestos work. Then talking with the GPs and the nurses and helping with compensation claims. So it was more than just the standard GP work. And although there was a contract and a thing called 'the red book' at the time, we just did things that we thought would match the needs of the population.

Even in the early eighties, Irish Travellers were coming to us. We realised that their health was pretty poor. There were relatively few older people, lots of young people with small children. Our health visitor realised that they weren't getting immunised, as there was a lot of resistance to immunisation. There was one family with 17 children, and they would all be living in trailers. Looking after these families was really difficult. We were campaigning and lobbying for funding and better facilities. Eventually, a health visitor post for the Travellers was set up. She was really good and visited families. We had a mobile clinic as well. But we worked with whoever we could, really, to deliver services. We got into having appointment systems then, like all GPs. That didn't always work out because people would just turn up and expect to be seen.

Tom and Jack are now retired, but during Covid-19 they both volunteered at the Sheffield Community Contact Tracers' project, helping to set up a contact tracing service for Sheffield residents before the government had one in place, and then working with communities to raise confidence in the vaccine.

ILLORA FINLAY

Cicely Saunders had started St Christopher's Hospice in 1967, pioneering new approaches to end of life care. Around the same time, Illora's father became terminally ill shortly after she'd qualified in medicine. The family cared for him at home, which was uncommon at that time. After qualifying as a GP in 1972, Illora became increasingly interested in taking care of the dying.

I took the decision to jump into what was called 'terminal care' and 'hospice care'. Palliative medicine as a specialty didn't exist. I'd managed to get myself appointed to the charity Marie Curie, and I was the first consultant in Wales to run what had been a nursing home and basically turn it into a modern hospice in Cardiff, 1987. I had 38 beds and a day centre. The first day I arrived, there was no provision for prescribing. I had to negotiate how we got medication. I discovered that there weren't proper case notes. I went and bought a pad of A4 paper and clerked all the patients in properly, because I needed to know what was going on. Then I needed to train the staff, so I used to run lunchtime training sessions. I was on call all the time.

An amazing GP called Dr Harry Rapport came along one day, 'I just want to help; I'm happy to come as a volunteer.', he told me. That was amazing because he would come and see patients in day care, so at least I could leave Cardiff. It was so novel to prescribe morphine in what looked like relatively high doses to get on top of people's pain. It wasn't really particularly high, but the drug squad came in one day because they thought I must be supplying drugs because of the quantities of morphine we were using. That was pretty terrifying.

We turned a couple of the side rooms into family rooms, so that spouses or partners could stay and sleep over. We got beds that joined together – because if you've lived next to somebody for 50 years and had a cuddle every night, you don't want to be alone, stuck on a hospital bed away from them. The family want to be there, but if they can't cope at home, then it was bringing home into the hospice. We set up a room with a big toy box for children and lots of videos in a day room.

We had fantastic catering staff who would do imaginative, tasty things that people would like. Tasty morsels to eat. We got a drinks trolley and had a happy hour. And the nurses were great. These were the auxiliary nurses, the care assistants. They made a restaurant menu of different cocktails, alcoholic and non-alcoholic. If you haven't got much of an appetite, a little glass of sherry or something can titivate your appetite and get you going. We always had wonderful flowers around.

We also had a hospice cat. The cat was very interesting because the cat would go and curl up on the bed of somebody who was dying. It was as if the cat sensed … whether it was the person was lying very still or what it was, but it was quite bizarre. We'd say, 'Oh the cat's gone in there.'

When we took the first HIV patients, some of the staff were terrified. The husband of one of the auxiliary nurses was absolutely terrified and said he wouldn't sleep with her if she was looking after HIV patients. We had a huge amount of education to do to get over the fear and stigmatisation. But we did.

We had some really memorable situations. One I'll always remember was somebody who was clearly dying, whose daughter was coming from Australia. She'd flown in and got a taxi from Heathrow at huge expense, and arrived. Obviously jetlagged, tired, emotional and the whole thing. We took a four-bedded bay. Her father was in one bed, we put one bed next to him and one bed across the bottom of the beds that made a huge square for his wife and his daughter. They all tucked down, you know, lots of cups of tea and things. In the morning, only two of them woke up. He'd died in the night. That's the right way to look after people – not get people sitting on chairs by the bed, because 'We don't put relatives in the hospital beds.' Just do what people need.

If you're in pain or you feel sick, you can't concentrate on anything else. So you've got to get that sorted out in order to be able to address all the psychosocial aspects. I quite often would say to patients, 'Look, this is Plan A, but I've got a Plan B. And if that's not working, I've got a Plan C.' At what point do you say, let's chuck the whole lot up? I think the reason that assisted dying worries me so deeply is I've had so many instances where the unexpected happens. Let me give you a specific example. A young man dying said, 'I just don't want to go on. I can't stand every day. I just want to die.' I said, 'I'm not going to give you lethal drugs, but if you want to be sedated and sleep your last days away, well, that's fine, I'll sedate you.' He signalled after a day or two that he wanted to communicate. So we switched off his medication, and he woke up. 'I just remembered something that I wanted to do.' He was writing a book on artistry and he hadn't written the last chapter. He was very ill, very frail, not able to sit up. I said, 'Well, do you want to borrow a Dictaphone and borrow my secretary?' He dictated the whole of the last chapter of his book. At the weekend, I was with his girlfriend in the room, and we were looking out the window. There were some children who had climbed over a garden wall and were climbing up a tree. We saw them and we laughed out loud. And as we turned around, he died. I thought, 'He'd completed his life's work. He could see that his girlfriend wasn't alone. And he just let go and died.' I've had people who've had amazingly important conversations that have meant a lot to the family for the rest of their lives. That would never have happened if they cut their life short with lethal drugs. So those moments are precious. They're completely unpredictable. But they are important for life to carry on. Life is so precious and so fragile. What's the rush to cut it off? I'm not saying we should strive officiously to keep alive at all. But it is precious.

Illora was appointed to the House of Lords in 2001. 'I've had several attempts with an Access to Palliative Care Bill and each time it hasn't got anywhere, but I will keep going.'

ROBERT DOWNES

Bob grew up with five siblings in a working-class Liverpool family, living in a house with outside toilets. His memories of childhood are 'amazing and positive'.

I'm known as Bob. I was born in Liverpool in 1956. I believe it's important to leave a verbal account of my experiences of working as a nurse, particularly from 1976, when very few men went into nursing. The assumption was that if you were a male nurse, then you were gay. Nursing has played an amazing path in allowing me to lead a very open life as a gay man since the age of 19 in 1976. An incredible thing to be able to do.

Bob has lost three siblings – two died as children with congenital problems and his younger brother died of leukaemia at the age of 40.

I applied to do nurse training in 1975. I'd never sat any educational exams at school. I had to sit an entrance test. If you'd got a certain level, then you could do SRN [State Registered Nurse] training. Otherwise, you could do the two years State Enrolled training. I got good scores because I was selected to go and do the three-year course.

Bob started his first post in 1979 as a staff nurse and worked his way up the ranks to ward manager. He then gained a specialist qualification in district nursing and has been a community nurse since 1987, with time spent caring for patients with HIV/AIDS. As a gay man growing up in the 1970s, he is deeply aware of the social stigma experienced by HIV/AIDS patients.

One particular memory I have was an HIV/AIDS patient whose dream was to die on a beach in Thailand. He applied for lots of different credit cards, maxed them all, and went to the place of his choice in Thailand, first class. I still have a letter that he wrote to me from the beach. He passed away in Thailand during that break. I remember, afterwards, his relatives having to try and sort out all the mess that was left behind from all the debt!

Relatives have commented that it was incredibly important that their relative was looked after by another gay man, because they knew that there would be no prejudice. A privilege was being asked to carry the coffin by relatives. Relatives have said to me afterwards that because we treated patients with dignity and respect, that made an impossible situation tolerable. The biggest problem was around HIV being a category-three pathogen. There are different categories of pathogens, graded by their life-threatening nature. Ebola, for example, would be a category one. There are guidelines about how each category is treated so that there is no risk of cross-contamination, or cross-infection from it. Category three is bloodborne viruses. HIV was categorised as a category-three pathogen. The guidelines after death for category-three pathogens are: the body isn't viewed or kissed; bodies should be placed in a body bag in a sealed coffin; and embalming shouldn't take place because of the risk to the person doing the embalming. Back then, a lot of the funeral directors stuck to the letter. Even in death, these people were identified as being contaminated as if it was a plague.

We were fortunate to negotiate around that with a funeral director sometimes. It sounds bizarre talking about it now, but we arranged for a lady's body to be kept on ice, so that it wouldn't decompose as quickly, so that a relative away from Liverpool could come and see the body. Another occasion was an embalmer agreed to embalm somebody's head and hands, so they could be viewed in their coffin. They were dressed in the coffin and had a polo neck on, with long sleeves. I guess black humour helps people to work through those things. I was heavily involved in that situation with the family. There was lots of laughter around it saying how the person who had passed away would really have enjoyed the experience. That person was buried and was viewed after death. No body bag was involved and the coffin wasn't sealed.

Liverpool's culture meant there was an expectation that bodies would be viewed after death.

In keeping with the Irish tradition of wake, there is that culture within the city centre. Not necessarily having the person in the coffin propped up in the corner, but in some cases, having the coffin in the house and having a party

– and the whole street will come and view the body. The problem was, if that wasn't allowed to happen because of the regulations, people started to ask questions about why that wasn't taking place. That was always a difficult one for people to get around. There were suspicions cast as to the cause of death, and often based on how people looked physically before their death. Many people with end-stage HIV disease told people that they had cancer that was terminal because the physical appearances are very similar. Most of the work was around helping people to have peaceful deaths in a place of their choice. There was psychological care involved, as well as all the physical stuff around making sure that people were as comfortable and as pain-free as possible.

What impact has the NHS had on your life?

Sometimes I think it's good. Sometimes I think it's incredibly sad that the NHS almost defines who I am. But also, HIV defines who I am because I've worked in it for so long. I talk more about HIV than anything else in the world. The thought of retirement scares me shitless, really, because if I retire, who am I? So, although I'm 63, retirement really isn't on my agenda – for the foreseeable future, anyway.

Bob concluded his interview by reflecting that it would be better for the NHS to be taken out of party politics and managed as a national institution.

LINDA LAMONT

Linda first got involved in patient advocacy when she joined Brighton's Community Health Council (CHC), newly established under the 1974 NHS reorganisation. She was the CHC's representative on Brighton Health Authority, chaired by Julia Cumberlege, Conservative MP.

In '85 I was in Washington, DC, with my husband for three months. He was doing a term of seminars. We were staying at the Folger Institute, which is pretty much at the bottom of Capitol Hill, and I offered to Julia Cumberlege that I would look at American healthcare. At the time we were looking at the NHS moving more in the direction of America, whereas we thought we could see signs that America was beginning to be interested in a more socialised system. The beginnings of it, anyway. So I was interested to see what they were doing.

I was lucky enough to be able to listen in on Senate hearings and to interview quite a few people at the time. I've got a box full of papers. I was impressed by the standard of healthcare for those who had the right insurance, and I visited at least one public hospital where the standard was much lower, but where you had to go if you hadn't got insurance.

It was all in the Washington, DC, area and the area itself was distinctly divided. For instance, the metro didn't go into the Black areas, but the buses did. So if you went on a bus, you'd be with the Black community. If you went on the metro, you wouldn't. I did go to a couple of clinics run for the Black community by the Black community, and talked to people there. I did get a broad picture of what it was like, and the haves and have-nots were very clearly defined.

The Patients Association was set up in 1963 in response to concerns that NHS patients were being used in medical experiments without their knowledge.

Coming back to England and I joined the Patients Association in 1988 as the director, following on from Dame Elizabeth Ackroyd, who had just died and who had been a remarkable civil servant. She had her own kind of computer system, which I wish we'd kept. It was in a filing cabinet. She had cards with holes in different places and she could put a knitting needle in and that would connect with the holes that were similar. So if she wanted dentistry, for example, she could find the right hole and put the equivalent of a knitting needle in and get through to all the cards which were to do with dentistry. It was pretty amazing, in '88.

I arrived up from Sussex never having done anything like this. I thought it was exciting. I was a bit nervous. By then my daughters were all at university and away from home, so I felt I could do something I wanted to do. I was going up to London for three days a week and earning just an honorarium and my train fares, really. I found that the office of this national organisation was just two rooms in St Martin's Lane in an Edwardian building with an antique mahogany and brass lift, which was a bit shaky. You went to the second floor and there were other organisations in the other rooms. There was Peace for Afghanistan and then there was the Women's League of Health and Beauty.

The Patients Association was representing the interests of patients. In those early days, it was a fairly new concept, in a way. It wasn't well known, probably, outside the usual circles in London. When I joined it, we just had the two rooms. We had a part-time secretary on an old typewriter who answered the letters. A very fierce woman – very sweet, when you got to know her – who answered the phone for complaints and helped to deal with complaints. And a retired army colonel. And that was the staff, and there was me. Then there was the council who met once a month and were quite prestigious, but I had to get sandwiches for their lunch and we had to try and fit everybody into this little office. They all were very helpful. I think they did wonder who they'd taken on, but I got to grips with it fairly quickly. We had a fortnightly newsletter and I wrote a piece, the 'Director's Diary', for that. So I was quickly into writing things. I was used to writing things. So that was something that I could do without too much trouble. But obviously, it was a different world.

The Thatcher NHS reforms came in 1989, very soon after I was there, and we had to give a response without being political. As a charity, we couldn't be political. You had to just be critical in clinical terms. You had to tread a fine line.

As my workload grew, I went up to four days a week. I was taking a lot of work home with me at weekends because there was a lot to do, and it was a time when the idea of patient representatives was very new. The Department of Health called on us, along with the Consumer Council and the Association of Community Health Councils, when they needed to say they'd consulted patients. That's as much as they did, as far I could see. We had to be diplomatic, but if the government was preparing a new complaints procedure, they would send it and I would have to comment on it. Occasionally, we'd go to a Select Committee on health. I commented a lot for the Audit Commission, which produced really good reports on different aspects of the NHS. It doesn't exist now. There was also the health ombudsman, who had never really talked to a patient's representative before. He was a really nice man. But it was really me making the running at that time, and with the Royal Colleges, who hadn't really had patient representatives. We got the idea of patient representatives going and we also set up a patients' forum. Toby Harris, Association of Community Health Councils, was instrumental in the ideas behind this with me. We wanted to unite all the special health interest groups like the Diabetic Association, the Asthma Association, different patient groups. So we set up the patients' forum, where they would meet regularly and I was responsible for helping to set up the programmes.

The Patient's Charter of 1991 was published by the Department of Health and set out patient rights in NHS services. But it was not widely welcomed by many patient groups, for fear that it undermined collective action around issues such as health inequalities.

When the Department of Health brought out the Patient's Charter 1991, we did our own Patient's Charter, which was a bit better than theirs. We included information on how to get the best out of your visit to the doctor. This was something that helped people who'd rang up with problems. In one way it was an open door, in that the Department of Health realised it had to have some patient representation. When I took part in some of their working groups, I made them pay the Patients Association £350 a day, which is what they were giving to the doctors on the group. They seemed to think because we were a charity, we didn't need to be paid. The patient was still seen as a lower form of life, in that sense. The doctors were the ones who were listened to more. I would be invited to speak at a BMA [British Medical Association] conference or workshop and, after I said my piece, the discussion would always include a doctor who said, 'We represent the patients. We know the patients and we can represent their views.' There were plenty of those who felt that the Patients Association wasn't necessary. On the other hand, I met some very forward-thinking doctors.

Linda left the Patients Association in 1995. She then became an honorary fellow at the University of Sussex and did a series of interviews with patient groups, patients and NHS staff to get a picture of what people's actual experience was. This became the backbone of a report produced with Fran McCabe for the sixtieth anniversary of the NHS in 2008. 'The individual patient's experience is gold. It's still my hope that there will be a proper patients' history of the NHS.'

LIONEL JOYCE

Lionel was born in 1947 in Wandsworth, London, to a Catholic family that was 'sustained by their Catholic faith, by their belief that there was a better world'. 'I became an atheist when I was 14 and have never deviated from that intellectual position since.' From his late teens Lionel was seriously involved with alcohol and was admitted to hospital in the early 1970s after a suicide attempt.

I was taken into Springfield Hospital. A 3,000-bed psychiatric hospital in Tooting. I was taken into the locked ward and put into pyjamas, banged full of Largactil and on 15-minute observations. I was there for three days before I got my clothes back. I started to get psychotherapy sessions with the Sister in charge of the ward. The case conference is one of the more mortifying experiences of the NHS in the 1970s. You would be taken into a room. There would be 20 people sitting in this room, including the consultant. The consultant would say, 'Right, now, Mr Joyce, we see you've made some suicide attempts and we've talked about your case and we've decided this is what's going to happen. In your case we're going to send you to the Cassel Hospital. In the meantime, Sheila will give you some psychotherapy. Goodbye.'

I was dressed in hospital pyjamas, which meant that the fly didn't button up. I had put my dressing gown round my shoulders. When I get into the room, the only thing I can think about is, 'Has my fly fallen open?' I hear not a fucking word anyone says. They look at me, so I say, 'Yes.' I'm dismissed and that's my treatment plan. I carry on getting this psychotherapy for a month and then I'm due to be transferred to this new hospital.

Lionel was transferred to a new hospital which focused on psychotherapy treatment rather than drugs. He continued to drink, as there were no restrictions on leaving the hospital. A friend suggested he applied to the NHS, so he created a 'fictitious CV', which left out his psychiatric admission, and joined City Hospital in Nottingham in 1973 as an administrative assistant. He was rapidly promoted, despite his alcoholism. In January 1975 he became sober and joined Alcoholics Anonymous.

At South Nottingham District Health Authority, we had a guy called Brian Blissett who was outstanding, probably the most principled and outstanding man I've ever worked for. He offered me the job effectively as his principal admin assistant. I had got sober in January that year. I didn't really believe I was going to stop drinking but, a day at a time, I didn't drink. I went and said, 'Look, I just want to come clean, I've been lying through my teeth about my job description, about where I'd been, what I've done. This is the real story.' He looked at me with the sort of look you'd get from someone who is so confident in their moral certitude. 'Do you really think I would think less of you because you've been in psychiatric care?' I was the one that felt ashamed that I should have doubted that he would be a person of such moral worth.

What's useful to know is that I'm slightly below average as a manager but I'm a genius. Just every now and then, I am brilliant and I see things in a way nobody else in the world sees them. I go, 'Well, why don't we do that?' Everybody goes, 'What the fuck?' I'd say, 'Well if we did that, we'd save £100,000.' That was how I got a reputation, but I was pretty shit at running the porters and the domestics. And we did do some extraordinary things.

Like David Rothberg, Lionel witnessed the advent of general management in the NHS.

They introduced a thing called 'general management'. Until this point, doctors were gods. They were the ones that made the decisions. They were responsible to themselves; they were accountable to God for what they did. General management meant that there was going to be a manager to whom the doctors were accountable, and who would ask the doctors questions. Why did you prescribe this? Why did you do that? What's this done for? It was introduced overnight. Margaret Thatcher, with Roy Griffiths from Sainsbury's supermarket chain. They were looking for general managers to run psychiatric services.

I was offered a couple of jobs, and one of them was in Newcastle. I describe it as one of those moments in my life – when I stood outside St Nicholas Hospital, which looks like Lenin's mausoleum but to the power of 10. It's a huge, monstrous building that's been there for forever and doesn't look like it has a useful purpose other than to store a dead body.

I stood outside thinking, 'I am now the boss of 700 nurses, of 50 consultant psychiatrists, including several professors. I've not even been to university. What the fuck do I know about any of this? The good news, Lionel, is you're just a drunk, your job is to not drink today, just to stay sober for one day and do the best you can, so just let's do that.' And that's what I did. I went in there and I didn't drink and I stayed sober and I did the best I could. I cared a lot. It mattered a lot.

There was quite extensive use of seclusion. There was quite a lot of violence. There was exploitation. The place was run by nurses. The nurses were third-generation nurses, so their grandparents lived on the site, their parents lived on the site, they were born on the site, they were brought up on the site. They heard all the gossip about patients and how patients were managed. A social club was where the decisions were made. The nurses' social club decided how the hospital would be run. I was going to change this, and I did.

I recruited some really brilliant managers. It was a bit of a swizz. I offered them a job, half-time lecturer at Newcastle University in health management, half-time manager of my mental health service at St Nick's. I was attracting these people with first-class honours degrees from Oxbridge. They would just go, 'What are you doing that for? Stop it, we're not going to put up with that, this is unacceptable. We're going to change the culture here. This culture is not on.' And they really got stuck in. The only people who'd been doing thinking previously were the consultants, and the nurses were stepping behind them doing nursing-type things. Suddenly, you had these managers who were really bright and challenging and clever enough to know more than the doctors. It was a dramatic change in which we were trying to give power to patients.

I don't know how long I kept my own history secret for. It was a period of time. Particularly, I was ashamed of alcoholism. I was less ashamed of mental illness, which is, after all, the business we were in. The next 15 years, from 1985 to 2000, was a journey in a number of different ways. How do we give power to patients? How do we see them as the people who should be determining what we're doing? How do we diminish the power of consultants as people but increase the power of their thinking? Because if their ideas are good enough, we should be implementing them.

One of the great tragedies of mental health, as I sit here now, is that the progress we've made in new thinking in psychiatry over the last 50 years is almost non-existent. What is mental illness really about? Even the simple question, is this biological or is it psychological? We don't know. We do know there are some biological elements. We can prove some probability of genetic component. Psychologically, we can demonstrate if you've been raped as a child, throughout your childhood, the possibility of you being, firstly, anorexic and dying, secondly, schizophrenic and completely destroyed as a person is higher. These are real. But the causation, what's going on? What could we do to intervene? How could you repair the damage that's been done? It seems to me we are still a million miles away, and we don't have an overarching theme for – how does our brain work? How does our psychology work? Who are we? What does it mean?

Lionel was made an OBE in 1998 and a CBE in 2012 for contributions to legal services and health and well-being. He is currently chair of the charity Dementia Matters.

At the end of the 1980s

The 1980s was a pivotal period which saw the earlier decades of political consensus around the NHS diverge. In response to the global financial downturn of the 1970s, public services everywhere were coming under pressure from right-wing ideologies that promoted business principles and techniques as the means of achieving efficiencies and improving outputs. A move to an insurance-based health system, along the lines of the American model, was considered by the Thatcher government, but there was too much opposition. Instead, a series of reforms introduced more business-like models of managing the NHS, including general management, as recounted by David Rothberg and Lionel Joyce.

The NHS reforms created a clear division between left-wing and right-wing politics. Campaign groups, including London Health Emergency, were established, raising public awareness of the threats to the NHS from ideologies including privatisation and neoliberalism, which put self-interest ahead of collective interest. Public activism around the NHS shifted significantly during the 1980s, introducing the idea of 'Save the NHS' and moving to campaigns that promoted the NHS as a single entity. In earlier decades, activism had focused on the closure of specific hospitals or issues and was local in focus.

Within the NHS, the racism experienced by overseas staff and the barriers they encountered in training and career development were brought to light in the first major study of nurses' experiences. Carol Baxter, featured in Chapter 4, published *The Black Nurse* in 1988, which was the first study to evidence the extent and nature of racism in nursing and its effects on future recruitment.[14] It came at a time when the NHS was struggling to retain and recruit staff. Nursing as a career had declined in popularity, and around 30,000 nurses were leaving the NHS every year on account of low wages and the pressures of the job. Immigration controls continued to present barriers, although the work-permit rules for overseas doctors could be sidestepped through seeking postgraduate training in the UK.

The HIV/AIDS epidemic played out across the NHS through the 1980s. This previously unknown disease provoked social stigma because it

was mainly understood to be transmitted through sex, and directly associated with gay communities. But survivors like Jonathan Blake became
activists, and their fight for access to drugs and appropriate care created a
new model for patient advocacy.

In January 1988 Margaret Thatcher was interviewed on the BBC
Panorama programme. To everyone's surprise she announced a review of
the NHS, prompted by increasing concern over its finances. The outcome,
published as the White Paper *Working for Patients*, set out a new model in which
all procedures would be costed and an internal market created through
making hospitals independent trusts. These trusts would charge for services,
which would be bought by local health authorities and GPs who opted to
be fundholders. The proposals were to produce the most ferocious backlash
from staff and the public in the 1990s. And in the longer history of the NHS,
the introduction of an internal market stands as a watershed moment, which
threatened the NHS's future as a universal health system for all.

Chapter 6:
1990s

'In the early nineties, the really big change came. It was when NHS Trusts were first formed. It was called "opting out."'

CAROLINE BEDALE

'One of the real positive advantages of being a female surgeon is that a lot of the patients felt they could open up and talk to the surgeon about how they felt.'

ANNE BRAIN

'I became the first person from a non-Christian faith to lead a chaplaincy in the NHS.'

YUNUS DUDHWALA

'[GPs] took on a lot of the work that had previously been done by general physicians in hospitals.'

ED BYLINA

'... you think doctors have all the answers, but they were very open that when it comes to the brain, they don't always have the answers.'

SARAH OLDNALL

'When the internal market came, it was a bombshell.'

RAJAN MADHOK

'Overall it was just a horrible experience, but it was made better by the caring people that were there.'

TERRY STOODLEY

'I say you either love the NHS or you hate it. It's either for you or it isn't. To me, it felt like it was in my blood.'

HUGHIE ERSKINE

'They would look at me a bit funny because they hadn't seen a woman porter before.'

BARBARA O'DONNELL

'I came to think that to really help people to improve their lives, we needed to be a lot more socially focused, we needed to be a lot more people-focused.'

KENYE KAREMO

'What really fired us up was when you took a parent to the mortuary, there was nothing there that was childlike.'

JOAN STEVENSON

'… the perpetrators knew that the woman had no escape routes through the NHS.'

MONICA MCWILLIAMS

'We were the first group of Filipino nurses that arrived in Hastings to work in the local hospital.'

DENNIS SINGSON

CAROLINE BEDALE

Caroline's mother had bipolar disorder and Caroline has memories of 'dreadful mental hospitals with big wards, patients wandering around, not enough staff'. She studied social administration and politics at university. In the early 1980s she got a job in the NHS on a short-term contract, doing research into people's housing experience and how that affected their mental health. She became active in NALGO (National and Local Government Officers' Association) in 1982.

I worked in the NHS for 35 years and I was an active trade unionist. Funnily enough, I was never that interested in the NHS when I was at university. I was much more interested in housing and planning and broader social policy. Because at that time, I thought, 'Well, the NHS isn't very political.' How wrong I was. [*laughs*] But this was in the early seventies. And really, all the battles hadn't started at that time over the NHS. It wasn't so political in those days because it seemed to be established. I certainly had no idea in the early seventies of what we would face in the next 20, 30 years.

In 1987 we had action in Manchester. A number of nursing auxiliaries walked out of work from Crumpsall Hospital [now North Manchester General Hospital]. They were night workers, and they weren't getting the right allowances. That broadened out into a much bigger campaign around pay – not just for nursing staff, but for all NHS staff, and in 1987/88 there was quite a lot of action in Manchester. We were quite a lead in the country. We campaigned around people's working conditions and hours of work and negotiated quite a lot of family-friendly policies. The union work fitted quite well with my day job, which was about trying to promote people's health at work.

NALGO joined with National Union of Public Employees (NUPE) and Confederation of Health Service Employees (COHSE) in 1993 to become UNISON.

NALGO had been mostly white-collar staff, although we did have some nursing and technical staff. When we merged the three unions, it meant that, as a steward, I was then representing a much wider range of people. I became branch secretary of North Manchester. We had had various campaigns from the late eighties onwards about policy changes nationally. Before this interview I was trying to think, 'Well, which government was it?' And there wasn't a lot of difference whether it was a Conservative or a Labour government. People used to accuse the trades unions of being left wing and tied in with Labour. But we were just as ready to campaign against things that a Labour government was doing as we were about a Conservative government if we didn't think it was right for the NHS. Some of the policy changes happened to be under the Conservatives. In fact, you could say that's where some of the rot set in, in the early eighties, when they started outsourcing.

The NHS and Community Care Act 1990 was the outcome of the Thatcher government's 1988 NHS review. The policies were based on the idea that the money in the healthcare system should follow the patients. They created an internal market in the NHS, which built on previous policies to establish business and market principles in the running and delivery of health services. The assumption was that competition would drive improvement, quality and efficiency. District Health Authorities and GPs who became fundholders would have budgets to buy services from providers and be known as 'purchasers'. Acute hospitals, ambulance, mental health and community services could apply to become self-managed NHS Trusts and would be known as 'providers'.

In the early nineties the really big change came. It was when NHS Trusts were first formed. It was called 'opting out' and, in a sense, for us campaigning, that made it clearer because it was about opting out of the NHS structure nationally. It was allowing them to set up trusts. In Manchester, we had two. We had the MRI [Manchester Royal Infirmary] and we had the Christie that both wanted to be part of this first wave of opting out. We had a big campaign locally, a lot of demonstrations outside the two hospitals. I remember our branch secretary in an open-top car holding banners high, as we had this slow cavalcade from the MRI to Christie's about 1989, 1990. We didn't win that one. Trusts were formed. [*laughs*] They were the precursor of what happened in the late nineties, 2000s, which was the split between purchasers, or commissioners, and providers. You can date it back to when those trusts were formed, because it's setting up an organisation which is outside some of the control of the NHS. If you allow organisations to become semi-autonomous or completely autonomous, it starts questioning the whole structure of the NHS. If they're autonomous as providers, who's going to buy their services? You have to have an organisation to purchase and commission.

In 1990 when trusts were set up, there were still health authorities, but it really set the basis for what we saw later on. The purchaser/provider split, the internal market, and then the external market, whereby health becomes a commodity that you buy. And it doesn't matter who you buy it from. You might buy it from an NHS trust, you might buy it from Bupa, you might buy it from Spire hospital or BMI Healthcare hospital or some private company – Virgin Care. It doesn't matter who you buy it from. You're just buying health services. That was set in the 1990s. So that campaign we had in '89/'90, we lost – and we lost nationally, it wasn't just a local campaign. But that really allowed what then happened throughout the nineties and 2000s. And a lot of people don't know that. They see the Lansley Act [Health and Social Care Act] in 2012 as being this big thing of purchasers and providers in the internal market. No. That was set more than 20 years earlier with the setting up of trusts. The Labour government after '97 extended the role of trusts and called them 'foundation trusts'. A lot of people don't realise that that was based on the earlier trusts. Foundation trusts were even more autonomous and could borrow money on the open market. So those were the sort of campaigns that were going on throughout the nineties and 2000s. That were nationally based but with a local focus if we had something happening locally.

The key message of campaigning was that this is about privatising the NHS. This is about opening up the NHS to competition. This is about turning the NHS into just a business that can be run by anyone. In 1989 the government White Paper was called *Working for Patients*. These sort of slogans come out nationally. In a sense, they are completely lies. *Working for Patients* wasn't working for patients at all. It was starting to open up the NHS to the private sector, being able to do more actual provision of health services, which had been really minimal up till then. Back in the early seventies, when I was at university, the NHS didn't seem that political. Yes, there was Bupa and there were a few other private hospitals, but you only used them if you had private health insurance. There was no real incursion of the private sector into the NHS. What we could see in 1990 was that this was what the long-term plan was. To really sell off the NHS by setting up these new organisations. By laying it open to becoming a market. That was what our fear was and what we were fighting against. It was really hard to explain to the public because the government policy looked as if this was about making things better and more efficient. It was coupled with all sorts of management revolutions within the NHS. Reports about making it more effective and efficient and bringing good business methods into the NHS. That's what we were arguing against. We feared that it was going to turn the NHS into just another way of making money for private health companies – which is what it's done.

Staff generally were supportive, but we never got that many people. Whereas on pay, we could get people to demonstrate – or when there were big, obvious cuts to the NHS, we could organise big demonstrations locally or nationally. But on *Working for Patients*, on the beginning of trusts, and then foundation trusts, it was much more difficult to get staff or the public to really see what was happening. We weren't good enough in our communication methods. We produced newsletters, we produced leaflets, both locally and nationally. I think a lot of people, when we explained it, could see what was happening. But I think that was the beginning of this feeling, 'Well, what can we do about it? It's the government and they've been voted in. This is their policy. So long as the NHS is still free at the point of use.'

It was difficult to get people to see that who provides those services, or how they're provided, is really important. We did get support from staff. We did get support from the public. But not enough to be able to combat that. What's interesting is in 2012, when the Lansley reforms were going through [*laughs*], there was about a six- or nine-month pause in Parliament over the legislation because there was a big groundswell of publicity. There was a lot more public understanding of just what these would mean. But they went through in the end because they were a continuation of what had already happened. They weren't that new. They weren't that different. But yes, we did get a lot more public involvement in the 2010s than we had done in the 1990s.

We were a microcosm of the NHS as a joint union committee. We had to find ways of dealing with any differences we might have and try and work together to represent our members to the best we could in relation to management. Underpinning all of that was our commitment to the NHS. I think we were always more keen to find a way to work together than perhaps we might have been if we'd been producing widgets or washing machines that we wouldn't have had that emotional attachment to. I've always been an eternal optimist. I live in hope that we won't lose the NHS and we will be able to make improvements.

Caroline is now retired, but keeps lots of material in her attic. 'I do intend to carry on trying to archive and catalogue this material so people in the future can have a glimmer of what it was like to be an activist.'

ANNE BRAIN

Anne was appointed consultant surgeon in Manchester in 1991. Before taking up the post, she spent three months on a 'tour of various plastic surgery units to get a feel of what other people were doing around the world in breast reconstruction'. The unit in Melbourne, Australia, was 'really pioneering' and a 'wonderful eye-opener'.

Then it was back to the real job. Half my work was at the Christie, which is the cancer hospital, with a lot of head and neck work. There wasn't much joined-up thinking to start with. Surgery was quite gung-ho. They felt, 'Well, we can do everything.' Maybe being a female was helpful in that way. I think, naturally, women are better at trying to broker relations across specialities and listen to what other people have to say. The multidisciplinary culture started in the 1990s, which helped treatment a lot. Patients were given more in the way of choices, which, in one way, was good. But some patients, especially from Lancashire, they worship the doctor, which was quite embarrassing, but that was just how they'd been brought up. 'Yes, doctor, if that's what you think should be done, then that's what we'll have.' So multidisciplinary working provided a much better context where you could go and have a discussion.

Some patients still found decision-making quite stressful. They wanted someone else to make the decision for them. I was trying to find that skill of getting a sense of how much they wanted you to advise on their treatment, and how much they wanted to be part of that journey. Now, of course, people really want to be part of that journey and not feel that someone's imposing a treatment on them. But in the nineties, there was still this old school thinking. I was 40 years old, but patients were 70. A completely different era of person that were having all these awful problems. They just expected the doctor to say, 'That's what we're doing' and hardly bother to tell them what the complications were. I didn't want them to think I was on a pedestal at all. We're all human beings at the end of the day. Now, it's gone the other way around in that the patients almost despise the doctors. It's a culture of the opposite where they assume that doctors are going to do something wrong.

Surgery started to become much more subspecialised and, as the maxil-lofacial surgeons started to do their own reconstructions for head and neck cancer, we were not needed so much. I went more into breast reconstruction, which was still very much the domain of plastic surgery at that time. One of the real positive advantages of being a female surgeon is that a lot of the patients felt they could open up and talk to the surgeon about how they felt. Up till the early nineties, I think they'd always felt they should be this grateful person – because they didn't have cancer anymore. At that time radical mastectomy included taking part of the pectoral muscle as well as the breast, which was real blunderbuss surgery, you could argue, in terms of treating the cancer. Then patients had radiotherapy. It was a very deforming process. With a female surgeon, patients could start to talk about how that was impacting on their quality of life. How they felt. Their sexual feelings towards partners and husbands. And so much about feeling whole, which they often felt they couldn't say to a man – or not to a surgeon. I'm sure their husbands would certainly understand. I think it probably caused quite a lot of marital breakdowns and break-ups because it was just so traumatic, and women didn't feel responsive to their husbands, who perhaps couldn't understand why not.

We were in the early stages of understanding the psychological impact of some of these treatments. We had huge challenges in terms of breast reconstruction because of the type of treatment that they'd had at that point. The radiotherapy on top of the very radical surgery. You had no skin to play with, and you can't just push implants in, because the skin doesn't work – it all breaks down. That was when microsurgery tissue transfer came into its own. Suddenly, you could start to offer a reconstruction with their own tissue, so-called 'autologous reconstruction'. And it was usually abdominal-wall fat based on the rectus muscle, and the little blood vessels that come through that, which supplied that whole area with blood flow. Then you had to find something to join up the blood vessels to the chest wall.

You could preserve more of their normal skin, so the results were much better. And that was the way of reconstruction after the early days where we were only reconstructing patients that had already had mastectomies. We were starting to do it at the same time, but in the multidisciplinary setting, with the oncologists and the breast surgeons on board, because one key thing was never, ever, to compromise the oncology treatment purely for the reconstruction. Now, oncology treatments have become much more sophisticated, much more targeted. I think the days of mastectomy being the default treatment are over, and most patients are offered something much more precise.

To start with, we did delayed reconstructions. We felt if they'd been cancer free for two years, then it was unlikely it was going to come back. If we had done a reconstruction and they had a recurrence, that would have set the whole thing back probably 10 years. We were extremely ginger about how we approached reconstruction in the early days. Women's groups started to get together and the breast care nurse role took off. A lot of women were feeling really down, so they banded together. As a pressure group, they helped to push forward breast reconstruction from a patient perspective. They said, 'A breast is a part of the body, it's not just some disposable bit that can be chopped off and forgotten about.' I used to go around and do lots of talks to say what can and can't be done, and that helped promote breast reconstruction. It was nice to lead that as a consultant.

In 1995 researchers identified the breast cancer susceptibility gene – BRCA2 – which led to genetic testing in breast, ovarian and prostate cancer.

As genetics came into the mix they started to identify the genes that made certain women more predisposed to getting breast cancer. I think we were one of the first in the UK to develop a multidisciplinary group to look at the genetics and to advise patients about having potentially risk-reducing mastectomy, i.e. having mastectomies as a preventative measure. But we did it within a very controlled setting. The research needed to go on for 10 years to assess whether it actually made a difference at the end of the day. So we had to be really careful. Everything was really well-documented all the way through. So after about 10 years, we could start to advise that 'Yes, this is effective, and the lifetime risk is reduced if you undergo this very devastating type of surgery.' Again, with microsurgery and autologous transfers of tissue from other parts of the body, it could be done immediately. But it's a

10-hour operation. So it wasn't peanuts for the patient, foremost, and for the surgeons and the anaesthetist and the teams doing it.

Anne retired in 2009 and moved back down to Devon, where she'd grown up. She was determined not to be an older surgeon that colleagues looked at and thought, 'Maybe you should have stopped a year ago.' I do miss the camaraderie and the colleagues, and the interview was a useful way of summing up what I've thought I did in the NHS.'

YUNUS DUDHWALA

Yunus was born in Blackburn in 1971, a time when a lot of South Asian families from India and Pakistan came to Lancashire and Yorkshire to work in the cotton mills.

Life growing up in Blackburn wasn't easy, initially. There was a large South Asian community where I used to live. Then we moved to an area where there was mainly English. I went to a predominantly white school. That helped me in learning how to interact with people from different communities and be much more comfortable in being part of the British society. We always used to go to a mosque in the evenings to learn Arabic and to learn the essentials of our religion.

My parents bought a corner shop in a predominantly white area, and it wasn't too far from the local football ground: Blackburn Rovers. Every week, we had to shut up shop when football fans used to go past the shop, because they used to be not too friendly. I think it was a little bit intimidating, scary. We used to board up the windows a couple of hours before and then open it again after the game.

Yunus was in the second year of secondary school when the family moved down to London. While at school in Blackburn, he'd started memorising the Quran and had completed six out of the 30 chapters.

London didn't have a system of evening classes where I could continue, so I started losing some of those chapters in terms of memory. I said to my father, 'Look, I've done six chapters, and if I don't continue, then I'm going to forget. Is it possible for me to go to seminary?' My dad agreed, and the most famous seminary in the UK at the time was in a village called Holcombe, near Bury in Manchester. I moved there in July 1985.

This was a boarding school seminary with students between the ages of 13 and 23. Initially, although I wanted to be there, I was really upset. You're away from your family, your parents are not there. Your brothers and sisters are not there. But I think that was the formation of becoming who I am today. One of the things that I learned there which stayed with me is service to people. You are not an individual. You are part of a community. That definitely stuck with me. Because you're staying in a seminary, you don't understand how the world works. 'What do you do as a religious scholar who's coming out into the world? What are the opportunities out there?' I wasn't too sure. The normal route for many was to become an imam in a mosque. I got married. But I still wasn't sure what I'm going to do.

In 1998 the local hospital, Newham Hospital, was looking for a voluntary imam. That's when I thought, 'Okay, this could be a good place to be.' It was exciting. I used to go one day or two days a week. 'Yes, this is really, really good. This is something that I want to do.' Within a few months they gave me a contract to be the official Muslim chaplain for half a day a week. Then that increased to one day a week, and then two days a week. I knew that the only vocation for me is chaplaincy.

I became the first person from a non-Christian faith to lead a chaplaincy in the NHS. I was the only person there, initially. The hospital didn't have enough money for Christian chaplains. I used to contact the local priest to come and support me in visiting the Christian patients. It was as if I had to prove to myself that, yes, it doesn't matter what faith you are, you can do this post. In November, I was told that I needed to organise the carol service. As a Muslim, organising a carol service for the hospital wasn't the easiest task, but I did get some help from my colleagues. The carol service was led by the Christian priest from the community. I think that's when the hospital board members who are Christian turned and accepted that Yunus can do this job.

It was a steep learning curve. There was resistance, which I found out later on, within the hospital. One of the directors, who was a Roman Catholic, did not want the chaplaincy to be opened up to all faiths because historically it's been Christian. I never felt the resistance because there wasn't any open discrimination. In fact, the person who was resisting became, after a few years, my biggest supporter there. I believe the chaplaincy should always have those relationships with leadership so that the hospital trust knows that the spiritual care is important.

There's been ups and downs, but I've always felt welcome. I've always felt valued. I've always felt it was a privilege and an honour to be in that kind of position. There's been lots of staff, colleagues who I've valued their companionship and their support and advice. Then patients and families. When somebody's dying or somebody's clearly ill, and they need somebody and there's nobody else there, and you've been given the opportunity to be there for somebody, you can't put a value to that. The advice that you're able to give at that particular time and how it's received, again, there's no monetary value to that. I can only say it's a privilege to be at the bedside of somebody who's let you in at their most vulnerable time. Then you are able to say some words of comfort, which leaves them with some hope or with some peace in the heart.

Yunus shares his experiences of supporting patients and staff during Covid-19 in Chapter 9.

ED BYLINA

Ed's parents were Polish refugees from the Second World War who met in the West Riding of Yorkshire and worked in the textile factories. Ed did a science degree before studying medicine at Dundee Medical School, which was one of the few to offer graduate-level entry in the 1970s. He began training as a GP on a training scheme in Hull and qualified in 1986.

The world was rather different then. The expectations of one's spouse was quite different and very misogynistic, as the wife of a GP would have the responsibility of manning the telephone when I was on call. My wife, being an accountant working full-time, couldn't answer the phone on the afternoons that the surgery was closed. I was told to buy an answering machine. During the evenings and nights, my wife did take the call if I was already out on a call and we developed a system where she would bleep me – no mobile phones at the time. If the bleep went off, I'd have to ring home and get the details of my next visit. One particular weekend covering practices around Hull, I ended up clocking over 150 miles.

By chance, a GP locum opportunity arose in Ed's home town of Elland, West Yorkshire.

A single-handed GP in my old home town had gone off sick with a heart attack and they needed a locum. I thought, 'Well, why not?' Being an older child, my mum wanted me to be around to help her, which was difficult when I was a student, and when we were living in Hull. She couldn't speak much English. I had to do a lot of the admin and financial work for her. I kept saying, 'Look, Mum, I'm not going to end up working at the bottom of the street.' But that's what happened, so she had the last laugh.

Ed was appalled by the standards of care in the practice he joined.

This was in the 1980s. The GP was still working in the 1960s, maybe even beyond. He wrote very little in the notes. The hospital letters and blood results were stuffed in a drawer. They weren't even filed. It was a complete mess, really. The thing that I stopped was the receptionist would automatically write the patient's name and address on the prescription. Between each patient coming in, she would come in with a prescription already with a patient's name and address on. I thought, 'I don't want to do this.' This automatically assumes that I'm going to give the patient a prescription, which is not what I was trained to do. So I told them to stop doing that straightaway.

Over time Ed joined forces with other doctors in Elland who had similar ambitions about becoming a training practice.

Within four years we built a new surgery and became a training practice. I was the GP trainer, which was quite rewarding. We immediately instituted changes. We introduced an appointment system, we hired more staff, we started getting the medical records in order, because the records had to be at quite a high standard in order to become a training practice. There was a good vibe at the time in general practice in Halifax and Calderdale.

The good changes were that there were brighter people coming into general practice. Some hospital doctors, even to this day, have this thing that GPs are second-rate and often come in for criticism. But, of course, we're not specialists. We're generalists. That's one of the important things in general practice is you get to know the patients. You get to know a lot about various medical conditions, but not to the degree a consultant specialist was, obviously. Over my career we took on a lot of the work that had previously been done by general physicians in hospitals. We increasingly managed more patients with depression, diabetes, heart disease, chest diseases, gastrointestinal diseases. We took on a lot of work that had previously been done by generalists in hospitals, which allowed the specialists to become even more specialised. General practice were early adopters of computer technology in terms of prescriptions, medical records, laboratory results, etc. Things improved. But unfortunately, as time went on, the screws were being turned.

The NHS and Community Care Act 1990 introduced the notion of an internal market in the NHS, which separated the roles of purchasers and providers of services. GPs had

the option to become fundholders and gain a budget that they could use to buy services from
providers like hospital trusts. But only large GP practices could qualify for the scheme.

When the Tories introduced the GP fundholding practice scheme in 1991, that was very divisive because you had to be a practice over a certain size. I think over 12,000 or 11,000 patients. You'd end up with more money as a practice, and great clout. And then competition came in – so the idea was the money would follow the patient, so the GPs could decide where the money went. The fundholding practices took priority over the non-fundholding practices. Our practice only had about 7,000 patients, so we couldn't even become a fundholding practice, which was frustrating.

Since 1948 GPs had been contracted to provide 24/7 services to patients. By the 1990s
the face of general practice was changing. There were an increasing number of women
working in general practice, balancing work and family commitments, and few GPs had
stay-at-home partners willing to provide a phone-answering service. A new GP contract
was imposed on the profession by Kenneth Clarke, Minister of Health. Payment by
results gave GPs incentives to carry out health promotion, immunisations and screening.
This allowed a £6,000 payment for out-of-hours services. GPs were motivated to
campaign for changes, and this led to the development of cooperative organisations that
provided out-of-hours cover across localities.

We were responsible for our patients 24 hours a day, seven days a week. That became much more onerous as patients became increasingly demanding of services out of hours. The older patients, if they had a bad cold or a sore throat, they'd wait until they either got better, or they go and see the GP. The younger patients with younger families wouldn't wait. They would ring all times of day and night, saying, 'Little Johnny's got a rash, or a sore throat. He needs to be seen.' It was very difficult to persuade them to wait and come to the practice, because you didn't want to get a complaint made against you. So doing on call was increasingly burdensome. In 2004 when we were told that we could have a pay cut of £6,000 to get rid of the on-call burden, it's no surprise that the vast majority of GPs decided they didn't want to do on call any longer. The government told us this 24-hour commitment is only worth six grand. That made us feel cheap. So we thought, 'Stuff it, you can be responsible for on call.' That's when things started to go down the pan from the patient's point of view.

I have had a long career in the NHS, an organisation which I love, and which has saved the life of my wife and my eldest son. I want people in the future to listen to a typical GP's experience with a twist, in terms of the fact that I was the first person in our family to attend university. In some ways, I'm proud of what I've achieved, but in other ways, I'm frustrated that I couldn't have achieved more. One of the best things about being a GP is caring for people of all ages. When I was on duty a few years ago, I visited my eldest patient, who was 103, just before lunch, and the first patient I saw after lunch was a three-week-old baby. To go from one extreme of age to another was fantastic.

Ed retired in 2015.

SARAH OLDNALL

Sarah grew up in Bootle, Liverpool in the 1960s. 'It was quite a happy time. We're a working-class family, so we didn't have much, but as a child, everybody was the same.', she recalled. She moved to London and after university went into academia until she had her son. She then became ill at the end of the 1980s.

It changed life quite a bit. I have multiple sclerosis. It was a long process to get diagnosed. I started limping a bit and was sent off to see orthopaedic specialists. I even went as far as having some knee surgery, because I used to ski a lot when I was younger. They thought there was a hangover from an accident I'd had. The surgeon said, 'We couldn't find anything wrong.' I started to go downhill. They sent me back to see a professor at the hospital, who was an orthopaedic surgeon, because they were trying to figure out what's wrong with me. I remember he made me walk up and down this corridor where they have their consultancy rooms, and watched me doing it. He got me to do it again. And he sat me down, 'I'm going to refer you to a neurological hospital.' At that stage he thought I had a brain tumour. He could tell that just from the way I was walking that something wasn't right. I was 31.

You think, 'That's the end of me.' Also back then, the internet hadn't proliferated. I was backwards and forwards to the library trying to find medical books to look at, trying to self-diagnose myself. I went over to the Walton Centre in Liverpool, which is possibly the best neurological hospital in the country, I would say. They ran all sorts of tests. This went on for about two, three years. They just really weren't sure what was going on with me. Even though I have MS, I don't have the classic scar tissue on my brain like other people have. So it took them quite a long time to get to a diagnosis. Even now, I have a differential diagnosis, something called PLS [primary lateral sclerosis], which is a motor neurone disease. I found it interesting because you think doctors have all the answers, but they were very open that when it comes to the brain, they don't always have the answers. They said, 'We don't always know what's going on – all we can do is test and eliminate.'

So how did you cope?

Not very well, to be honest. First of all in my head was, 'I'm going to die. I'm going to leave these two children behind.' Even when we got to a diagnosis of MS, MS was something you died of. That was what was fixed in my head because I couldn't get hold of the knowledge to find out more about it. In those early days, it was quite difficult because I had no idea what path I was gonna go down. Would I be able to work next week or not? It was quite challenging. At the time my husband worked away. I was with the children by myself all week long. I look back now and I think, 'Gosh, that's hard work.' My son was only little. I didn't have the strength to pick him up. Even walking them backwards and forwards to school was tiring me out. Initially, I had a stick, then I moved to a crutch and then I moved to a walker. Taking two small children to school when you can't physically hold their hand – you're relying on them to hold on to the walker – was quite interesting. Two years into that I wasn't allowed to drive because of problems with my vision and my reflexes. So it was quite difficult, actually.

At the hospital, you are designated an MS nurse who you phone if you have got any problems. They can look at medication, or how they can help that medical issue. But practically and emotionally, there wasn't really any support at all. Unfortunately, I don't have a family that's very supportive either. So I was on my own. There were MS groups and I did go along to one support group, but people just sat around moaning about the fact they had MS. I was quite young in comparison to most. I didn't feel I had anything in common with them. So I used to do a lot of reading. My consultant said, 'When you're diagnosed with something that's chronic, long-term, quite often you go through all these emotions of being angry, being sad, until you level off.' I think, eventually, I levelled off. I thought, 'Well, I've got to deal with this and just do the best that I can.'

I think I self-manage really well. I found a charity that I wish I would have known existed 20-odd years back: the Brain Charity in Liverpool. They offer the emotional and practical support that I was missing. It's an umbrella charity, so you get people who have all sorts of different neurological conditions together. It's quite nice to sit down and talk and say, 'Gosh, I feel absolutely worn out today, or I just feel like I can't function today.' They know exactly what you mean. So that's been good for me, I think.

When I first started going to the Walton Centre, it was very clinical. It was about the diagnosis. It was about the condition. Over the years, and particularly the last five years, it's become more holistic in its approach. It thinks about the whole person now. In the old days I'd go in and they'd test your reflexes, check your Babinski reflex sign, do your bloods or whatever. Now you go to the doctor's room, they get up, they shake your hand, they say, 'Hello, Sarah, how are you doing?' They chat to you about your life in general. It's not a doctor behind a desk anymore.

Sarah became a volunteer for the Brain Charity, working to support other people suffering from neurological conditions, and she contributed regular interviews through the Covid-19 pandemic to the project.

RAJAN MADHOK

Rajan's parents were refugees from Lahore in Pakistan, and moved to Delhi, India, during the Partition. He trained in medicine in the early 1970s in Delhi before coming to the UK.

I'm very passionate about the NHS. I often remind people, as somebody from India, I chose to work in the NHS. I came from India and didn't go anywhere else once I'd seen the NHS because I was really impressed with it.

It was my great-grandfather who influenced me in terms of choice of my profession. He always wanted me to become a doctor – and not just a doctor. He wanted me to become a surgeon. I think it was because civil surgeons in India were the senior people in the locality. He wanted me to be the equivalent of that. The first hurdle was getting into medical school. The second thing was that I had to go to Britain to get my surgical qualifications – the FRCS [Fellowship of the Royal College of Surgeons]. So it was not an option, in one sense. I left India immediately after my preliminary training to do my PLAB [Professional and Linguistics Assessment Board] test and come into the system here.

What ideas did you have about the NHS in the UK before you came?

Frankly, very little apart from the very basic stuff I've read. All the focus was on passing the General Medical Council exam, because we thought the system would then take care of us.

It was never the intention that I'll actually stay back here. Now, almost 39 years later ... [*laughs*] At that stage I was going to do my FRCS and go back to India. I was going to use the NHS as a training ground for myself. But once I got into it, it really hit me what a powerful system it was. Remember, I'd come from India, and in the seventies, it was largely public hospitals with poor infrastructure. In other words, cleanliness and all those issues were a big problem. People used to worry about going to hospitals, and the private sector hadn't taken off in India at that stage. So I saw how good the NHS was compared to what was in India, and also the fact that you didn't have to pay for it directly – we paid for it through taxation. And what a difference it made to people's lives in terms of being a safety net and the peace of mind. In the early days as I was talking to people, it struck me, we never talked about Health Service. We took it for granted. We knew it was there. Unlike in India, where as soon as something happened, you'd say, 'Oh, where will you go? How much will they charge?' All that stuff. That is what really made me more and more convinced about making the NHS my home.

The vast majority of my contemporaries did not stay back here. And that's another story to do with how foreign graduates are treated in the NHS, because most of them then went off to America, or to the Middle East and then back to India. But I was very, very clear. I did not want to work in a for-profit system. It's a personal choice. I'm not making comments about people who feel otherwise. It certainly is not a criticism. I was never, ever comfortable about taking money directly. I wanted to be paid. Yeah, that's for sure. I wanted to have a decent life as well. But I was never comfortable with receiving money from patients. I did not want money as part of my relationship with the patients. I also did my American exams like my contemporaries, but then when I researched more about the American system, I realised, 'No, I didn't want to go to America, I wanted to stay back in the NHS.' That was the big change. So although I'd originally started life wanting to become a doctor, wanting to come to the UK to get my FRCS with a view to going back, I realised that even if I went back to India, it will conflict with my values. And the only safe place where I was comfortable as a person was the NHS. So I ended up staying here.

My claim to fame is that I ended up working in the four corners of the UK. My first job was in the Shetland Islands; then I worked in Southend, near London. I also spent time in the Isle of Wight and then I went to work in Ireland and then came back to the UK, to Edinburgh and the north-east. But Shetland is where it all started. I was in a new society. I didn't know how to relate to a different culture. And I made some faux pas. [*laughs*] You know Indians nod their heads in a different way. Sideways doesn't mean no, it means actually I'm agreeing with you, or it could be I'm disagreeing with you, and you're left completely flummoxed. All of those things are part of learning to get used to a new society and to get integrated. So although I'm a Hindu and have always been a Hindu, I'm also quite British in my outlook. I always found it very disturbing to have ghettos – to stick with your own. I've always found the value is to learn about a new culture and take the best out of that culture.

So Shetland provided me with a safe place to start experimenting and start learning, and that stood me in good stead over the years. Being an Asian person, I was a curiosity. I had a friend who was a Sikh with a turban. He came over to Shetland and they all thought I was royalty because my friend was seen as the maharaja.

Most people found it very bleak. I loved it. In the Shetlands gale force 6/7 is like a breeze. The winters could be taxing for people, but I was really curious about it and would go out in all weathers. By the time it was April/May, it would be light till 11/12 o'clock at night. I found it fascinating, the nature, the people – and the job was good as well. I don't think they ever thought of me as different. I was a doctor, so I fitted in. I like to think it worked really well from both sides. I went for a month as a locum and got extended for a year. Then I said I was having too much of a good time and I had to get out and concentrate on doing my FRCS. You had to do a number of jobs and your exams were in two parts, your primary and secondary FRCS.

Rajan passed his exams and trained in orthopaedic surgery.

In 1988 I hit the the glass ceiling. I could just not break through it. I wasn't alone. Even the local graduates got stuck as senior registrars. There were no consultant jobs. It wasn't the kind of manpower you see nowadays. Orthopaedics was one of the premium specialities. So I did various jobs, I did the right things with consultants, tried to do additional qualifications. At that stage I decided to change careers completely. The only given was that I did not want to leave the NHS. I did not want to go to the Middle East. I did not want to go to America. So I was, in one sense, stuck in the NHS and I was stuck professionally. I didn't want to get defeated. I said, 'I'm not going to do substandard jobs, travel around, or keep doing whatever is necessary.

I'm better than that.' In my life, there was only one thing I wanted to do, which was to be a surgeon. So if I could not be an orthopaedic surgeon, I decided to leave clinical practice completely and started looking for training in public health. I was fortunate enough to get a training place and went to Newcastle to go to university again. Basically, I started my life all over again.

After gaining his public health qualifications, Rajan was appointed a consultant in public health in 1991.

I still remember *Working for Patients*, the first White Paper, in 1989. When the internal market came, it was a bombshell. We were all struggling – what is a 'health needs assessment'? We got into discussion about need versus want versus demand versus supply. How do we know how many hips we need? No idea! Even today, we can't cost anything. So it completely threw us off. But it was also very good for public health. Because, for the first time, you could demonstrate the value of the discipline. Why it is important to study the epidemiology, which is basically the study of distribution and determinants of health. So you had to rise to the challenge. But it was also the weakness. The policymakers, once they made a policy, they want the results yesterday. There was an initiative called Project 26, which was led by people in Bristol. Let's start quantifying how many tonsillectomies we need because we have to purchase these. We had some historical data because they were health population-based systems, unlike today's systems. But we could not say how many of each we want. And that opened up other conversations. 'Okay, let's do block contracts.' We slowly started chipping away. A block contract is basically, we'll give you the money that we used to give you, but we'll take away 5 per cent. We also had to work hard to find out what the communities want.

We became these clipboard people. I remember standing on the street corner, 'What do you want?' When they said, 'I want you to clean that dog litter up from over there?' I was thinking, 'what do I do?' We discovered there's such a big gap between what the communities were saying and what we as bureaucrats are imagining. Their stuff was real life: damp housing, crime on my street, vandalism, litter, drugs. I'm talking about Teesside, Tyneside,

Middlesborough and the deprivation. For me as an individual, it was an inter-esting answer, but as a manager, it was terrible. Because we could not deliver and that is when things started going wrong. Margaret Thatcher wanted it done yesterday. Ken Clarke was the secretary of state then, chomping his cigars and with his orange suede shoes. They were impatient, you see. The worst of them was Tony Blair, who was more impatient. He made it worse because he started throwing money at it without solving the problem, and money made it worse to some extent. But health services were never a market in the sense of a retail market. I'm not at all anti the private sector. I think there's a role for it, but there's a time and a place for things. And to make the internal market the default way of working was wrong. There's clearly room for that sort of approach, to bring discipline, etc. But not as the default option. Now, every service has to be tendered and we are struggling. Organisations are failing because they can't do it. Health is much bigger than that.

In 1994 Rajan became director of public health in Gateshead and South Tyneside.

I joined in the last days of the Major government, and Tony Blair got in in 1997. It was a time of real austerity. As a group of directors, we were really innovative. 'What can we do differently?' We were one of the first places to do a smoke-free initiative, including the Metro centre, which is the biggest mall in Gateshead way back in '96/'97. We tackled neonatal mortality and maternal mortality. The reason why I think it was most satisfying was that I was able to, for the first time – for me – to demonstrate the value of public health for health services. Every time a decision was made, we'd say, 'Okay, what will public health do?' We were able to integrate it to everything. It was also the first place where I managed to convince people that the NHS was not there to count money. You only got this much money. Yeah. But don't spend money on counting money. Spend money on doing the job.

I'll tell you another story which was transformative, and which is why Gateshead and South Tyneside are so prominent in my thinking. I was the last director to be recruited and we had an awayday with the board. At the end of our session, one of our non-executive directors said, 'Okay, Rajan, you're the new kid on the block. What are the two takeaway messages?

What should I take away from this conversation?' I said, 'Two things. Think health. Don't think ill health. Think about health in the broadest sense – primary care, mental healthcare. Don't make these artificial distinctions. Think holistic health. Keep people well. Secondly, don't get involved in running hospitals. It's their job. It's our job to hold them accountable. So be true to your role. Do your job – which is asking for performance reviews, taking corrective action and all that stuff.' The chief executive said, 'No, no. Forget that. Number one, think money. And number two, think regional office. Because we're not in control.' I'm glad I had that experience early on.

What happened then was I started by zooming in on these two things in my work. The financial redline and the regional office redline. So, feed the beast. The beast wants you to do this? Do it. And that became our slogan in the department: 'Feed the beast.' So, every time, what are the absolute must-dos?. Because unless you do your must-dos, you don't have the scope to do what you want to do. I was able to convince people like my finance director that you're safe with me. That is why it became such an important part of my professional life.

Because first, it was the place where I learned how to be good at my job. My job was not about complaining or moaning. I could not afford to be a critic. I can't stand outside and throw stones. It is up to me to get better at it. And second, I actually did manage to break into some of the very wicked public health issues and solve them for the time being. So, professionally, it was very satisfying. To have started some new things. Because that's all you can do. I benefited and I hope I left something which benefited others. And that is how life goes. It also personally developed me in the art of gratitude and all those other things that I learned as part of living and doing the job, which then helped me with my life subsequently, both professionally and personally.

Rajan is currently a non-executive director at Wirral University Teaching Hospital NHS Foundation Trust. He continues to promote leadership development and reflective practice at www.ramareflections.com. 'I stood on the shoulders of giants, and my way of thanking them is to share my learning with the next generation.'

TERRY STOODLEY

Terry was born in Bristol in 1964 and joined the NHS as a healthcare assistant when she was 18. 'It was quite scary to go into a ward, and everybody was in bed in them days. I bit the bullet and went for it and got the job.' She continued working until she had her first baby in 1989.

I was a nursing assistant for quite a few years. When I had my children, I suffered from pre-eclampsia with each pregnancy. My first son was born at 27 weeks, weighing one pound 11 ounces. He's now 30, living in New Zealand. He was in special care for 10 weeks. They had to put me in an induced coma, I was so poorly. I remember my husband saying he didn't know who to sit with, as he was told both myself and Luke probably wouldn't survive.

Once Terry had recovered she was able to visit Luke.

We arrived one day and it was a bit traumatic. Luke was in the incubator facing the door and the incubator was all smashed. He'd stopped breathing. They'd tried flicking his feet but he didn't breathe. We arrived at the worst time because as they'd opened the incubator, they'd smashed the door and taken him to the next room to resuscitate him. But he survived.

He came home to me and Carl, and we were terrified. We had this four-and-a-half pound baby that had had all these monitors and alarms. The staff gave us the confidence to take him home, but it was still scary. We basically watched him for two hours because we didn't know what else we were meant to do. We'd never had a baby before. Luke was only home a week and he had a strangulated hernia. So we took him to the medical centre, who immediately sent him to Dorset County Hospital for a hernia repair. He was still so tiny. He didn't cope very well with the anaesthetic. He had to have the other side done, and we were told we had to go to Southampton the following week. If I'm perfectly honest, this was horrendous because it was such a big hospital. Luke came back from theatre screaming from his procedure. It was not a good experience. But it did what it had to do. And then we got him home.

I went back to work on nights, and we didn't live far from the hospital. One night my husband thought he'd stopped breathing. So he phoned me at work. Said he was taking him to the ambulance station, which was at the bottom of the hill from the hospital where I worked. I ran down in my uniform. My husband was shouting at the ambulance crew to take him to Dorchester, which they were quite happy to do. I ended up in the back of the ambulance with the baby, with two very calm paramedics, driving to Dorchester with my husband overtaking the ambulance every 10 minutes, asking them to get a move on. We arrived at Dorchester and all was good again.

Five years later I was pregnant again and was showing signs of pre-eclampsia again. I was taken into hospital and monitored. I was very naïve. I just thought I'd sit there for 40 weeks and then I'd come home with another baby, but unfortunately, things deteriorated and the baby – Jake – was born at 25 weeks. He only survived for 20 minutes. Luke had been born at 27 weeks. I thought it was going to be fine because I'd got away with it with Luke. Work was very supportive and said I must have my full maternity leave, which in them days was 18 weeks. The personnel people visited me at home, which I thought was really nice.

Three years later, I was pregnant again. But that one didn't go well at all. Again, I was sat hoping things would go well but, at 23 weeks, the baby died. So they tried to induce me to have the baby – which, because it was so early in pregnancy, it didn't really go very well. And the nurses were just unbeliev-able. [*becomes tearful*] There was a wonderful consultant called Mr Dooley. And he came to see me because we tried for two days to pop me into labour but it wouldn't happen. He said, 'If you haven't had this baby by the morn-ing, then we will take you into theatre and do a caesarean.' Which I didn't want because they thought it would be harder for me to recover. I think they pumped me full of pethidine and Carl stayed with me. At five o'clock in the morning, they rang the consultant to say things were happening. I remem-ber the nurse saying to me, 'You won't need that nasty operation now.' I had the baby in the morning but unfortunately, it was stillborn, very tiny. 'We'll ring Mr Dooley.' Even though it was his day off, he was gonna come in to look after me especially. That was quite precious. Overall, it was just a horrible experience, but it was made better by the caring people that were there.

I came back to work after the maternity leave, and I was working on the wards, trying my best to look after the patients. I was doing a shift with our matron and we were laying a patient out. I couldn't do it. I didn't expect to react like that. It shocked me. I thought I could do the job still. I think I just had no more energy for anybody but myself. I knew I still wanted to work in the NHS. I was very proud to work for the NHS, but I knew I couldn't look after patients. I wanted to work with the people I work with because they were good people, they were caring people. And I loved what I did, but I just didn't have any more energy for anybody else. The Sisters had meetings with the bosses and said they could create a role for me which was the ward clerk role. I knew nothing about filing. [*laughs*] But I think because I had the experience of working with all the nurses and the doctors, I knew what they wanted on the paperwork side of things. I made it my job that they shouldn't need to ask for too much. That I would make sure it was there for them, which gave them more time for patients. I felt like I was doing a good job, so it worked out really well.

Interviewed in 2020, Terry has worked for over 30 years in the NHS. If she had a magic wand, she would double the number of staff. 'That would be amazing, because staff could sit with patients, they could spend more time with end of life patients. Staff feel terrible they can't always do that. We have pamper boxes with bits and bobs in to do patients' nails and wash their hair. It's not used enough.'

HUGHIE ERSKINE

Hughie was the thirteenth child in a family of 14 and grew up in Bathgate, West Lothian, Scotland. He joined the NHS in 1984.

I started at Altrincham General Hospital as a cleaner/porter on a fixed-term contract. It was a job that I was just passing through because I'd done a lot of painting and decorating, and the wintertime always brought layoffs. I was there about a month, two month, and I just did not want to leave. I literally fell in love with the place. I loved what I was doing. I was cleaning the wards. I was doing a bit of portering and I done that for three month. I say you either love the NHS or you hate it. It's either for you or it isn't. To me, it felt like it was in my blood. You felt like you were achieving something – even though I was just mopping floors – and you felt you were part of a team.

In 1989 Hughie applied for an administrator's job but was turned down because he didn't have relevant qualifications. He was then asked to support the new administrator and decided to accept, as it was a way of getting better skills. Outsourcing of ancillary services like cleaning and laundry had been encouraged by the Conservative governments since 1979.

I took it on board, took it on the chin, and I done it for four months and, just before the four month was up, I got a phone call asking me if I wanted to apply for the linen services manager's job at Trafford General, the renamed Park Hospital. I got the job. What had happened was, they'd outsourced the hospital laundry. They had just got a new contract with a company in Blackpool and was taking it away from Hope Hospital because of the issues they were having. I trained there for 10 weeks, at Hope, learning all about linen and the washes, and then I come back and I started. I spent the first 18 months literally working day and night, because there was no processes. There wasn't sufficient linen. There was horrendous problems, with the wards crying out for linen. The theatres crying out for blue scrubs. The only way I could resolve it is to look at every issue, step by step, bank holidays, weekends, and how we could ensure that the linen was there. I identified the losses, what we had, and the trust did support me in getting as much as they could financially to get new linen in. It was never sufficient.

There was one thing I learned very quickly: in a hospital environment, you lose something like 20 per cent of your linen on a yearly basis. That is the stuff that's stolen. The main reason is misuse. You know, somebody has an accident on the floor, a nurse grabs the sheet or the pillow, the towel, and they wipe it up and then, because they're embarrassed, they throw it in the bin. So, it never goes back in the system. The big thing identified was that the theatre blue scrubs, nurses like to make them into designer little suits for their self, when they're in theatre, so they never go in the system. They're always with the person. I've seen photographs with people on the beach with their blues on. I had photographs of people who had used them for painting and decorating on their homes and I used to be arguing with all the management consultants and them saying, 'No, no, you've got it wrong' and I'd say, 'Well, that's the evidence, that's what's happening to your blues.' It was an ongoing problem, linen, massive headache. Just before we were due to renew the contract, I looked at building a laundry or hiring an area in Trafford Park and having our own laundry, with a view to bringing in work from other hospitals. It was something like two and a half million pound to do all this, with the equipment. I felt it was a massive investment, but a worthwhile investment, because I could see that there was lots of hospitals struggling with the providers and I just felt that we could guarantee a lot better service with having that inside knowledge of the NHS. But there was no money to be had. So that was put on the back-burner and never to be brought back out again.

I then took over a bit of the security and car parking, and the biggest challenge I got with that was we had no car parks. I was challenged with building a new car park because we had lots of land around Trafford General. I put together a programme with the engineers and, you're talking something like a £1,000 per-car parking space, and we needed something like two 300-space car parks. The final bill was like £100,000. We had no proper security in the hospital, no access control, no security guards, no car park people. I suggested that we borrow another £50,000 and put a completely new access control system in so that the wards, the corridors, were all locked at a certain time at night and staff were to use a card to get in. You couldn't just walk into the hospital, you had to use buzzers, or you had to have swipe cards. That went down well with everybody.

Car park charges for patients and staff were introduced to cover the costs of the new security system.

It got a lot of bad press. The MPs, all the national papers were all over it, having the audacity to charge patients to come to hospital and staff to work in a hospital. But my logic was that if I couldn't pay it back by self-financing, it would have to come from patient care budgets – and that was my reason for continuing with it. A security system was essential for the hospital as a whole. The type of crimes that were happening in hospitals at that time, baby-snatching, all sorts of things were going on across the country. We had to do something, and I could sleep at night knowing that, even though I was being blasted for it by everybody, that it was the right thing to do, for us, at that time. Once we paid the money off, that money was then invested in improving the car parks, improving everything, as we went along.

It is not as easy as people think to run a hospital with the money you've got. We get paid on activity, so whatever activity you do, that's what you get paid for. But the whole set-up is not funded properly. For instance, you can close a ward tomorrow, but before you close that ward, for whatever reason, it may be that you've not got enough patients, you have to cost up how much it costs you to run that ward. Then that gets taken out of a budget. Six weeks later, they ask you to reopen that ward. Then you spend the next two years fighting to try and get some money back to fund that ward. That happened through my whole career.

You said you were grateful for the opportunity to tell your story. Why was that?

I've worked in the NHS for 30 years and I have seen so many changes. I've seen so many things that I believe were just not the right way forward for the NHS – and because of my position in the hospital, I couldn't speak out. I could speak out if I was in the boardroom, I could speak out if I was in an office. I couldn't get off my chest things like bringing in private consultants to tell us how to run the NHS, who get paid mega money, and we're still in debt. I couldn't get that around my head. That we're in debt to £6 or £8 million pounds, but we'll pay £6 or £8 million pounds to bring somebody to tell us how to do it differently – and it didn't work. I've seen that so many times. I enjoyed the relief at getting some of the stuff, that I felt, in my heart, had to be said and that gave me a great deal of pleasure. I do think that the public, if they hear it from the staff and people, like myself, who are retired, and are willing to share their experience, I think they get a better understanding. It doesn't matter if they agree or disagree, but they will have listened to somebody else, instead of a media that is pushing their own agenda to put a story out there.

We talk about the consultants and the doctors and the nurses, but the whole hospital only succeeds if everybody is working together – the porter, the domestics, the cleaners, the caterers, the linen staff, the switchboard, security. Everybody working together makes a hospital work. That's what never gets portrayed by the press. I got so much pleasure out of working within the NHS and I recommend it to anybody.

I would like to just say to the public: support your NHS no matter what. Because if you don't, it will go and we will have a two-tier service, for those who has got and those who haven't. I say, from the bottom of my heart, support it. Nye Bevan will be turning in his grave; he will be literally turning in his grave. I'm filling up here. [*becomes tearful*]

Hughie was interviewed in 2018 while he was being treated for cancer, but has since died.

BARBARA O'DONNELL

Barbara grew up in a pub in Bantry, County Cork, Ireland. 'When you grew up in a small rural town on the edge of the Atlantic Ocean and the next land mass is the States, things that come in from the outside are very important to you. I was a very curious child.'

In Easter 1994, my sister sent me an advertisement for a music assistant on the Holloway Road, London. On the back was a job advertising for health-care assistants in the operating theatres at the Whittington Hospital. I said, 'I want to go for that.' Those first few days in theatres, it's still as clear as a bell.

I would go up to the wards to pick up a patient and the nurses would stare at me. 'I'm Barbara, I'm the porter from theatres.' Portering was a large part of the theatre healthcare assistant job at the time. They would look at me a bit funny because they hadn't seen a woman porter before. There was four of us ladies taken on. Two had gone to the day surgery unit and two of us had gone to main theatres. Other staff would kind of look at you a bit strange, but it was fine. You get over it and you do your job.

The end of my first week, we got word that an emergency case was coming. Even if I hadn't understood in myself that it was very serious, the sense of extreme seriousness of literally life and death was added to by the amount of preparation that was going on inside the operating theatre. People rushing around. Nurses gathering swabs and sutures and trays. The patient came down the corridor with an anaesthetist at the head looking after their airway. Somebody kneeling on the trolley, doing chest compressions. It was absolutely like something on television. It was a life-or-death situation.

I was told by my mentor, a lovely West Indian, extremely experienced theatre nurse, to stand in a specific corner in theatre and just watch. She was trusting me to look after myself, but also not get in the way. The operating theatre environment is very different than any other healthcare environment that you would ever work in. Our processes are so specific. There's scrubbed people and there's not-scrubbed people. I slid around the corner with my back to the wall, into the room where the surgeons and the nurses wash their hands. One of the vascular surgeons came in and was washing his hands.

'I want size seven gloves, please.' I couldn't speak for a moment, because I didn't know how to explain to him that I didn't yet know how to open those bags. He got his gloves himself and went and operated. I can remember huge portions of that scenario as clear as if it were yesterday.

I found out about the operating department practitioner training. They were called operating department assistants back then. I was fascinated with what they were doing. I would be trained in anaesthetics, scrub and recovery, which are the three areas of practice within an operating theatre. The idea being that then I could later go and work in one of those areas.

I handwrote 20 letters to 20 hospitals. 'Dear X, my name is X. I would like to apply for your operating department practitioner training programme.' The programmes were still run in-house then. I got replies from several of them and took up the position of trainee operating department practitioner at the Middlesex Hospital, starting in September 1995. The training at the time encompassed anaesthetic, scrub and recovery, across what would be considered basic theatre specialities: general surgery; gynaecological surgery; urology surgery; ear, nose and throat;, obstetrics; and orthopaedics.

We get the first patient down, introduce ourselves. The 'Hello, my name is' is very important. Check them in, make sure that we are safe to proceed for surgery, that the patient has consented. That's really important. We document all of this and then we will pop some monitoring on. These are very routine processes that are in place to keep people safe.

The development of keyhole surgery (operations through small incisions) and shorter-acting anaesthetics supported the introduction of day surgery.

Day surgery was a relatively young speciality in 1995. Theatres and admissions and discharge areas were not in any way aligned. Patients were admitted via wards and discharged via wards. Everybody brought in for an operation stayed in at least one night and went home the next day. Now, we have what's known as diagnostic treatment centres, with surgical admission and discharge areas. That is a huge change in how we do things, because it allows you to put surgery through, without constantly having to find beds for patients.

The system that I grew up with in Ireland, I watched my mother, year on year, save the receipts for the voluntary health insurance scheme, so that she could do the annual return – you had to pay at the point of use. But if you can't afford that, you're looking at being means-tested for a medical card. What happens if you fall in between those two groups?

When I first came to the UK, my sister said to me, 'You must make sure you sign up for your GP. This entitles you to free care.' I said, 'You what? Are you crazy?' It took me a good while to comprehend it. It's an astonishing thing. It's the cornerstone of a really civilised society.

Barbara continues to work in the NHS, now as a resuscitation officer.

KENYE KAREMO

Kenye grew up in London and her father suggested that she should consider going into healthcare because she was good at science, and she was the only one in the family to enjoy maths, chemistry and physics.

I was always intrigued and interested in how and why people make choices about health. I knew that I wanted to be someone who helped people to be well and healthy. Pharmacy was my first degree at Bradford University in 1988. Can you imagine being in London and going all the way to Bradford? It was a bit of a culture shock, but it was one of the only pharmacy schools that offered a vocational degree so you could gain hands-on experience of working with pharmacists and being in a pharmacy environment as part of your degree. I really wanted that because I wanted to hit the ground running. I was always hands-on.

One of my first placements was in community pharmacy. We call them 'customers' more than 'patients'. I knew them. I knew their lives. I knew what medicines they were on. I knew a lot about their social history, the homes that they lived in. For people with diabetes, I learnt what it was like to really live with diabetes. The impact it had on their health, on their family, how they needed to change their diet. What I was taught in university, in terms of how you would treat and manage a patient with diabetes, I learnt how difficult it was to do that in real life. And how medicines really weren't the key to sort out everything. There was so much more that affected people's lives than just medicines.

The most valuable piece of learning from the placements was I would dispense the antibiotics for customers, and then they'd come back in a week with the same cough or cold. I'm thinking, 'But I gave you those antibiotics, and I told you how to take them. You didn't follow my instructions.' Then I realised that there were so many reasons customers may not take the antibiotics that were prescribed, apart from the side effects. If you've got to take an antibiotic four times a day, for five days, that's quite intrusive. It disrupts people's systems. It's not easy to remember. It's not easy to do. That was a

powerful learning lesson for me. Just because we understood the pharma-
cology doesn't mean that's how life truly worked. I came to think that to
really help people to improve their lives, we needed to be a lot more socially
focused, we needed to be a lot more people-focused. We needed to meet
people at the point where they were. I loved being in the community. I loved
being part of the solution. We interacted with a whole wealth of people, the
suppliers of medicines, local GPs, local communities, mental health nurses,
local nurses. It was just a big experience.

I worked as a community pharmacist for about five to six years. Then
I got tired, bored and disillusioned. I became a healthcare professional
because I wanted to help people get better and be healthy. And very few
of them became healthy. Most of them remained unwell. I used to think
it was me, and that maybe I wasn't a very good pharmacist. Especially in
the early years of my career. I hadn't really fully appreciated how people's
social lives had a greater impact or just as great an impact on their health
and their ability to follow health promotion advice. That was one of my
motivating factors. Secondly, in local chemists, they're a linchpin in the
communities in terms of health promotion and health prevention and
looking after people, but they are businesses, and I wasn't always comfortable with the commercial side of it. If I felt perhaps that you would be
better off going to the GP, I would strongly recommend that. But there's a
bit of tension in the commercial setting that you should recommend something anyway, so that they have something at least until they get to see the
GP. I felt I wasn't having the kind of impact that I felt I should have had,
and I was curious to understand how I could do that better in hospital.
That's how I joined the NHS.

I've always loved learning, and I went into teaching in the NHS. I found
that although I wasn't saving lives in the way that I had initially intended, I
was saving lives and contributing to healthcare via another route. I was also
contributing to the learning of other colleagues. It gave me, as a pharmacy
professional and as a person, a new meaning and a sense of purpose.

What was very clear was that because I'd had my earlier experience as a
community pharmacist, I was used to interacting and working with people.
I was used to interacting and interviewing patients and understanding the

social issues that affects people's lives and their health. And I'd become good at doing so.

I started teaching how to work with patients at ward level. I knew all my patients and all my patients knew me. I applied my community pharmacy skills in a hospital setting. So whenever I go onto the ward, I know them, who they were, where they came from, why they were in hospital, and explore the factors that were influencing how they manage with their conditions at home. I was able to use my experience of having worked in community pharmacy with the students and the staff that I was responsible for mentoring or supporting. To make them understand that people come into hospital for very small, specific periods of time. No one really likes being in hospital. But whilst they were there, it was our obligation to understand them. It was our obligation to ensure that we tried to make sure they had access to the right services so, when they go home, they could still continue to be independent and look after themselves.

Kenye now works as an NHS director of education and workforce development: 'I do my bit helping others to remain healthy and safe. It's such a big responsibility. And it's such a big privilege. Every day I meet patients, I'm humbled, and I feel lucky.'

JOAN STEVENSON

Joan was born at St Hilda's Hospital in Hartlepool. 'My mam had a lot more children after me. I did a lot of caring for me brothers and sisters.' Joan looked up to her aunt, who was a midwife. 'She used to come home with stories of delivering these tiny little babies, one and a half pounds, the size of a bag of sugar, and them surviving. She was the real inspiration, as I wanted to be like her and wear the white apron and the white hat.' Joan became a community nurse in 1989.

What fired us up was when you took a parent to the mortuary, there was nothing there that was childlike. There was no cot. There was just a baby on the slab, more or less, in the box. Me and a couple of sisters on the premature baby unit and on children's ward had been going to the counselling course in Durham with Tim Bond, one of the first counsellors in the northeast of England.

That helped us more than anything because you did a lot of soul-searching yourself. How you felt when you had a death in the family and things like that. So we went back and got a crib specially made to go in the mortuary. The mortician and everybody were absolutely fantastic. We got the baby palm prints and footprints and things like that sorted. Around 1990 we started a service for bereaved parents at St Hilda's Church, Hartlepool, which we did in conjunction with their lady vicar. We used to do it on the Saturday before Mother's Day and on Christmas Eve, for parents who had lost a child. We have a great big memory book in the church that the parents can put the baby's name in. We had a calligrapher who used to write the names and everything on the month that they died. That rounded everything off. Made it that the parents did have somewhere to go after the hospital. I used to go to the homes as well for a while after. I still have coffee with a couple of the mothers that I used to go to.

As a newly qualified nurse, I had a thing about uniform cuffs. If I forgot my cuffs, or I didn't wear them, I nearly always had a death. On children's ward we had the sash windows that used to lift up and birds would fly in. Of course, on a children's ward, especially in the late sixties, we used to have quite a few deaths. If a bird flew in, it meant a soul flew out. So I always kept the windows shut just because I didn't want a bird to fly in. I didn't want a child to die. That was just my feeling. We had a death book and, as a cadet, I used to look in it, because I used to be interested. These ledgers were kept meticulously in order. They were written in with the age of the child, the diagnosis and everything was in there. I wrote a few entries because anybody that was on for a death, that was a part of their job.

Constipation was something I was very passionate about as well. Children came into hospitals with swollen tummies, poor little things and skinny legs. They were constipated. They were toxic. They were ill.

So when did you first notice constipation?

It was always there. I can remember doing an enema on a little boy called William. He was only about five. We did a soap and water enema in the treatment room. He literally exploded. There was faecal matter all over the treatment room. It was just a blitz. He came in pale, nervy and frightened. He went out pink-cheeked, smiling and a different little boy. A lot of children are constipated for silly reasons. Like one little boy had been pushed in the toilet when he was three years old by his older brother, who pulled the chain on him. He thought he was going to go down to the sea and was horrified of sitting on the toilet and having a poo just for that simple thing. It was getting past the fear.

In the early days, we listened to the consultant and we weren't equals. But as time went on, we became more equal. We knew something and they knew something, and we joined together and it made a whole. And children respond better to nurses than they do for doctors. We didn't wear uniforms in the community. I was just somebody popping in and having a chat and doing this.

In my clinics, constipation and diabetes – it was all nurse-focused. Constipation was just such a big problem. I don't think any of them really realised until I started getting patients referred to us from here, there and everywhere. The GPs were even starting to refer into me. The consultant was saying, 'If you've got a constipation case, refer to Joan first, let her skim them and see what's needed.' We had a good relationship.

I would say nine times out of 10, constipation was psychological. Sometimes it was after an illness, when it had hurt them. It was getting the confidence back. I used to go into the schools. If it was children that didn't dare ask to go to the toilet, I used to talk to the teachers. To say, 'You have to listen, because it's causing a big problem.' The teachers were fantastic. But I was treading on school nurses' jobs. I used to get a lot of flack from going in where I shouldn't. I said, 'I have to go in, because I'm passionate about it. I know what they need to do. If they don't do it, the problem will grow.'

From 1990 paediatrics changed, with more complex-needs-children with tracheotomy, and gastrostomy, and all that kind of thing. They used to be in Newcastle Hospital after having major surgery and major things done to them. We used to have a multidisciplinary meeting with the council and social workers on how to get them home, back into the community. That's what we did. We got them home, come hell or high water, we got the equipment there. We got them home.

Joan retired in 2010. 'I think prevention in the NHS is definitely on the up – I've just been for a blood pressure check.'

MONICA MCWILLIAMS

Monica was involved with the women's rights movement in the early 1970s in Northern Ireland. 'We set up some rape crisis centres and various things in the voluntary community sector. There was no difference if you were being beaten up, whether you were Catholic or Protestant.' She struggled to get recognition for domestic violence as the Troubles continued to rage but eventually succeeded in establishing training programmes to raise awareness of the issues.

The police couldn't go into many areas because of intimidation, or they had to be accompanied by the army. Working-class Loyalist and Republican areas didn't want the police near them because of what was going on. The police didn't see domestic violence as something they should be policing. When I was training the police, they would say, 'I joined up to fight terrorism, not split up families.' The Catholic Church didn't see it as an issue. We had an organisation called Gingerbread, which was to ginger the government up for more bread. It was for one-parent families, and most of those were prisoners' wives. Again, a cross-community effort, because it didn't matter which side they were on – they were having to make ends meet. More women were being killed in their own homes than killed by the Troubles. I documented the level of the violence by sitting in police stations and counting all the incidents, because there was no computer data. They were being referred to as ordinary crime and ordinary murders.

None of the perpetrators got convicted for life. I was taking the testimony from over 100 women in all parts of Northern Ireland. They had nowhere to go. There weren't shelters for many of them. This was as late as the early nineties. In 1992, I published the first report and the second in 1994. It led to the first policy and the first piece of legislation on domestic violence in terms of the civil law. And criminal law was asked to take it much more seriously. We started doing the training of the judiciary and the police.

Women were contained and controlled in a more powerful way by perpetrators because the perpetrators knew that the woman had no escape routes through the NHS, or through police. If women go to casualty, they would worry because they were so crowded with the victims of bombs and assassinations. They didn't want to take up the time. To be honest, the doctors and nurses didn't want to know much about it either, and would send them straight back into the situation that they were coming out of. When I traced some of those deaths, I could see that the woman had been to the health service, but not sufficient attention was paid.

The police, to be fair, when the peace agreement came about, reoriented themselves. They stepped up and started to do a great deal more work on domestic violence. The doctors, I would say, still haven't changed. I used to recommend that doctors meet the woman at the end of a busy surgery. But they too often saw it as a legal issue, rather than a health issue. Sometimes a woman just wouldn't go back. Where I got a success was with the midwives. The midwives all got organised and they started bringing in the training to antenatal care. They asked of everybody, 'Is there anyone hurting you?' The woman might not say 'yes' now, but she knew there was someone there if she ever wanted to come back.

The biggest damage of all that's been done is the huge level of prescriptions that they medicated men and women with. Predominantly women. Women would go and say, 'It's my nerves,' during the height of the conflict. They would be handed out prescriptions of Valium, antidepressant sleeping tablets, to the point where the woman could hardly make decisions. It was also what they did in domestic violence cases. Women would be on them for 25 years. Their mental health was deteriorating for every year that they were taking large doses of prescription drugs, and they became addicted. Then, suddenly, when the conflict was over, the mental health service decided they couldn't afford these and told them to go cold turkey. That's when the real trouble started. There was no serious intervention to help them come off it. All they would do is divert them to other kinds of medication. So they started buying all kinds of different alternatives. It was a form of self-harm. What I find is women turn the harm on themselves, rather than turn the harm on others. That's why they were dying.

By the time the peace talks were declared in 1996, Monica and other activists were ready to form a political party.

When we discovered it was going to be all men at the peace talks, we said, 'We'll write to the government and ask if they would consider including us as a party.' They asked, 'What's your name?' 'Women's Coalition.' Then we stuck Northern Ireland in front of it, because 'WC' would have meant two things: a joke, and we'd have ended up at the bottom of the balance sheet. That's how we became activists in 1996, with six weeks to get organised, no money, no office, no nothing. We did it and we got elected. And we were the only two women at the table.

It was a baptism of fire. No one thought to explain to us all the previous negotiations. The details, the technical format, logistics. But we brought in trainers ourselves and got ourselves well prepared, as women usually do. We also benefited from the fact that we weren't seen as such a big threat. All the parties would speak to us. If some didn't like us, because of where we were coming from and what we were saying, we kept on talking to them. Occasionally, we'd bring some of them here for dinner. It was all about relationships.

There were different moments when things were going badly. There was a lot of violence outside the room. And there were times when you didn't feel safe. When, eventually, Sinn Fein walked in, I felt this is going to work because we've got the two prime ministers. We've got everybody here. I guess the most momentous occasion was three nights and days before the agreement was signed, when we didn't stop working or sleep. We signed the agreements at quarter past five on Good Friday 1998. It was pretty memorable.

Monica served as a member of the Northern Ireland Legislative Assembly from 1998 to 2003 and as Chief Commissioner of the Northern Ireland Human Rights Commission from 2005 to 2011. She is one of the three per cent of women in the world who have signed an international peace treaty.

DENNIS SINGSON

Dennis did a BSc and master's degrees in nursing in the Philippines and also spent time working as a nurse during the Gulf War in the Kingdom of Saudi Arabia. He decided he wanted to work abroad and came to the UK in 1999.

I don't have a Filipino name. My only name is Dennis Singson. I was born in Manila, capital city of the Philippines. I was the youngest in seven. Mum and Dad were really supportive; they always made sure that there's food on the table. Philippines being a poor country, my parents always inculcated in our minds that the only thing they can leave us is education. All seven of us are professionals. Look after the family, look after the community, earn well, work abroad. I have a brother who's an engineer, a sister who's an air traffic controller, another sister who's a lawyer. My parents would always say, 'Your job is to study, our job is to provide for you, pay for your tuition.' Remember, in the Philippines, you have to pay for everything. Nothing's free, unless you get scholarship.

I heard from one of the local employment agencies that they needed to hire nurses for the UK, which was almost unheard of then. When Filipino nurses think of going abroad, the first thing would be the Middle East, as a stepping stone. I thought, 'That sounds like a good idea.' We had numeracy exams. We had tests for written and spoken English. A chief nurse came to the Philippines to do the final interviews. They stood in front of us and they talked about the price difference of a McDonald's Happy Meal. That was so surreal. [*laughs*] I think the message was, 'You will get this certain amount of money, but don't get too excited. Because you won't be spending it back home. You'll be spending it in the UK. And £500 is nothing because you have to pay rent. You have to pay council tax. You have to pay to watch TV.' I thought, 'If I've already bought the TV, why do I have to pay a TV licence?' I thought, 'Yeah, let's still go for it.'

I arrived on a cold, grey, rainy morning – 4 October 1999 – to begin at Hastings and St Leonard's. The hospital was small compared to the hospitals that I worked with back home. Other Filipino nurses were already working in the hospital, so they're like our second mum in the UK, showing us around local places. We had a week-long induction period with different people from the trust talking to us. First thing was about opening our bank account, which was exciting. How to get to places. Reminding us of the different English terms that we've only come across in movies. That we should stop calling 'elevators', and say 'lift'.

There were four of us guys in one house, two small double bedrooms. We didn't even have a bedside table because there's no space for it. We did have a garden. But it was always raining. It was so funny, all the linens and all the towels in the house had *NHS property* printed on them. I thought, 'If the neighbours didn't know that we just arrived in the country, they probably thought we stole everything from the NHS' – because everything in there was from the NHS, even the kettles! So it was like an extension of the hospital.

To begin, I worked in the stroke unit. Four bays, four side rooms. Busy, but not as busy as the Philippines. If you can work as a nurse in the Philippines, you can work anywhere. In the Philippines, you'd probably have about 20 patients to look after for a 12-hours shift. Here, I was only expected to look after six, so that was easy – bearing in mind that these are just post-stroke patients; most of them are incapacitated or have some form of limited mobility and dexterity. You give them a full bed wash. I was really quick at it because I was used to doing more. I'd be finished with my drug rounds and washing, helping the patients get dressed and get ready for the day. We did an hour or so when some of my colleagues are still having their cup of tea. That was also the thing I was never really used to – having a cup of tea every hour, couple of hours. My mentality was: I need to do my work first. I'll have my drink later. Patient first. By the time doctors come in for their rounds, 10 a.m. or whatever, my bays are ready. Sparklingly clean and my patients have been washed and dressed, and ready for the day and their visitors.

Nurse education had changed significantly in 1989 when university-based training was introduced. Nurses attended higher-education institutions which offered diploma- and degree-level qualifications. Students were removed from hospitals and instead, healthcare assistant roles were created. By 2009 nursing was an all-degree profession. But nurses from overseas like Dennis have struggled to have their qualifications recognised by the UK regulatory bodies.

When I arrived in the country, all my academic qualification was just equivalent to diploma level. It was disheartening and disappointing. My ward manager was really supportive. We spent countless hours in phone calls trying to find out how I can make UKCCNMHV [The UK Central Council for Nursing, Midwifery and Health Visiting] acknowledge my BSc and my master's degrees. My ward manager said, 'Dennis, this is getting really annoying and exhausting. We've been doing this for two years. I know you can do it. Unfortunately, you have to prove it. We need the paper.' (When I started in that ward, I was a D-grade nurse, entry-level qualified nurse. Five months into the role, I became a senior nurse. But my managers told me, 'That's the only thing I can give you, because you can't progress further.') She said, 'Go back to uni. I know this is not what you want to do, because you've already done this, but we're just wasting our time. Just do it. You need to do a year and a half of full-time education so you'll get your RMN [mental health nurse] registration.' I went to University of Brighton. Because I was seconded, I was still getting paid the usual basic rate. I liked studying. It was just disappointing that I was studying the same thing. I'm a fully fledged RMN and an international nurse. So I had two qualifications after five years of being in the country. It took ages.

Dennis later set up a staff network for Black and minority ethnic staff.

I saw the need for it. We need more than equality within organisations, we need equity. If we're talking about equality, we'll give 10 nurses 10 uniforms of the same sizes – that's equality. People are saying equality is looking after people, regardless of age, race, sex. That's so basic. That's so passé. We need the equity. We need to be seeing people differently. We can't treat people equally. There's still a lot of issues. I mean, white people don't see it. But we do, I do.

In 2018 Dennis was nominated by his trust's chief executive for a national Windrush Achievement Award for 'clinical excellence' in nursing.

The bulk of clinicians within the NHS are nurses. You can imagine the number of nominees nationwide. I just came from a small town in Hastings. I won. Imagine. I was proud. NHS had been really good to me. It gave me a lot of opportunities. I wasn't planning to stay. My end goal has always been to work in America. I thought, 'This is my home now. NHS has provided us with the support to establish UK being our home.'

Dennis continues to work in the NHS and advocate for Filipino nurses.

At the end of the 1990s

The decade began with the onslaught of change brought by the NHS and Community Care Act 1990 and the introduction of an internal market to the NHS. Hospitals had to decide when they would apply to become independent trusts and develop business plans and projections to support the bid. GP practices had the option to become fundholders but, as Ed Bylina experienced, the rules prevented smaller practices from taking advantage of the opportunity. In 1995, Leslie Turnberg, dean of the University of Manchester medical school and president of the Royal College of Physicians, spoke of the 'uncertainty, frustration and even despondency' of many NHS doctors who feared the changes were detrimental to standards of care. Caroline Bedale speaks to the long-term consequences of these policy changes and reflects on the difference between public support in the 1990s and the 2010s. Hughie Erskine's experience of involvement in hospital management illustrates how innovations in services depended on staff, rather than policies.

Public expectations of the NHS had also changed. By the 1990s the idea that patients had rights was well established. It reflected the difference between earlier generations, who had vivid memories of healthcare before the NHS, and generations who had been born into an NHS. It also reflected a full awareness among the public that the NHS was paid for out of public taxation, so people who paid tax had a right to use services. The shift in language to talking about patients as 'consumers' emphasised the culture shift – although, as Anne Brain testifies, many patients felt more comfortable in being advised by clinicians rather than making choices themselves.

The pressures of an ever-expanding, ageing population, new technologies and rising patient and public expectations left NHS staff feeling more under pressure than ever before, as they coped with staff shortages, underfunding and poor facilities. In 1997 New Labour won the general election and a new era of NHS reforms to address these apparently insoluble problems began.

Chapter 7: 2000s

'What you get when you're in a national role is a helicopter view of what's going on all over the country.'

YVONNE COGHILL

'We went to the airstrip where they filmed Top Gear, did a lot of driving exercises.'

KEVIN DADDS

'We tried to keep the focus on the chronic harm [from alcohol].'

PETER RICE

'Broadmoor being run by the NHS, that's when they started checking things out.'

JOHN B

'Whilst you're the neonatologist, you're also a mum and a wife.'

NGOZI EDI-OSAGIE

"I just need a new liver and someone to sort me out."

PAULA WIGG

'I searched for 14 years for a job.'

PATRICK PETERS

'… It was that period where we were all going to have these ridiculous targets.'

GILL HOLDEN

'… the emergency department is like a portal to the world where you see the best and worst of the general public.'

LALITH WIJEDORU

'The staff were so supportive of me. They've shared my best times … They've shared my worst times.'

YVONNE UGARTE

'For that role, I felt really passionately about preventing young people becoming pregnant if that's not what they're wanting.'

ALICE WISEMAN

'We got [Callum] home five weeks later. For three weeks he had been on full life-support.'

DAWN ADAMS

YVONNE COGHILL

Yvonne was born in Guyana, the only English-speaking country in South America. Her father died when she was young and her mother decided to come to England. 'Lots of people took that opportunity, bought their tickets, got on the boats and came across to the mother country in the hope that it was the land of milk and honey.' Yvonne joined her mother later and the family settled in Bristol.

She was a wonderful woman, my mother, and tough as old boots. Wanting absolutely the best for her kids. People say I've got a strong personality – and I'm strong, but I couldn't do what she did. Growing up in the sixties in Bristol, my brothers and I were the only Black children in a school with about 1,500 children. That was really tough. You got into your huddle with your family and your cousins because it was safer. I remember seeing signs saying 'No Blacks, no dogs, no Irish'. But my mother was tenacious. She wanted her children to be well educated, and to have the very best that she could get for them.

I started my nurse training in 1977. I became a general nurse, a mental health nurse, a health visitor, a family planning nurse and so on. My career was on an upward trajectory. There wasn't a problem. If you'd said to me, 'There's an issue with race in the NHS,' I'd have said, 'Not really, I haven't experienced it.' It was only when I wanted to become a director of nursing that I began to realise that something was not quite right. I thought it was me, not the system. I went for five directors of nursing posts after getting two master's degrees and all my nursing qualifications and experience. There was always somebody better than me on the day. I decided I was going to leave the NHS. It wasn't working for me. I had a really huge sense of self-worth, which was, I suppose, infused in me by my mother always telling me how brilliant I was.

In the early 2000s the permanent secretary at the Department of Health and chief executive of the NHS, Sir Nigel Crisp, was launching something called the Leadership Race Equality Action Plan. He was looking for a Black and ethnic minority person to mentor and to have in his private office as his private secretary. I was about to leave the NHS. I said, 'No, I'm not doing that, I'm not interested.' My son said, 'Well, what have you got to lose by talking to him, and seeing what he's like?' I'll never forget my first trip to Richmond House, opposite Downing Street. All the ministers and senior civil servants were on the fourth floor. Nigel was lovely because he listened to me. All the stuff that happened to me, all the difficulties I'd faced and all the rest of it. He just listened. At the end, I will never forget what he said to me. 'Well, Yvonne, you've told me that story, and it's really interesting, and so on. But are you any good?' I stopped in my tracks, because nobody had ever asked me that question before. He said, 'Because what you're saying to me is that people have been awful to you, terrible to you, not given you opportunities. But the question for me is, are you any good?' I couldn't answer the question. I couldn't say, 'Yes, I'm fantastic. And brilliant. And wonderful.' I said, 'I think so.' Then he said, 'You only think so?' I said, 'Well, I hope so.' He said, 'The thing is, Yvonne, you have to know yourself, whether you're good or you're not good. You have to own it and know it. When you own it and know it, other people will know that about you as well.' So I left. I wasn't the only one he was interviewing. But he said he wanted me. I didn't know whether I should take it or not. I was a bit frightened because I was a hands-on nurse. I'm a health visitor. Everybody said, 'You've got nothing to lose.' And it was the best thing I've ever done in my life.

Nigel was my mentor and I was his mentee, but I was also his private secretary. What you get when you're in a national role is a helicopter view of what's going on all over the country. He was the chief executive of the NHS and permanent secretary at the Department of Health, which meant that he was accountable to the secretary of state, but he was also responsible for the NHS – a massive job. His private office was made up of around 10 or 11 of us. The post was coming in constantly. Every minute of every hour of every day, he'd have meetings and discussions. From about seven o'clock in the morning till nine o'clock, 10 o'clock at night.

My job was being his private secretary for health. Letters and notes that were coming in about health, I would deal with. I got to see documents and all sorts of things I wouldn't otherwise have had the opportunity to see. I could see very clearly there was an issue with race. It was in my face that there were only 12 executive directors of nursing from Black and minority ethnic backgrounds at that time. Yet we had thousands of people from Black and ethnic minority backgrounds that were nurses. The wheels start to rotate in my head, telling me that something's going on here. This is not right. The fact that there were only 12 executive directors of nursing, and five chief executives from Black and ethnic minority backgrounds that could sit around the board table and make decisions. The documents and data evidence showed very clearly that if you were from a Black and ethnic minority background, your chances of progression in the NHS were poor.

What we did then is not what we would do now. But in 2004 we launched the Breaking Through programme, which I ended up leading and managing. Nigel had a group of people around the table to talk about holding the NHS to account. He did the mentoring programme. All of which was great at the time. But it didn't do very much in terms of changing the culture in organisations, and that's what we really need to do, change people's attitudes, their beliefs, their behaviours. We didn't focus on that. To be fair, we didn't have the evidence that we have now about making things work for everybody and how it is the culture of the organisations at the heart of the problem. We trained and developed and supported Black and ethnic minority staff to be better so that they would get the job. So again, we were focusing on the individuals as being the problem, as opposed to the system being the problem. Those people had a really wonderful experience, I have no doubt about it and 68 per cent of them went on to higher-level positions. But that was just a handful of people. What we didn't take notice of was the system that they were working in. So you put them back in the system, and they get chewed up and spat out again. People were astonished and shocked that the issue wasn't these Black folks over here needing to change and be more like us. It was actually our system needed to change, to be more accommodating of difference. That was back in 2004 and I think that's what we've been trying to do ever since. We're not there by any stretch of the imagination. But I think the system is beginning to understand now the complexity of the issue around race because it's not something you can address with policies or tick boxes.

We have to be attractive to young people, we have to be attractive to ethnic people, we have to be attractive to everybody, so that people want to work in our NHS. It's folly for us to imagine that we can have a wonderful, world-class service without treating all of our staff really well.

Yvonne is director of the Workforce Race Equality Standard Implementation.

KEVIN DADDS

Kevin grew up with his family in Battersea, London. His first memory of healthcare was disliking having a plaster cast on his leg after he'd broken it by climbing out of a first-floor window and falling into his neighbour's garden.

I've always been London based. Dad's been a bus mechanic for longer than I've been alive, and Mum's a cleaner. I've always been a bit dubious when people know exactly what they want to go into. 'Cause I still don't really know where I'm going and I'm 35.

I was a prison officer, so I was shutting the doors, doing the counts, breaking up fights, all that usual sort of malarkey. I just had enough. I was in Wormwood Scrubs and, due to cuts, it was just getting ridiculously more and more dangerous as time went on. I did look into going full-blown paramedic but I couldn't afford to just drop everything and go to university.

The one role I initially went for was non-emergency ambulance care assistant. It was brand new at the time. It was predominantly older patients. People that literally there was no need to get 'em in, in any kind of hurry. Then I wanted to do more. I got bit by the bug. I went up to the technician role, which was starting basic drug administration, more life-support techniques, driving bigger vehicles, which involved another licence. The driving course was what everyone liked the most. We had to pay and learn to get the C1 category licence. Then we spent a solid week driving. We got to put the blue lights on, which is always fun. We went to the airstrip where they filmed *Top Gear*, did a lot of driving exercises on there, like manoeuvring, and then I got in trouble. We didn't realise it was still a live airport, and they didn't tell us that. So I went over the line by about six foot to turn around and I got told off a little bit for that. The hardest bit was the ambulance was wider, whereas non-emergency, it was essentially just a long van.

On my first day I remember being nervous. Luckily enough, the guy I was with was really nice. We just took things slowly. The first one we would call 'Nana down'. So a little old lady just fallen over at home. It's probably not a very nice term, but it's what we use if an old person can't get them-selves up and family members can't always assist.

I know it's a bit clichéd, but the funny jobs were always sex-related jobs, just by the nature of them. Someone's partner had put a screwdriver where it shouldn't be – handle first. The reason this one particularly sticks in my mind is 'cause they put a line on the paperwork which said, 'Due to the nature of the incident, they transported the patient face down,' instead of sitting, as they normally would! A friend of mine went to this couple. The gentleman was on the bed with two fractured, dislocated ankles. 'Well, what's gone on here?' They were both being very cagey and eventually revealed they were having a little bit of role play. He was dressed as Batman. She was dressed as Robin. He climbed onto the wardrobe in the bedroom and was gonna jump onto the bed, but the top of the wardrobe gave way. That's how he's ended up with two broken ankles. We ended up cutting him off dressed as Batman. They're the ones we always remember, 'cause the job itself can be a bit dark and not nice. But jobs like that do make the day in the nicest possible way. Weekend nights weren't fun. My bugbear was dealing with drunk people – and obviously, I'm not gonna lie and say I've never been drunk, 'cause I have. But I never got myself to a point where I needed an ambulance to take care of me. And it was annoyingly common, especially Saturdays or Sundays, for that to happen. People that literally got so paralytic they were falling asleep on the street.

Kevin was planning his move through the ranks to qualify as a technician, then as a para-medic, when he discovered some of his own medical issues.

It did come out the blue. I was with my girlfriend and we were at a comedy show in Hammersmith. When I turned my head one way I had double vision. When I turned it back the other, my vision was fine. I put it down to being tired. I was driving home and I still had the double vision. I went in to hospital and they couldn't find a reason. 'Cause my blood pressure's fine. My thyroid's fine. I don't have asthma or diabetes or anything like that.

'We're gonna send you for an MRI just to rule everything out.' I had the MRI, which wasn't the most enjoyable thing in the world. Then I got the phone call I'll never forget. 'Is this Mr Dadds?' 'Yes.' 'We're forwarding you to St George's 'cause we found a lesion in your scan.' That was literally how the whole phone call went up. I was at St George's two, three days after that phone call. I had something called a dermoid cyst, which is common. It's where skin and hair cells get trapped. They're quite often found on the backs of people. Mine just happened to be on my brain, behind my right eye. The consultant was quite confident. 'I don't think it's anything vicious, but due to the scans and symptoms, this is what we think it is.' I had it removed and I spent a whole Easter with 55 staples in my head 'cause they literally peeled my face down, moved part of my skull on the right-hand side, removed the cyst and put two plates in it. But that is where the problem came in, because it was brain surgery. It means my basic driving licence for my car was suspended for six months. And the C1 category licence is suspended for minimum five years.

Without a C1 category licence, Kevin was not able to return to his ambulance work. He did light duties for a few months, but then had to leave.

I was unemployed for about a month. I wanted to stay with the NHS, 'cause it's where I already had my feet and I was happy. I got an admin role for St George's Hospital. It was difficult for me, but that's purely 'cause I don't have any admin experience 'cause I've always been more of a hands-on person. I'm a cardiac investigations administrator. So for example, echo-cardiograms, which is basically an ultrasound of the heart, or 24-hour monitors, or general queries with regards to appointments. Unfortunately, people come on the wrong date, the wrong time. I've had someone come in a year too early. I feel really bad pointing out something like that to them. I'm looking for promotion opportunities at the moment. I've got a few applications for higher bands in admin roles. But as I said, it's a bit of an uphill struggle just 'cause I don't have admin experience. Like, when I see the role, I know I can do it. If I can get myself to the interview, I've just gotta sell myself, really.

NHS is probably the best thing about being in Britain. I've looked at hospital bills for people in America. This one gentleman, he got bit by a rattlesnake. But his medical bill was I think 150 grand just for something that he can't help. I've had to use the NHS and my family have had to use it. I dunno what we would do. I mean it literally is holding this country together at times.

How has it felt being interviewed for this project?

It was quite an honour, actually. I don't think I've been interviewed for anything other than for jobs before.

Kevin continues to work in the NHS as a cardiac investigations administrator.

PETER RICE

Peter's youngest sister, Joan, had cerebral palsy and was severely disabled. She spent the first few years of her life at home and then she moved into a small disability hospital in Lanark, East Kilbride, in the late 1960s. 'She was aphasic. She communicated through smiles and stuff like that, but needed full nursing care. She was in a unit with children with similar disabilities. Mum and Dad were very happy with the care. We had a pretty good feeling about it.' Peter had become a consultant psychiatrist by the time that the drive to move people out of institutional long-term care and into the community began with the NHS and Community Care Act 1990.

We started to get all this information on the benefits of independent living for Joan and how it would be better for her to move out of the hospital. It felt like we were getting sold this ideology. I remember the example given to us was that people who are living in hospitals don't have choice. If you want to have custard for your breakfast, you should be able to have custard for your breakfast, which is fair enough. But Joanie really wasn't in a position to choose custard for breakfast.

I remember going to this public meeting where evidence of the harm of institutionalisation was produced from Ashworth Hospital, a high-security psychiatric hospital in Liverpool. To apply learning from Ashworth Hospital to this wee learning disability hospital in Lanark was just nonsense. I remember feeling very angry about that. You were meeting NHS managers whose job it was to sell the plan to the families. It felt dishonest to me. The irritating thing was you felt you were dealing with a sales force. People were out to sell you something, whether you wanted it or not.

Joanie had lived much longer than she was expected to live, but while these plans were afoot, she died. We saw a very good side of the NHS with her care. But for that phase, you were in the middle of a machine that was trundling on with its own momentum. What you said didn't matter. That was frustrating as a family member, but enlightening as well, just how the system can grind into action.

About 2004/5 I was invited to join an advisory committee for the new Licensing Act to control the sale of alcohol in Scotland. I was starting to work on this and it suddenly dawned on me that all the talk was about pubs. But none of my patients were drinking in pubs anymore. Until the mid 1990s the majority of drinking was done in pubs. Now, three-quarters of drinking is from off-sales. It's a huge shift. You would never have known that from sitting on this licencing committee. The talk was all pubs and fighting in the streets and stuff. People dying quietly at home from home drinking were not on the radar at all. So that became my mantra. I was irritating people, going, 'We're missing the target here. You are putting all this effort into regulating pubs. Having a fit and proper person. Making sure that the licence holder doesn't have convictions and giving licencing boards guidance on how to do that. Meanwhile, you're nodding through Tesco, Asda, Morrisons – all these superstores that's shifting thousands of litres of alcohol that's going to end up causing a lot of damage to some people's liver and brain. Never mind the family impact.'

I didn't get very far with that licencing committee. I remember asking, 'Why are the supermarkets not here?' The poor civil servant said, 'We didn't think they were relevant.' That brought home to me there was a big explanation that needed to be done to the wider community, including policymakers, of how the nature of Scottish drinking was changing. We're seeing all these cheap white ciders, cheap vodkas. That's what the heaviest drinkers are drinking. The rising rates of harm were in 40-, 50-, 60-year-olds. Not 20-year-olds fighting in the street. What's happening behind the net curtains of Scotland was where the health harm and family impact was increasing.

There was an alcohol interest group run by the Royal Colleges that was a great chance to get together with other people. We decided to take on a campaigning edge. We started to get some really good analysis to show that rates of liver disease in Scotland had trebled over about a 10- to 15-year period. A striking rise. A paper came out in *The Lancet* in 2006 that showed Scotland was on a cliff edge in comparison to other countries, particularly Mediterranean countries that had moved away from the 'drinking at lunchtime' culture. Their liver rates had fallen a way down. The Scots' liver rates were climbing their way up. We absolutely hammered that message. That the home drinking of middle-aged Scots was really harming our communities. The group managed to get some funding from the Labour/Lib Dem coalition in 2005, so we set up a campaigning arm of our Royal Colleges group. That's what became Scottish Health Action on Alcohol Problems [SHAAP], established in 2006. The funding enabled us to appoint a director and a researcher, just two posts. I'm now chair of SHAAP.

People see their countries or communities having a history with alcohol. They think that history is unchanging. 'Ach, well, that's just what Scotland's like.' There's a sense of inevitability. 'It's such powerful, cultural, historical, agricultural forces here that you'll never change it.' That isn't true. I became very interested in the 1920s/1930s temperance movement, and the huge declines of alcohol harm. That was the first thing we needed to get over. That there are levers. We can pull them and that will make the difference. We needed to get the message over that it wasn't disorderly young people fighting in the streets, because there had been big declines in those kind of problems from alcohol. We tried to keep the focus on the chronic harm.

We've now got to a place where Scotland's a world leader in alcohol policy. A mortality fall of 30 per cent in less than 10 years. There were various things fell into place that enabled that to happen. The epidemiology coming through of liver disease was really the platform. The reason that was important was, if you asked how many child protection cases in Scotland are alcohol-related, people would say loads. 'Right, well, how many?' 'Don't know.' 'How many of them now compared to five years ago?' 'Don't know.' If you're making a case for things changing, you need robust numbers. In 2007 there was a new political party in power who were keen to do things differently. They were persuaded that there were some levers of power that they could use. Scotland set up the alcohol brief intervention programme in 2008. The first in the world and it's still running. There were restrictions on multibuy promotions, the 'six bottles for the price of five' offers.

There was a very interesting study of the changes in the NHS across the four nations of the UK by American political scientist Scott Greer. He said that England had moved and taken a market consumer system. But in Scotland there was still a legacy of professionalism which dated back to the Enlightenment. That the professions and the institutions still have a respected place in Scottish life – and if you speak, people will listen to you.

In Scotland there's still the sense that you've got a responsibility to the wider community. But if you do that properly, then you'll also have the opportunity to have influence. I kind of like that idea.

Peter has retired from NHS work but is still involved in alcohol charity and policy work: 'I do things when I get that chance of making a difference.'

JOHN B

At the age of six, John had a major car accident. He was thrown through the windscreen ('1970s, you had no seat belts') and spent 18 months in hospital recovering, and needed daily injections of morphine until he was about 12 to manage the pain.

The consequences of the accident, it damaged my short-term memory. It's very hard for me to learn things and it's progressively got worse over the years. Speech impediment, dyslexia. Before I had the car accident, I could tell the time in three different languages.

After returning home, John was taken into care because of abuse from his stepfather. The care home was 'even worse than being at home. I was sexually abused.' After a few years he returned home to his mother, who had a new partner. 'Home life was perfect. Summer holidays every year.' John's family were pagans and he went to the US where he spent time in the wilds, 'learning the Native American ways'. He returned home in 1989.

That's when my rebellion started big style, where I started thieving, breaking into houses; I also didn't have a lot of confidence, so I started drinking … taking more drugs. I started glue-sniffing and everything. The reasons was to get high and to have confidence and things like that.

Got my life sentence in 1990 with the conditions that I seeked mental health treatment, which from that time on, I did do. But it took me 13 years of being in prison to get that. I went to my personal officer, and I said, 'You read my notes and everything and I'm supposed to be receiving some form of interaction with psychology and psychiatrists, and it's not happening. Can you do something about it?' My personal officer then contacted Broadmoor, a high-security psychiatric hospital. Broadmoor interviewed me on three occasions and turned around and said, 'Yes, you do have this, this and this. We believe if you volunteer to come to our place, we can help you.'

Since the late 1870s, prisoners had received healthcare through the Prison Medical Service. A 1996 report from the chief inspector of prisons highlighted the poor standards of care in many prisons and led to responsibility for prison healthcare being taken on by the Department of Health. For the first time, prisoners were recognised as members of local populations, with healthcare needs to be met by the NHS.

Broadmoor being run by the NHS, that's when they started checking things out. Broadmoor said that I was a psychopath, and my scale at that time was just on the border of curable. They knew I definitely had paranoia and antisocial behaviour, but I would have to go to Broadmoor to finalise what everything else is. They said, 'Was I willing to go there?' and I said, 'Yes.' Getting that diagnosis actually proved what I always thought at the beginning, so it was a relief to find that what I had believed for so many years was right and I could start to engage with therapy.

John moved to Broadmoor in the late autumn of 2003.

It's big. It was daunting. It smelt like a hospital … don't ask me to describe the smell of hospitals, please. [*laughs*] All I can say, it smells like bleach gone wrong, everything sterilised everywhere. The staff there were welcoming, engaging and treated you like a human being.

We had our own rooms. In hospital they call them 'rooms'; in prison they call them 'cells'. We all had en-suite rooms and the rest was a big, open ward with two group rooms, video room, lie detector room, ECG room. All different rooms for different things. Most of the staff that walk around, the day staff are in the NHS uniforms, the only ones who aren't are the psychologists. The psychiatrists and the doctors are usually just in suits, the actual day-to-day nurses on the ward always wore nurses' uniforms.

I can recall all my time at Broadmoor and the daily routines. Monday, get up at eight o'clock, go and have your breakfast, finish at half past eight. You then have a group, which could be dilemmas, stress management, anger management, men's group – which consisted of men talking about day-to-day what's going on – that would be in the morning, that would finish at 11. From 11 until 1.30 you would have an assigned psychologist. Dinner goes until 1 to 1.45, then you have then till 3, just to relax, coffee and everything. Most of the time you'll be doing in-between session work from the groups. Then three o'clock you would have another group for an hour and a half, which could be recognising things that could trigger your personality. You'd do diaries between session work. At 4.30 you'd have tea. Then you would have another one-to-one with your psychologist until five in the afternoon. Then you would have your supper, which consisted of a drink, chocolate or something like that and a sandwich and a cake. After that you would have another one-to-one with the nurse on everything you'd done that day and then you'd go back to your cell between 8.30 and nine o'clock. After that you're locked back in your room and you'd do your in-between session work [*laughs*] and that's every day.

When I say intense therapy, I mean intense therapy, I'm not joking, no – and that's Monday to Friday, every day. Saturday and Sunday you'd have tons and tons of between-session work and diaries that the psychologists would have set for you during your one-to-one sessions. By the time Monday comes, you're starting all over again – and I was like that for seven years.

How did you find that sort of routine?

Challenging, anger-provoking, tedious but worthwhile. Psychopaths, which a lot of people don't realise, cannot receive medication. Schizophrenics can have medication, to stop the voices that they're hearing in their heads that can cause them to do stupid things to their selves. Psychopaths can't. Psychopaths' mentality work in a totally different way.

Medication will not work. Only intense therapy, for you to understand the disorder that you have, will help you. All the therapy is behavioural, teaching you how to have empathy, 'cause psychopaths don't have empathy. To describe … I could pick that cup up and throw it over at your gentleman over the way, hit him on the head and it wouldn't bother me in the least. Or that's the way it used to be, because I've been taught how to have empathy. In other words, put myself in his shoes. How would I feel if someone done that? You take that consideration in.

In 2010 John moved to a Category D open prison.

It was decided that I don't need therapy anymore 'cause I know what there is to do with my therapy. I don't need alcohol or drugs to have confidence anymore. If I did, I wouldn't be sitting here. That's one of the good things, doing all that intense therapy – that it give me my own confidence. I don't need to have a drink to be confident. I don't need a drug to be confident. So, mentally, I'm fine.

If it wasn't for the NHS, I'd probably be dead, or if it wasn't for the mental health system, there'd probably be more people dead. If I had not got my sentence that I asked for then I could have gone on to do a hell of a lot worse because I wouldn't have known about being a psychopath. I wouldn't have known how to cope with the paranoia. It would have just got worse and worse and worse, which was happening just before Broadmoor. Like I said, I was on the cusp when they caught me, so it was close.

What does the NHS mean to you?

'What does the NHS mean to me?' They're lifesavers and they deserve more money than what they get. Firstly, take all the money off the politicians 'cause they're not worth a scrap, and give it to them. For all the people of this country, the NHS is immense. How do we thank them? We don't. We don't thank them at all. They slave their guts off, from when they're 20 years old until they're in their late fifties, sixties before they retire. What thanks do they get? Apart from the patients. What does this government do for them? Nothing. I know fully well if my ancestor was still alive to this day to find out what happens to his NHS, he would go ballistic. I'm on about Aneurin Bevan, my countryman.

The therapy John has undergone means that he no longer needs alcohol or drugs to feel confident. 'The diagnosis will be with me for ever. I've had all the treatment, it's just that I have to carry on doing it.'

NGOZI EDI-OSAGIE

Ngozi was born in Manchester in 1964. Her father was Nigerian and her mother West Indian. The family returned to Nigeria in the 1970s, as her father believed the work and education opportunities were better there. 'I don't think I'd have been a doctor if I'd stayed in the UK,' Ngozi reflected. She qualified in medicine in Nigeria in 1989, the same year that her dad died and the family came back to the UK, where she discovered her passion for paediatrics.

I wanted to do paediatrics. I liked seeing where children had come in really unwell and, all of a sudden, they'd be well and you felt that you did something. I like the feeling of seeing that your intervention had meant something. Within paediatrics, we do different bits. I knew I didn't want to do oncology [cancer] – I found that much too sad. I liked neonates, which is newborn babies. 1995 was a fabulous year. I thought to myself, 'Can life get any better?' I've got my registrar job in Manchester. I had my baby. I passed my exams. We bought our first house.

Ngozi became a consultant in the 2000s.

I knew that I wanted to be a neonatologist on a unit that does intensive baby care – neonatology. I felt I was good at it. I was really good at putting in lines. The size of the baby didn't faze me at all. It was the fact that you could have such a huge impact in a family's life. Parents come into the ward and most have never seen a baby that small. Their concept of a premature baby is a small, cut-down version of a normal baby. But premature babies are not like that. It's always a big deal. Most people don't start off their pregnancy, when they see the little sign that says 'you're pregnant', thinking, 'I'm going to end up in a special-care baby unit.' It's always a loss of a dream in that sense for them to come here. And most people come here fearing the worst. Irrespective of what they're told. You look at a baby who is under a kilogram in weight and is so small and fragile. No matter what we tell them, it is really difficult for them to conceptualise taking this baby home. To be able to do that is wonderful.

When I was a junior doctor in the 1990s, we'd have babies who'd come in at 26 weeks' gestation. I'd say about 50 per cent survived. That has improved dramatically. About 70 to 80 per cent of our 24-weekers survive now. There's no one thing that has happened, but I think the level of care has just gone up. Attention to detail, nursing care, things that weren't considered to be very important before. So developmental care and maybe noise levels on the unit that we didn't consider as much when I started, but we do now. There are various aids that we put into the incubator to keep the positions of the babies steady. We didn't do that before. We're very careful with the length of time we keep the lines in and how they're handled. It's not that we didn't care before, but we know now that if you do that, the chance of getting the infection in the lines reduces. If the baby's not getting infected, they're most likely to do better. So lots of little things have improved the standard of care. No massive new innovation, no brand-new drug, but from when I first became a consultant in the early 2000s to 2018, the babies I look after are doing better.

Parents' expectations are so much more because everybody's heard of the baby who only weighed 500 grams and survived. There are lots of baby programmes on TV. More and more we're seeing babies who are unlikely to survive, but parents will still say, 'We want you to do everything.' That can be quite tough. We've had babies who are 22 weeks' gestation. When we go to the delivery, the parents want you to do everything. We'll look at the baby to see if it's viable, and by viability – is the baby active? Is it moving around and breathing? We will intervene if that's the case, but even so, the outcome's not going to be very good. We have more and more situations where parents will not accept that the baby's that ill and is probably not going to survive. We have long conversations about the ethics of this. It's one thing to say, 'Okay, you've got parental rights', and we do listen to parents. But what's our obligation to the baby, if we know that the treatment we're providing is not going to end up being of help to that child, and we're just delaying the inevitable? What is a moral standpoint in that situation?

The balance between home and work is difficult sometimes. You don't know when these difficult conversations are going to happen. Then you think, 'My daughter's got a music lesson. I can't be late. If she doesn't get there on time, she'll miss her slot.' So when you're talking to parents about a life-and-death situation, how do you extricate yourself from situations like that? Those are the bits I find hard. Where you truly have empathy with your patient, but you need to manage the situation because you've got other competing interests in your life. Whilst you're the neonatologist, you're also a mum and a wife.

Ngozi continues her work in Manchester and is currently chair of NHS England's Clinical Reference Group for Neonatal Critical Care.

PAULA WIGG

Paula remembers having a lovely childhood growing up in Ely, Cambridgeshire. When her younger brother was brought home from hospital, she thought, 'This was grand. I had somebody to boss about.' From the age of 18, she worked for her father in his jewellery shop, but life took a dramatic turn when she was 37.

New Year's Day 2007. We'd had some people around, but it had not been a rowdy party. I woke up and didn't feel great. I thought I'd got a flu or something like that. Working in retail, over the Christmas period, you work and work. As soon as you stop, you become ill. I struggled on for a couple of weeks, then went to the doctor's. 'My throat feels like I'm swallowing pins. I'm hot and cold.' 'Have some antibiotics and go away and get better.' After a week of antibiotics, I woke up and I was yellow on my face.

The GP sent off for blood tests and then referred Paula to Addenbrooke's Hospital.

The consultant said, 'I don't know what's going on. We know it's nothing to do with drink. You must be taking cocaine.' 'I've never even seen it. I don't take any drugs apart from aspirins.' 'Well, you must be taking something, because your liver is completely shot. Whatever happens, you're not going home. You're too ill.' That was beyond weird. I got a bed about eight o'clock. Sent my partner home and said, 'Find me a toothbrush and a nightie and all the rest of it. I won't be in for long.'

They needed to do a really urgent biopsy on my liver. Apparently, I was supposed to lay flat in bed for six hours. Nobody told me this. I got up and went into the hospital concourse, because I couldn't get mobile phone signal to tell my other half I was still alive. People searching everywhere. [*laughs*] 'You've got to lay down! We assumed you'd be too poorly.' They hadn't met me by that point. They still couldn't work out what was going on. I had scans, I had MRIs, I had CT scans and daily blood tests. By this point, I was ensconced on the hepatology ward. A ward full of old ladies with dementia at one end. At the other end were patients drying out.

My mother-in-law described it as *Gormenghast*. That was pretty accurate. It was hard going. A complete shock to my system. The food was pretty grim. They kept saying, 'You've got to keep your weight up.' I was desperate because I didn't want to stay in a bed. They didn't want me to leave the ward because they were worried something was going to happen. I was like, 'I've got to get out. I've got to get some fresh air.' They had to lock the doors of the ward because of the people being brought in various states of trying to die through drugs overdoses and the rest of it. I got no sleep whatsoever. I invested in some noise-cancelling headphones and lots of lavender oil to try and make my little bed-space as calming as possible.

'You're not well enough to go home. But you're not ill enough to have a transplant. So until something changes, we're not going to do anything. Because the liver can regenerate.' We never did get to the bottom of it. The educated guess is that it was some sort of virus, because of the cold symptoms. Basically, I was sat in bed. Bloods every day, weekly stool sample, urine samples. Take your temperature every two or three hours to make sure you weren't getting anything fever-wise. I taught myself how to crochet. I read a lot to start with. But as I got sicker and sicker, I couldn't really do anything. When your liver's packing up, you sleep all day and you're awake all night. It was always quite exciting because you never knew which old lady was going to try and get in bed with you. [*laughs*]

I got poorlier and poorlier. My ankles swell up. My stomach started to swell up because my liver wasn't flushing out the toxins. At the end of April, my bloods suddenly got a little bit better. 'Right, we're gonna let you out. We'll see you in the middle of next week.' I was huge. I went into hospital a size 10. When I left I was a size 20. It was so much fluid. I needed to eat because although I was so enormous, I was just skin and bone. My liver wasn't able to store any sugars. It was basically burning my muscles to keep me going. I went home for the weekend. On the Sunday night, I said to Steve, my partner, 'I really don't feel very well. I'm going to bed.' I can't remember this but two hours later, I woke up and was completely bonkers. I was screaming at him and I'd got the most massive temperature. And I remember being brought in to A & E by an ambulance. The doctor came in and said, 'Oh, so your liver's packed up.' I said, 'Has it? Nobody told me my liver's packed up.' 'Oh, yes. When did you stop drinking?' I was ragingly angry because she'd assumed that, rather than reading my notes. We had a bit of set-to. She apologised. Another consultant came in, 'Do you think the patient is suffering from HE [hepatic encephalopathy]?' 'I just need a new liver and someone to sort me out.' They put me in a coma to start with. I kept pulling my breathing tube out.

I woke up and I was in a room by myself. They were feeding me through a nasal tube. I was completely blown up and my liver was so poorly that I couldn't keep any fluid in my body. It's all leaching out through my skin, so they're having to wrap me in absorbent towels to try and stop me getting cold. At one point I woke up and I'd got something on my legs. I thought they'd chopped my legs off. I remember laying there thinking, 'Oh, my God, I only came in because I've got a poorly liver, now I haven't got any legs.' [chuckles] I was so ill. It's all like a soup of madness.

Then I got sepsis, pneumonia, all these hospital-acquired infections, because I had no immune response at all. 'We've got a liver. No, she's too sick.' 'Oh, we got another liver. Oh, no, she's too sick.' I don't remember anything else until I woke up. I couldn't see anything. I could hear a voice and I recognise the voice. [becomes upset] It was Steve saying, 'You've had your transplant, now you've just got to get better. But you've had your transplant.' I think he'd been there for hours. The operation was 10 hours or 12 hours. But then it turned out that the liver that they'd given me didn't work very well. One of the surgeons later said that they didn't really think that I would make it but they did it because they liked me. [laughs] Which is quite a relief. I was so poorly they reckoned that I'd got about two hours to live. I was on something called the super-urgent transplant list, which is basically get a liver from anywhere in the country. About a week later, they worked out that I'd had some sort of blood clot in the hepatic artery, which was why it wasn't working very well. 'Right, we're going to have to relist you, but we need you to put on a bit of weight and get a bit better, because you're not going to survive another surgery.' I weighed about 40 kilos. I'd been in intensive care for nearly two months. I couldn't walk, had this trackie – tracheotomy – so I had to learn to breathe by myself again, I had to learn to talk.

Everything hurt. When you start taking all the strong transplant drugs, they call it 'attack shakes', because you're literally shaking. I was so weak that everything was just exhausting. I was so thin that my coccyx stuck through my skin, so you couldn't sit up on a chair because literally your bone was poking through. I was desperate to get outside. They got me a wheelchair. I was doing wheelies around the hospital corridors in a wheelchair. Great fun. I wasn't allowed out of the ward because I was still too poorly and I needed my oxygen cylinder with me.

Steve was absolutely brilliant and remains so to this day. My brother who was alive then was also excellent. They rallied around and kept me going. I had a goal, I wanted to get better to get home. I wasn't going to get home until I could go upstairs. The physio would come around and most people in hospital beds try and hide. I'd be like, 'Me, me, me. Can we do it now? Give me extra homework.' That took a surprisingly long time to just have the muscle mass to walk. 'We think you're well enough to go home. But you're gonna have to come in two or three times a week to keep an eye on you.' It was hard going to start with for everyone because I was still a very poorly person. I had to be brought back in here three times a week and everyone was absolutely terrified that I was going to catch something.

Paula eventually went home and remained well until 2010.

In 2010 I went a bit yellow again. I had my second transplant. They told me that I would probably be in for three months, because of complications. Second transplants are so much more difficult than first transplants because of all the scar tissue and plumbing factors. I woke up on a high-dependency unit, one-to-one care. This lovely nurse, I think his name was Martin – anything he could do for me, he did. I was only there for a day because I was too well. Chucked me out on the normal ward. I was out after 17 days. Everything was going swimmingly.

I felt so much better straightaway. So much better than I had done for years. I can't stay awake for more than about four hours at a time or I suffer with migraines. My lungs still are shot to pieces, and always will be. There's nothing that they can do about it. To keep the actual mechanism of the lungs going they said do singing, which is something I always loved doing, but had never dared to do it. I joined a choir and then ended up doing open mic, which is my worst nightmare, getting up on stage, but it's like, 'Right, I can do this.' My adrenal insufficiency is a pain. I've never had a night's sleep that I've woken up and felt refreshed from and no one can work out why I feel so fatigued all the time. But I have a lovely life.

I'm still here. If there hadn't been two people that were willing to donate, or their families, then I wouldn't be here. I wrote thank you cards. Which was the hardest thing I've ever done. [*becomes upset*] Because how can you say thank you? That's not big enough, is it, for my life? It's a huge thing for somebody to do, so you're so grateful. But you can't put that into a letter. Because it's pathetic. But you need to do it. I thought it was very important to do. I've had to do it twice.

Paula continues to benefit from the transplant.

PATRICK PETERS

In 1990 Patrick was working at Sharp's factory in Wrexham, which manufactured appliances and electronics. He had a fall and went to be checked by the nurse on site.

The nurse said, 'There was a little speck on the eyeball.' I went to the optician. They sent me to a doctor. It took eight months, from January to August. I was registered blind in August 1991. I was 32. I can't remember the first six months. That's how bad I was. It was hard. I didn't learn to accept it. I learned to live with it. I've never learned to accept it. I went away to the RNIB [Royal National Institute for the Blind] college in Torquay for three months, on behalf of my company, Sharp. While I was down there, they phoned me and said, 'Job's gone. You're finished.' I felt even lower. I'd lost my job as well.

A guide dog was recommended to me. It took me about 18 months to think about it. Nobody understood what I was going through at the time, even the family didn't know. I went for a guide dog in 1993. You went away to Bolton for three weeks. Trained your dog there. And the dog knew its stuff. It was fantastic. My dog was Nimbus, a Labradoodle. I think I was the only person with a guide dog in Queen's Park housing estate. It was a strange thing to see a bloke with a dog with a harness on. I used to get some stick for that. But then we moved house and been happy here ever since. Well, as far as I can be, you know.

I searched for 14 years for a job. I was too much of a risk to take on for health and safety. They put me on a press in a factory in Wrexham. They asked me if I could get from this position to a fire door in 60 seconds. There's no way I could have done it, no way.

Then I met a lady from Remploy recruitment, who told me there's a job going in the Wrexham Maelor Hospital switchboard. That was 2005.

What do you remember about your first day?

Oh, God. It was just so much fun! It was calls, after calls, after calls. External. Internal. I could not believe why I applied for the job in the first place. [*laughs*] It was just so hard. But I learned the numbers. I learned to work alone.

We had a computer screen. Your external calls come into F1, your doctor calls come into F2, and so on. It would ask you for a bleep number or extension number, and you told them that. I had a CCTV-machine video magnifier from the RNIB, which had two cameras. One looked down to give the number I needed to ring out. The one on top showed me the fire and pathology lab alarms. So I can see two things at once. The emergency phone would ring and ask for a crash call – an emergency call to the nearest doctor to a certain area, and you put a code into a machine. There's different code for different emergencies. You have to do a hash tag for an emergency – #10 for a crash call, #20 for maternity. It was just so mind-boggling. But I picked it up so well. And it was fantastic. I had some peripheral vision then. Even though I could see the computer lighting up, I'd have a buzzer as well on mine. So it'd be audible as well.

At six months, I was working an afternoon shift on my own. I was really scared that day. I was glued to my seat. I wouldn't move to drink my cup of tea. I wouldn't even move to have a sandwich. I just sat there, glued to this machine. Every time it buzzed I answered the call and hoped to God it wasn't nothing important. I think I lost about four or five pounds in sweat. To be honest with you, I never felt so ill all my life. I couldn't wait to get home at 10 o'clock. It was really unbelievable.

One colleague lost her temper with me one day. I asked for a number. She said, 'It's on the board up there, you won't learn unless you try yourself.' I said, 'I can't see the board.' She said, 'That's not my fault.' I thought, 'Fair enough.' [*laughs*] I remember going there with a video camera and recording all the numbers and coming home, and I would learn them all.

One call, I had a young lady with psychiatric problems. Said if I put the phone down on her, she would kill herself. It was tough. I managed to get in touch with the site manager and told her I'd be taking no calls for the next five minutes until I got this woman under control because she's really upset. The site manager sent a psychiatric nurse across so I could transfer the call. Sometimes you're answering calls from the police saying that somebody is on his way up to the hospital with a gun and then putting the hospital on lockdown so nobody can get in. It was just never-ending. Don't get me wrong, it wasn't all trouble. It was really nice to work there. It really was.

I had a stroke when I was working there 2017. I was in resuscitation for 12 hours and the stroke ward for three days. The doctor said to the ward staff, 'If you need a number, this is the bloke to ask.' Then all day, they was asking questions. 'What's the number of the canteen?' 'What's the number of the restaurant?' I thought they were doing it to test me out.

It affected my legs, mainly. I was bit slow. I would answer very slowly or I'd have a rethink what I was going to say. My wife would take me for walks every night. We went to a beach last week on Anglesey. Newborough beach. It's just all sand. I run. Just run and run and run. It makes a change. The wife shouts to me, 'You're going too far right, you're going too far left.' It's fantastic. It takes you back years. To be independent. To do something you want to do. The wind blowing against you. You're so free.

Patrick is currently being treated for bladder cancer. 'I go to the clinic and the registrars are fantastic – "Good morning, Switchboard", they say.'

GILL HOLDEN

After a degree in psychology, Gill worked with psychotherapist Susie Orbach, well known for her 1978 book Fat is a Feminist Issue. *'She was a big influence on me.' Gill then worked in services that ran alongside the NHS, including the British Pregnancy Advisory Service. 'The whole gamut of fertility, from infertility to unplanned pregnancy to contraception.' In 2000 she decided she wanted to work in the NHS.*

Primary care is a very odd part of the NHS. It's the mix of GPs as business people and clinicians. The two are conflicting because what may be right for patients is not necessarily right for business. The way that primary care is funded is you are on contract to the NHS. You get the core contract to deliver core services, mainly acute services, and everything else is paid for on top. You sign all these extra service agreements. You've also now got QOF [Quality and Outcomes Framework], which is a quality framework and on top of that, you've got the PCN [primary care network] investment framework. If you do this, you get this much money. And if you do that, you get that much money. It's all carrots, and no sticks. That is the fundamental difference. I have worked in an acute hospital at several very difficult times. And that's all about sticks. That's about, 'We'll take it off you, if you don't do what you're told.'

Between 1997 and 2010 the New Labour government introduced centrally managed targets across the NHS. In 2004 a new GP contract gave GPs the opportunity to opt out of out-of-hours cover and also introduced a voluntary Quality and Outcomes Framework. This was intended to incentivise doctors to achieve clinical targets.

I was a GP commissioning and performance manager at a PCT [primary care trust]. I helped draw up the contracts for GPs and then I performance-managed them against those contracts. I remember one of the GPs drawing up a piece of paper with all of the pockets of money from the different service agreements. He put pound signs next to them. He had some sort of ratio whereby it was how much work for how much money. It wasn't anything about how good it was for patients. When I was in the acute trust and I worked in surgery, I would see consultants coming in to check on their patients that they were worried about at 12 midnight, or one o'clock in the morning. They would just appear and then disappear again. You'd never get a GP to do that unless they were paid for it.

Gill worked in the acute trust during the introduction of performance targets, including four-hour waiting-time targets for A & E.

I was complaints manager for surgery in a good old-fashioned district general hospital with all the old buildings and all the old corridors. I was there for about eight, 10 years. I worked my way up to being operations manager for surgery. It was that period where we're starting on the targets. Tony Blair had come in. Basically, he'd decided we were all going to have these ridiculous targets. So what would happen is you'd breach a four-hour A & E waiting-time target, and then it would be a game of where can you move somebody and pretend that you've admitted them. There were people on trolleys in corridors. I remember there being two massive issues that happened in surgery there: one was you parked people in recovery because you had nowhere else to park them. Recovery wasn't very suitable because relatives couldn't find them and there were no facilities – no toilets, no kitchen. The other place that they parked them was in endoscopy. But it meant that the endoscopy lists couldn't start the following day until you cleared out all of the patients that you admitted there overnight. And that then caused a riot because your endoscopy targets went down.

I loved being in secondary care. I loved being part of that team. It was stressful, but it was controlled. You knew what you had to do and you did it. My role was to support staff delivering the service. To make sure that they were okay and to make sure that complaints were investigated but that there wasn't blame attributed. There was learning, not blame. That was a great experience.

There was pressure on the waiting lists in the Blair days. There was a decision that you could outsource. But it wasn't just outsourcing to the private sector. It was outsourcing out of the country. There are two problems with outsourcing. One is they would take all the easy stuff. So all the hips, the knees, the eyes and the cataracts would go out of the general hospital, and you would be left with everybody who was really, really sick, and would spend three times longer in hospital than anybody else. Two, when they started outsourcing to places like Belgium, it was fine if it went well. But if it didn't go well, what would happen is you would have a patient who went and had a hip done, came back and the hip had gone wrong. The surgeon who is the most likely to be able to put that right is the surgeon that put the hip in. That's the surgeon in Belgium. The patient records are not in English. If you get them, you have to have them translated. Then you've got a surgeon who's in a general hospital saying, 'Why should I put this right? It's not my mess.' From the patient's point of view, that isn't the best surgeon to put things right for them. It would have been the surgeon who did it in the first place. Now they're saying patients are going to be able to elect to go anywhere in the country. Well, that's not going to work because the services that need to wrap around even a routine operation are local. Where are they going to get their physio and their occupational therapy? Where are they going to get the follow-up check-ups? It's just nonsense. It's just popularist nonsense. It doesn't make any sense. It's what will sound good to the general population, but not what best healthcare is about. This is my experience: that as these changes go on, and you go around in the same circles, it's never in the patient's best interest. It might be what the patients think they want, but it is not in their best interest.

Now that she is moving into retirement, Gill believed it was a good time for reflection. 'I'm at the end of my career. I'm absolutely passionate about the NHS. I've seen huge change and I've seen the cycles that the NHS goes through.'

LALITH WIJEDORU

Lalith was born in Hong Kong in 1979. His family are from Sri Lanka and his father moved to Hong Kong to take up opportunities for 'Commonwealth English-speaking engineers' to develop the city. 'My father, being a civil engineer, was very socialist in his view, and always taught us principles about helping others and advocating for those who don't have a voice. My mother, also working in health and healthcare management, advocated for promotion of health as well. There are a lot of influences in our family about being involved in helping other people.' Lalith came to the UK in the late 1990s.

The major advantage of coming to the UK was that it was still one of the few English-speaking countries that did medicine as an undergraduate course, as opposed to a postgraduate course. The United States, Canada, Australia, New Zealand – you have to apply for medical school after doing a primary degree first. I did not know what the NHS was. I had extensive understanding about how healthcare worked on a regional level in China, Hong Kong and Sri Lanka. I remember sitting at my medical school interview in London, and candidates were saying they're going to ask about the NHS. I leant forward. 'What's the NHS?' You could imagine the candidates thinking, 'There's no way this idiot's getting in!' [*laughs*]

Lalith was offered a place at University College London.

In the early 2000s I was focused on a career in paediatrics. I was in Sheffield for three years. Being a junior is exciting because you are frontline. Your experience is very different depending on the department. Starting your night shifts in the middle of winter. There's queues out the doors. Lots of coughing, wheezing children. You've got to firefight to manage them, stabilise them and refer them on or discharge them. If you're working in the neonatal unit, you'll be called to deliveries for premature babies, resuscitating poorly babies, and attending Caesarean sections.

2007 is a very important year. The training programme for doctors changed. In the old system, you had one year pre-registration house officer;

then two to four years of senior house officer; five years, roughly, in a registrar post; and then you become a consultant. You could apply to anywhere in the country, dip your feet into another specialty. The new medical training application [service] – MTAS – was called 'run-through training', where you apply to a certain geographical area. You apply for a particular specialty and it will be a competitive interview at national level. You enter as a specialist trainee and move through level one right through to level eight. You remain in the same geographical area in that specialty. Because the training system had been operating in the old system for a long time, as you can imagine, with any change, a lot of resistance was there. I was right at the end of my training when this new scheme was introduced, but we had to reapply for jobs at the senior registrar level.

I applied to Sheffield. That would be comfortable and easy. Then I was attracted to Leeds, which is in West Yorkshire deanery, because they were offering a master's programme as part of their senior-level training. I was successful. But the whole MTAS debacle led to a huge exodus of doctors who rejected this training scheme. Lots of UK doctors ran away to Australia. When I took up post in Leeds, they said, 'Sorry, no bums on seats on our rota. No master's programme. Do the job. Deliver the service.' That really affected me.

A Leeds trainee without promise of a master's degree. At Sheffield I had got very interested in the use of paediatric diagnostic tests, the use of treatments, antibiotic usage. I thought, 'Actually, I would like to do a master's looking at these areas.' Liverpool School of Tropical Medicine offered an MSc called 'tropical paediatrics'. I took the brave decision of resigning from my training. You can imagine, at the time of this new system when they're losing people, and I offer my resignation. The amount of grief that I got from people. They threatened me, 'You will never get a job in a training programme again.' I called up Alder Hey Children's Hospital, Liverpool. I said to the consultant, 'I'm looking to do some locum jobs.' He said, 'It's very strange, because you seem to have answered our prayers. We've been advertising for a clinical fellow and nobody's applied.' I put an application in and I wasn't shortlisted. 'I thought to myself, 'oh my God, what's going on? It's probably because of immigration changes and the changes to the training programme.' I'm not a UK citizen. I'm a foreign passport holder, UK graduate. I presume that HR said, 'not eligible'. I called the same consultant. 'I'm really sorry, I applied for this job and I wasn't shortlisted.' 'What? Why are you not shortlisted?' I said, 'I suggest you check with HR. The fact that nobody's applied may be because they're throwing everybody's application out the window.' Many healthcare professionals do suffer at the hands of the NHS HR from time to time. After the consultant contacted HR, I had an interview and I got the post.

I fell in love with the people at Alder Hey. It's about NHS healthcare teams. Whatever area you work in, the strength of your team is the most important thing. And you need to feel part of this team and the team needs to work. Working in a place like A & E, I think that the emergency department is like a portal to the world where you see the best and worst of the general public. You see great joy. You see relief. You see teamwork. You see efficiency. But you also see abuse, death, intense sadness, anger and violence. The thing that will hold you together is your team. Working in an emergency department team in Sheffield and in Liverpool is character-building and you grow together. I'm somebody who's very loyal. I can't forget the team building, or the kindness, or the support, or the shared experience that I've had working as a junior in this hospital. That goes a long, long way.

Throughout the pandemic Lalith contributed regular interviews to the project from his perspective as a paediatric consultant. He left the NHS in 2022 to work as a storyteller and facilitator, supporting organisations to develop authentic leadership and compassionate workplaces.

YVONNE UGARTE

Yvonne was born in Leeds in 1959. She was taken into care at eight months old. She had nine siblings, but they were split up and sent to different children's homes. In 1983 Yvonne gave birth to Tim, her first son. By the time Tim was a teenager, Yvonne had separated from Tim's father and was married to Tony, who also had a teenage daughter. The family was over the moon with the birth of a new baby.

When Emil came along he was the absolute sunshine of our life. At 15 months he was such a happy little chap. I was at university doing a part-time degree, my teaching certificate. He used to go to crèche when I was in college. He suddenly became very withdrawn. He faced away from us. (He was a very cuddly little boy.) He didn't want his milk. I said, 'There's something not right here.' We rang the emergency doctor. It took three hours for the doctor to come. 'There's nothing wrong with him.'

Before Emil was born I was a health visitor assistant. One of my last jobs was doing this big meningitis awareness campaign. I was giving all the cards out to parents. I'd got posters everywhere, what signs to look out for. So I was quite savvy with meningitis. At the back of my mind, I kept thinking, his little body is burning up, his hands and feet are freezing. It sounds like the pneumococcus meningitis. I might have been overanxious, but it could be.

I told the doctor, 'I've done this meningitis campaign.' 'No, it's not. I'll give you a prescription for some antibiotics. Put him in tepid bath.' And the doctor was gone. He made us feel like overanxious parents. We put Emil in a tepid bath and the water was warmer when I took him out than when I put him in. We wrapped him up in his towel and rang the local taxi cab. They whisked him down to hospital and he was losing consciousness in the back of the car. At the hospital they weren't able to stabilise his oxygen levels. It was an absolute nightmare. It was meningitis. He was in and out of consciousness, but he was stable. One day he just sat up and he said, 'Tubby toast, tubby toast!' He loved *Teletubbies*. I ran down the corridor and got the nurses, and they did all the blood tests and everything. They said, 'He's clear.' It hadn't affected his hearing or mobility. It was amazing. Me and Tony went to St Anne's Cathedral and lit a candle. 'Thank you for saving our son.' For seven months we had the most fantastic time. Emil loved creepy-crawlies. Loved flowers. Loved butterflies. He just loved life.

Tragically, seven months after recovering from meningitis, Emil died. The pneumococcus was still in his brain and spine, even though it was undetected in the tests. He'd aspirated it and it had burned the lining of his lungs.

After Emil died he went to Martin House Hospice in an air-conditioned van. I carried his body in my arms in the back of the van. It was like invisible arms supported me, Tony and Tim for the week that Emil was there. Emil was in an air-conditioned room. Me and Tony were in a separate room. They played music for him 24 hours a day. They had the windows open; you could hear the birds singing. They would go in every morning and say, 'Good morning, Emil.' The hospital staff and the health visitors came to his funeral, which was so wonderful. I've done loads of fundraising for Martin House.

I realised that our arms were empty. Our older children were growing up and we still had all this love to give. The only option was IVF. Because of problem pregnancies, I had been sterilised. I went to see the GP. He was really good. 'The only option I can give you is IVF. Because of your age – nearly 40 – they're going to charge you £1,800.' I thought, 'Okay, right, that's fine.' We thought about fostering or adopting but because it wasn't successful for me, I thought, 'I can't do that.' I said to Emil, 'If you want Mummy and Daddy's arms to be full again, you are really gonna have to help us from heaven.'

It was hard to find that money. I went to the bank. I thought if I say, 'I'm nearly 40 and I want to try IVF', it's like, 'I don't think so.' So I said, 'I'd like a new kitchen, please. About £1,800.' 'Yeah, that's fine.' They gave me the money and I went to the IVF clinic and paid for my treatment. Then I entered a competition and I won a brand-new fitted kitchen, to the value of £10,000 – laminated floor, Bosch cooker, fridge-freezer, everything. I couldn't believe it.

I started going through the IVF treatment. You had to snort drugs, inject drugs, physically take drugs. You're like a junkie, all the time. Then that overstimulates your ovaries. Once you've got all these eggs that are graded [*chuckles*] – like when you get eggs from a corner shop! They ring you up and you rush into the IVF clinic. They were absolutely amazing. I think because they knew about Emil, they were so gentle and understanding. They were really rooting for it to work for us. Instead of just putting two eggs back, they put three eggs back. For six weeks, I was potentially a parent to three human beings. And in IVF, the strange thing is, if you miscarry, they are absorbed back into your system to nourish your remaining embryo. I like to look at it like her potential brother and sister nourished her and sacrificed their lives for her.

I had the eggs put back inside me. I was lying there waiting. I was looking out over the playground of the staff crèche. I saw this little boy climbing up this slide. He'd got a red coat on and blonde hair. Emil used to have a red coat and trousers and blonde hair. I thought, 'I'm pregnant.' I knew that was it. I'm pregnant. I remember Tony and the IVF nurse saying, 'You know, you shouldn't build your hopes up.' I was sick as a dog. That phone call confirming the pregnancy was just – wow. Like I'd hit the jackpot. It was incredible. The weird thing is that the timing was just like Emil. His birthday was on the 10th of July and Amali's was due on the 10th of July as well. Which was amazing in itself. I asked if I could have Amali four days later.

The staff were so supportive of me. They've shared my best times, when my children were born. They've shared my worst times, when my son died. The bereavement counselling was second to none. Over my lifetime I don't think I've seen any changes at all in the NHS. I think the care has been constant. I think they've always treated me and my family as individuals. Not just a case number. Not just Mrs Ugarte. They've always treated us as individual people. They've always made us feel special.

Yvonne contributed regular interviews to the project through the Covid-19 pandemic.

ALICE WISEMAN

Alice studied for a degree in social policy at Newcastle University in the late 1990s and had the opportunity to work alongside sociologist Peter Selman, who was leading research into the Teenage Pregnancy Strategy. 'I knew that was what I was most interested in, but I didn't know quite what you could do with it.' Alice's passion for these issues was also driven by her own experience of teenage pregnancy. She became a primary school teacher, but after a couple of years an opportunity presented itself.

A job came up in South Tyneside: teenage pregnancy coordinator. It came out of the Teenage Pregnancy Strategy that I'd had the opportunity to feed into while I was doing my undergraduate degree. I thought to myself, 'I bet I won't get it, but I'm going to put my name in the hat.' I was really amazed I got it, and a little scared. It was completely different to teaching. But I was confident enough to apply for it. I had the best director of public health in the world, who was just amazing and said she saw so much potential in me. She supported me to do all sorts of further training in public health. I started there in January 2003. I was leading on the Teenage Pregnancy Strategy. I was in the public health team, but it was about the whole strategy and how it fits together.

I do think one of my strengths is my ability to engage with lots of people and bring people with me on the journey. I'm not perfect at all, but I try and make sure that people feel included. It's not about what I'm doing. It's about what we're doing together, and that's a really important thing for public health. You can't deliver any health outcome on your own, you need to have that collaboration. I don't need the glory for it either. I just need it to happen. For that role, I felt really passionately about preventing young people becoming pregnant if that's not what they're wanting. Also, if young people chose to continue with the pregnancy, then ensuring there was the best possible support for them so that they could achieve their outcomes at that stage.

When I was teenage pregnancy coordinator, I spent a lot of time not mentioning the fact that I'd been a young parent, because I didn't want people to think that I was being too subjective in the way that I was managing that work. I wanted people to take me on face value. I had a bit of a worry that people would think that I was only interested in it because it had been part of my experience.

Within a year I was a public health practitioner for children. I was given a day a week and a funded place to do my master's in public health, but I kept a hold of the teenage pregnancy [role]. I got resources to build a bit of a team around me, but I kept that strategic overview.

What are the most memorable things from that role and your job?

I copied the idea of an annual workshop from the teenage pregnancy coordinator in Northumberland, who was amazing. I'm not shy about taking things from other people and using them whilst crediting them for it. She let me shadow her leading this event which brought stakeholders together with young people to look at the four components to the Teenage Pregnancy Strategy: sex and relationship education, contraception, sexual health, support for young parents. We would have this event where I'd have the director of public health sitting next to a 16-year-old who's going to give birth in the next two months, or somebody who's got a young child themselves. They were my highlights. Seeing the buzz of people in the room discussing the challenges. Seeing people sat next to each other, and seeing young people having the opportunity to have their voices heard. From that we developed an action plan for the following year.

Alice herself had benefited from the opportunity to continue her education after having her baby. This enabled her to get the qualifications needed to go to university.

I did a couple of extra GCSEs, which meant I was able to go and start my A levels at college. I had a really challenging time, financially. I had nothing. I didn't have a home at points, and I thought, 'I don't want my life, or my baby's life, to be like that. I want it to be something different.' I knew that the only way that I would get around that was by going back to education and really focusing. At the point where my son was able to go to nursery, I went back and did A levels.

The thing I was most proud of in the work around teenage pregnancy was the support we created for young parents to be integrated into mainstream school once their baby was born. They had that choice of having them in childcare, which was part of the school, or in a different childcare, if that was what suited them. I think our support offer was more robust than some areas. I knew the impact that support would have on not only the young women but their children. It's at what point can you intervene to try and provide the best opportunities for both the young mum and dad, and the child.

It frustrates me when I hear people judging other people for what they see as their choices. My dad always used to say to me, never judge a man until you've walked a mile in his shoes. I always think of that as a really important principle in the way that I view and treat other people.

Alice shares her experiences of being director of public health in Gateshead during Covid-19 in Chapter 9.

DAWN ADAMS

Dawn grew up in Belfast and her first memory of healthcare was going with her dad to visit her newborn brother in hospital.

I'd never had any contact with the NHS until I was in my final year in Stranmillis University College, Belfast, and I was diagnosed with Type 1 diabetes in 1992. I ended up in the medical ward in Lagan Valley Hospital with a girl – Louise – who I knew. There we were, the two of us, side by side. The Sister in the ward was brilliant. She organised teaching sessions about diabetes, then she would come over and talk us through the options for lunches and dinners. What would be sensible food to have, what wouldn't be.

I had no idea what diabetes was. When we were diagnosed, the insulin pens that you could use had literally just been launched. We were the first people they trained in the Lagan Valley on the pens. Until that point they had been giving out syringes. You're only testing your blood sugar at that stage three times a day, because you injected three times a day.

I remember the consultant coming in and talking to us about fertility. She said, 'Girls, your chances of getting through a pregnancy and getting a live baby at the end of it are slim. Try not to get pregnant until your blood sugars are fairly good.' It all sounds incredibly negative and incredibly awful.

Roger and I had been going out together at that point for four years. He'd come in to visit that night. Louise's boyfriend Paul had come to visit her. We recounted the entire conversation. I said, 'Roger, right, if you want to call this relationship a day now, I totally understand because the chances of family are really limited.' Both guys said, 'No, it's okay, we'll see what happens.' Fair play to them. At that point in life, you have pretty much all of the options still on the table.

Both couples married a couple of years later. Dawn and Louise fell pregnant around the same time.

We had our first son, Connor. Everything was grand with him. Pregnancy went as well as could be expected for any first pregnancy. He was an elective [Caesarean] section because he was breech. Louise and I were involved in a research group. My group were just doing the traditional thing of only testing and injecting before your meals. Louise was in the intervention arm, where you tested your blood sugar two hours after you'd eaten. There were 61 of us recruited into the study; 57 of us had positive pregnancy outcomes. That changed global practice. Now the routine practice is a minimum of eight tests a day.

By the time Connor was seven months old, I was pregnant with Callum. My waters broke at home. We knew it was a boy and we'd already decided we were calling him Callum. We hadn't settled on a middle name. When he was born, the midwife said, 'Have you a name for this baby?' It just slipped out – Callum Josiah. Callum had Group B strep, he had a heart condition and, within six hours of his birth, he'd had three cardiac arrests. Whenever babies are born, ducts in the heart start to close and they transition from a foetal heart rhythm to a recognisable heart rhythm. His heart was still beating as if he was still in the womb, so they were quite limited in what they could do in the way of CPR with him. The Group B strep was complicating that as well. He has a congenital heart defect. Instead of having three aortic valves, he only has two aortic valves. The odds were not in his favour. Because I had a normal delivery, I was able to walk from my room down to the neonatal unit – about as far apart from each other they could as possibly be. We were told to get him baptised. We said, 'No. If we're meant to get him home, we'll get him baptised at home. If we're not meant to get him home, God's not going to say no to him. He's going to heaven.' We went back up to the room and the hospital brought a bed for Roger to stay because they didn't think Callum was gonna make it through the night. Our families went home. There were just the two of us.

The hospital had a Gideon Bible in the room. I said, 'We're gonna read the story – King Josiah.' It nearly finished me. [*sighs*] Josiah became a king in Israel when he was eight years old. When he was 17, he discovered the Ten Commandments and the books of the law, which had been lost. Whenever he read the Ten Commandments and the books of the law, he tore his robes and he cried. Josiah was lying on his face in tears, beating his chest and praying that he would die. God said to Josiah, 'Because you have humbled yourself before me, and wept in my presence, I have heard your prayers.' We just went, [*whispers*] 'That's our promise.'

The next morning [*chuckles*], having had this word from God, we went into the neonatal unit. 'How's he been?' We hadn't heard anything overnight. The staff were walking on eggshells around him because he was so ill. They said, 'We're not holding out any hopes – you seem very positive?' We're like, 'Yep, we've been given a promise. We're gonna get him home.' They're looking at us, going, [*puts on a dubious voice*] 'Okay, that's lovely, who gave you the promise?' 'We were reading the story of King Josiah last night in the Bible.' 'Great, fantastic,' but they were thinking, 'Fruit loops, complete fruit loops.' [*laughs*] One of the consultants came over. We said, 'Can we get him a football?' He said, 'I wouldn't be getting him anything at this stage. Do you actually think you're gonna get him home?' We're like, 'Yeah.' He said, 'I think you're the only people in this room who think that you're going to get him home.'

I couldn't face being at home. Connor was farmed out to my mum, or my mother-in-law. I went straight down the motorway every morning because I was expressing breastmilk like there was no tomorrow for this baby that nobody ever thought was gonna get drinking it. In fact, he was evicted from the neonatal unit the night that he breastfed. They went, 'That boy's fine.' [*chuckles*] We got him home five weeks later. For three weeks he had been on full life-support. The staff were amazing.

Dawn went on to have two more sons.

Chatting at home one night, my husband said one of his friends from work had applied to do midwifery at Queen's. I said, 'That's fantastic, she didn't need to do her nurse training first?' He said, 'No, they've started this thing at Queen's where you don't have to have been trained as a nurse. It's direct-entry midwifery.' 'I'd love to do that.', I said. I was still a primary school teacher. I had four children under the age of six and I thought this might be a good time to do a wee career change. [*chuckles*]

My first day going in, meeting the team, 'Hey, I know all of you.' The team leader had been my community midwife with Judah, my fourth son. It was just like walking into family. The first day was community midwifery visits. She was getting me to do blood pressures and pulses and temperatures. Feel how well down any of the women's wombs were, just by feeling their tummies. Talking to them about breastfeeding. I came back and I was on fire, thinking to myself, 'This is brilliant, and I've done the right thing.' In the office they were going, 'You're a lunatic, quitting teaching to come into this job.'

Teaching and midwifery have their own individual styles of politics. Both have the unwritten rules, and both have a lot of benefits. They're never the benefits that you think they're going to be. Everybody thinks with teaching, your holidays are the benefits. The actual benefit is when that child that has struggled with reading – the penny drops. When you're doing midwifery and working in the NHS, the golden moments are when you've looked after somebody who's had a very sad or tragic pregnancy outcome. They come back. You both have flashback moments as to what happened previously. But because you know what the history was, you don't have to go over the history with them. There's tears, and there's hugs, and it's, 'We're gonna get you through this today, and we're gonna keep it safe.' Those are the golden moments in midwifery. Those are the things that really matter.

Dawn used her own lived experience of diabetes to support the care of pregnant women with diabetes and is now studying for a PhD in the field of diabetes, pregnancy and technology.

At the end of the 2000s

The 2000s saw the biggest increase in NHS funding in its history. But experiences of patients and staff continued to be shaped by the persistent pressures of staff shortages, increasing patient demand, and expensive new technologies and treatments. New Labour was in government for the decade and the NHS was the subject of more new policies and reforms than ever before.

Despite New Labour's manifesto rejecting the internal market, the government retained the separation of purchasing from providing, and the move towards a primary-care-led NHS was reinforced. Much emphasis was placed on the introduction of national standards and the National Institute for Clinical Excellence (NICE, now the National Institute for Health and Care Excellence) was established to produce clinical guidelines and recommendations on new treatments and drugs. GP fundholding was abolished and replaced by primary care groups (PCGs). These included local doctors and nurses who would commission services for a local area. PCGs became primary care trusts in 2004 and were given increasing powers. Subsequent policies addressed the underfunding and staff shortages, promising extra nurses, new hospitals and extra beds. Private-sector involvement in NHS service provision was also included. New commitments were made to lower waiting lists and introduce new performance indicators of targets and standards. Foundation trusts (FTs) were introduced, and FT status gave hospitals the power to borrow money. Many hospitals keen to undertake major rebuilding projects became FTs, raising money through the Private Finance Initiative.

Power had been recently devolved to an elected Parliament in Scotland, and an elected assembly in Northern Ireland and Wales. From this point onwards NHS policies began to diverge, shaped by the local context of politics and patient populations.

The idea of patient 'choice' was introduced but the Community Health Councils, which had been highly effective at local level, were replaced by the Commission for Patient and Public Involvement in Health in 2003. Worryingly, the 2000s saw a series of scandals which raised deep questions about the persistence of paternalistic attitudes towards patients and issues of poor-quality care. The exposure of poor care at Mid Staffordshire NHS Foundation Trust during the 2000s led to the Francis Report in 2013, and recommendations included a review of all acute hospitals and staffing levels.

The recognition that Black and minority ethnic communities were underrepresented in executive, senior professional and support worker positions led to new initiatives to tackle issues of equality and opportunity; Yvonne Coghill describes how she was at the forefront of that change. The NHS continued to recruit from overseas, but immigration policy had tightened rules around visas, and doctors like Lalith Wijedoru struggled to develop their careers.

The NHS celebrated its sixtieth anniversary in July 2008, and this provoked many reflections about the future of the Service. The continuing popularity of the NHS meant that no political party could take the risk of uprooting its fundamental principles of providing care free at the point of access – and the injection of more money by New Labour had enabled waiting lists to be cut and services improved. But as with the oil price crisis in the 1970s, the financial crisis of 2008 was the trigger for a long period of austerity when, once again, the NHS would be at the centre of political efforts to cut public spending.

Chapter 8:
2010s

'*The role of a communications professional has
really changed over the past 10 to 15 years.*'

STEPHEN LIGHTBOWN

'*I suddenly had all these intrusive thoughts.
Of believing that there was a conspiracy against me.*'

LAUREN MASSEY

'*I'm transsexual and I had my reassignment
surgery and treatment on the NHS.*'

JULIET JACQUES

'*[The NHS] is absolutely part of the fabric of the country,
and I think will always be so.*'

ANDY BURNHAM

"*Can you think of anything that you can attach to a
smartphone that will replace care and compassion?*"

ETHEL ARMSTRONG

'It was a significant moment in the fight for women's rights.'
GRAINNE TEGGART

*'... my doctor had tears in his eyes when he gave
me the diagnosis.'*
ALFRED SAMUELS

'Addiction has not got a class. It will affect anybody.'
MAXINE BALL

'I've always been excited, a bit geeky about cybersecurity.'
LISA PETRYSZYN-EDWARDS

*'We got the choir together, chose the name –
B Positive – and delivered.'*
COLIN ANDERSON

*'It's a significant chunk of services, the acute care that
went from Trafford, so we just played merry hell.'*
JOANNE HARDING

*'When you get that thrill at the end of every day, there's
no wonder that you want to go back the next day.
Maybe I'm addicted to general practice.'*
PUNAM KRISHAN

STEPHEN LIGHTBOWN

Stephen grew up in Blackburn, Lancashire, and spent most of his childhood running around outside, building tree swings and swimming in rivers.

My first really big experience of the NHS came when I was 16. It was January 27, 1996. It had been a really bad winter and we'd had a heck of a lot of snowfall. I'd gone out sledging and I had a serious accident. I was sledging backwards and I hit a tree. I was very lucky not to have killed myself. I was taken to Blackburn [Royal] Infirmary and the day after was transferred to Southport spinal unit, where I spent six months. I'd broken my back. I'd snapped my spinal cord and became a wheelchair user, paralysed from the waist down. The NHS then became my life for six months. I could have lost my life on at least two or three occasions in the first few weeks due to the injuries. I had fantastic care.

The tens, if not hundreds, of other people I met in those six months in the spinal unit were a real leveller. The same accident that could happen to me as a 16-year-old could happen to a 55-year-old. We both had to reset. Go back to square one. Rebuild literally everything, from learning how to go to the bathroom, to moving about on your own, to getting dressed. It took a couple of months for me to get out of bed. I didn't want to get discharged. You can see how people can become institutionalised. Hospital was a comfort zone. Everyone around me was in the same boat. You cling to the normality that you've created in that unit. It's only when I left hospital – on day release, or to go back home for a weekend – that you realise how different everything is going to be. That was really tricky for me.

Stephen had looked forward to working as a fireman or a lighting technician in the theatre, but had to change direction. An A level in communication studies led him to a degree course in public relations.

By some weird twist of fate, I was sent on placement to Southport Hospital maybe five years after my accident. A really weird experience. I was in the press office looking through the press cuttings of a hospital that had saved my life. It made me think, 'I want to work in the NHS to help the reputation of the NHS.' That's what led me to a career in NHS communications.

The main part of the job was helping the hospital, or wherever I work, tell the positive stories that were happening. In my first proper job, at a large teaching hospital in Preston, there was two of us that worked in the press office. We were press-release machines. We would go out across the hospital and find as many good news stories as we could. One Christmas we wanted to do a story about some of the unsung heroes that work in the NHS.

We got a really good story across the local media, newspapers, television and radio about two members of domestic staff who clean the wards in the brain injury unit. We observed that they were integral to the recovery of the people in that unit because they were the constant faces. They were there five days a week. The nursing teams may have worked on different shifts, or different parts of the hospital. But the cleaners would be in a room or around a bed for 15, 20 minutes. They would not stop talking to the people in the bed, helping those people have conversations or a bit of chatter in the background. A porter, pushing a bed from one side of the hospital to the other, has a really important role to make sure that wherever that patient is going they feel safe, secure and comfortable. He's chatting to them along the way. Telling those stories lets people understand what we do.

But it is a really difficult job to get those stories out. You need to find a news angle or tell that story. In my first role in 2002, it was about how many press releases we sent out. We would phone the local media or newspaper at eight o'clock in the morning, and try and get something in the print edition by 10 o'clock. Now, we're much more in control of our own channels. Communications teams have got bigger because the number of channels is bigger. If you think of social media, every hospital trust has a Twitter, Facebook, Instagram account. There's YouTube channels. There's a whole range of different channels which I am not modern enough to know and that's why I employ better people in my team to do that sort of stuff! None of that existed in my first role. That's on top of dealing with the media.

The role of a communications professional has really changed over the past 10 to 15 years. It's a much more multidisciplined role. But also, I feel like public scrutiny of the NHS is much more than it's ever been. But maybe that's always the case.

Swine flu was the first really big thing that I had to deal with. I was in the London office in around 2010. You would hear that swine flu was going to happen. You would sit and wait for confirmation of the first case. That's always the first thing in any epidemic – you know the first case will hit. You have to be prepared for that. You have to make sure you've got spokespeople lined up. It is really important to make sure that people are media-trained, because it's nerve-wracking. It doesn't matter how many people you've operated on, or how many hospitals you've run, or how many ministers you've had to deal with. When there's a camera pointing at you and you're going to be beamed to a million people, you've got 30 seconds to talk to those people eating their tea or their breakfast and give them some reassurances. That is a pressure that people aren't used to dealing with.

I think there's a view that communications is about spin, but I've always tried to tell the truth. I've tried to give an honest picture of the NHS. And I've tried to be humble in what I do. That's the advice that I give to people, to chief execs that I've supported, or people that I've helped to do interviews. Be humble about the fact you get to work in the NHS. The NHS isn't an organisation full of gods who hold people's lives in their hands. It's a very special privilege to be given the chance to help somebody get better. It isn't recognised that most people who work in the NHS don't want praise or adulation. They feel really passionate about their job. But they feel like they're just doing their job. They're doing miraculous things every day. It's my job to help tell those stories. Equally, it's important to never lose patience with people and to never stop remembering that going into hospital for many people is quite an anxious experience. It's important to help people through that process.

The NHS has been a really key part of my life, personally and professionally. Without the NHS I wouldn't be here. So I'm really proud of what the NHS has done for me, in terms of my own health, and in terms of the things that I've seen through my career.

Stephen was interviewed in Bristol in 2019 when he was director of communications for North Bristol NHS Trust. He has since left the NHS to pursue his work as a poet, and has trained as a yoga teacher.

LAUREN MASSEY

Lauren didn't pass the eleven-plus for grammar school and went to a private school, later winning a place at Cambridge University to read history. At university she became much more aware of her mental health issues, and was prescribed antidepressants during her final year. She came off these after leaving university in 2008. 'In retrospect, I should have stayed on them. But I was ashamed of having had depression. I thought that it meant that I was weak.' Around 2011 the issues with low mood and stress returned and Lauren went back on antidepressants. By 2014 she was suffering episodes of depression every winter.

There was a lot of stress at my job. I felt under pressure that all the responsibility was on me. I had never disclosed any depression to any of my employers. I went to the GP again, 'Look, I don't think citalopram's working anymore. Can I try something else?' I changed to mirtazapine. That didn't make any difference, and possibly made it worse. Because I was so desperate, I was also paying for private counselling. It was the first time that it had such a serious impact on my employment. The GP never engaged. He was looking at the computer screen, hurrying you along and nodding. I never felt better after the appointment. After pushing again, we changed the antidepressant to venlafaxine. Two months later I had my first manic episode, which involved psychosis. Venlafaxine is one of those antidepressants that can cause people with a bipolar tendency to go manic. That is what happened to me in 2015.

I lost touch with reality. It all happened very quickly. I was under various stresses and I'd had a few friends to stay. I hadn't been sleeping that well. I was being very chatty, going off on different tangents. I suddenly had all these intrusive thoughts. Of believing that there was a conspiracy against me. That's when I started talking to one of my friends who's a doctor – and she had experience on a psychiatric ward. She picked up the signs and calmly persuaded me, 'Shall we go to A & E?' We were there overnight and I didn't feel safe being in the hospital. I thought it would be easier for me to be a target. I said, 'No, can I go back home?' I was borderline being sectioned at the time, but they couldn't force me to stay if I didn't want to. The idea was that a crisis team would follow up. My parents and boyfriend were trying to manage me at home. I was having various thoughts that they were all trying to kill me, which was obviously quite terrifying. 'We're under attack. We need to put wardrobes against the windows.' To the point when I smashed the glass and ended up cutting myself by accident. That was a shocking moment for us all. We drove to A & E and I was admitted. I remember going from A & E in an ambulance to the building where the acute mental health service was. I think it's unfortunate that when I was first admitted, there wasn't that immediate follow-up. It's very easy in retrospect to say, I wish I'd have just gone in voluntarily. That would have saved a lot of stress for everyone. It would have meant I got treated a day earlier. But it's very easy to say that now, whereas when you've got psychosis, everything feels very real. I just wasn't trusting things.

Lauren was sectioned under the Mental Health Act.

I don't remember my first few days in hospital. Because of how unwell I was, I was put on one-to-one care. I always had a member of staff with me. I had to eat my meals in my room rather than the dining area with the rest of the patients. I presume I would have been quite disruptive and confused. I am aware that there's gaps in my memory. I don't know whether that's because of the nature of psychosis or being medicated. I certainly felt very safe. Very well looked-after on the ward, to the point that I feel a lot of love for the staff that treated me, especially the nursing assistants, who were the people that I was on one-to-one with. I remember it as a very positive experience. It was very confusing. It took a while for me to get over my conspiracy theory. But I have nothing but praise for most of the staff, who treated me with a lot of kindness.

After a week or two in hospital, I was told, 'You've got bipolar disorder.' It was a big shock for me at the time. When I've heard other people being diagnosed with it, especially the 'highs' that they have, I could never relate to that. It was, 'What, me?' But I definitely had the issues with depression. But I think once I learned more about bipolar disorder – and I was quite proactive in asking, 'Can I have some information sheets?' when I was in hospital – I did come to terms with it quite quickly. 'Okay, I've had depression. I've also had a manic episode. That's what bipolar is. Let's kind of move forward.'

I was prescribed diazepam in the morning and evening, as well as an antipsychotic medication for people with bipolar. As I was getting better, I was given more leeway – they graduated the care. Every 15 minutes I was checked by someone, to the point where I could live quite independently in the ward. Go make myself a cup of tea. Do whatever I wanted. When you're under section, you have to get permission from your doctor that you're ready to be taken by a family member to the café in the hospital [and] to the point where you're allowed out on your own. Then I was discharged for a weekend, and when I came back for my next weekly meeting with my psychiatrist, that's when I was fully discharged and released from my section.

Lauren had been in hospital for just under a month. She was discharged into the care of the Tameside and Glossop Early Intervention Team and given a support worker.

I feel like she knows me. We had a full four hours of me going over my history with her. We discussed the things that you believe about yourself, coping mechanisms, big events in your life. Then we worked on the areas that we'd identified to improve my self-esteem, how I define myself and relate to other people. That process was massively helpful. It made me think that primary care of six weeks of CBT [cognitive behavioural therapy] is not enough for anyone. We identified that in the past, whenever I got stressed or depression, I would put a lot of pressure on myself to work really hard. And that wasn't the best way because that would often make me worse.

Lauren was discharged and then spent a year studying in Ireland before returning to Manchester.

I saw my support worker recently. She was really pleased to chat through my year of studying. 'You have learned from our sessions. You didn't go back into your bad habits.' That was really reassuring and nice for me to realise, 'I worked really hard at this therapy and it has made a difference.'

I think that I've only received such a high level of care because I had a crisis. I had full-blown mania and psychosis and was sectioned. It feels like you have to get to crisis before you get any in-depth treatment. In primary care, depression is a few sessions of CBT, antidepressants. If I'd been more closely monitored when I changed my antidepressants, then a doctor should have spotted, 'Wow, okay, she's gone from suicidal to super-excited about life. She's moving to Dublin. All in the space of a month. What's going on here?' Once I got this diagnosis of bipolar disorder, which people agree is a serious mental illness, it's like a magic ticket to really good care. I know a lot of people with depression and anxiety that perhaps haven't received as good care. I wouldn't particularly say that my depression is any worse than theirs. I never want to be dismissive of people and say, 'Oh, you just have depression or just anxiety', because they're massively life-limiting. But the NHS doesn't prioritise them as much. Because I do have this serious diagnosis that has opened a lot of doors to really good treatment for me, when I have friends that haven't benefited in the same way because they're seen as just having depression or anxiety and only receiving primary care for that.

I'm quite positive that I won't have another manic episode. It was a perfect storm at the time that led to it. I don't envisage that happening again because I have a list of triggers and warning signs to look out for. If I am feeling stressed and not sleeping, that will raise alarm bells. So hopefully the early intervention approach will work. I can't really envisage a future without depression. It probably will come back at various times.

Lauren was in the first group of volunteers to join the NHS at 70 project in autumn 2017 and continues to support the work.

JULIET JACQUES

Juliet was born in 1981. Her mum was a nurse, and Juliet worked as a hospital cleaner at the age of 16. 'Politically, the NHS is something that has always interested and inspired me. I think it's this country's greatest political achievement. Whenever anyone asks me if there's anything that makes me proud to be British, I say, "No, it's a stupid concept." But if I had to name one, I'd name the NHS. It's an institution that I have had an intellectual and political connection with, as well as an emotional and vocational one.'

I'm transsexual and I had my reassignment surgery and treatment on the NHS. Under an American-style healthcare system, there is no way I would have been able to afford it. The support I got from the NHS – that's pretty extraordinary. There's all sorts of problems with the reassignment pathway, but that was a very crucial experience for me. I became prominent as a writer by writing about that process for *The Guardian*. The NHS has been a huge part of my life.

Between 2008 and 2011, long after doing the cleaning job, I worked for the primary care trust [PCT] in Brighton and Hove. Through the period of Andrew Lansley's White Paper that became the Health and Social Care Act, which abolished the PCTs and turned them into clinical commissioning groups. I didn't know what PCTs were until I got a job with one of them. They felt like Blairite organisations. Very New Labour. That was where I discovered there was already quite a degree of privatisation. I hadn't been aware when I cleaned the hospital that I was a private, contracted worker rather than a public-sector worker. It was only when I went to the PCT that I realised there was quite a lot of private-sector involvement with commissioning and running healthcare services. Absurdly, I don't know why I thought this, but I thought everyone would be on the same salary. That it was going to be a socialist utopia where I would get paid the same as the chief exec. But everyone in the NHS has different pay bands. At one point, an email had to go around the whole organisation saying, 'Can you please not refer to your admin staff as "band fours"? They have names.' That was the culture of the place at the time, so it was not the kind of socialist culture that I was hoping for.

That experience made me realise that the organisation was very vulnerable to structural changes imposed directly from government. The 2010 election – a crucial plank of David Cameron's messaging was there will not be any top-down reorganisation of the NHS. The first thing they do when they get the support from the Liberal Democrats who formed the coalition government is to announce that top-down reorganisation.

In March 2012 the Health and Social Care Bill came into force, with the abolition of strategic health authorities and primary care trusts and the introduction of new health and well-being boards.

A strength of the NHS is the type of people it attracts. Very interesting, intelligent and creative people. Brighton and Hove is not a huge city. It was a town that had high prevalence of people with mental health issues, a big LGBT population, quite a high proportion of drug users, a comparatively large homeless population. There were a lot of unique challenges in Brighton and Hove, and I was around a lot of good people. It felt like being at a university. It felt like a creative environment because my job was to take minutes at the meetings. I did get involved with a transgender working group there. The PCT would link up with a local LGBT advocacy group and other voluntary organisations providing support to trans people and they would link up with the SE Commissioning Group, who were responsible for the sexual reassignment services at Charing Cross Hospital. So the PCT was at the centre of this integrated, city-wide healthcare culture, managing hospitals and other health services, but also taking a more holistic approach to different types of healthcare. I found it quite stimulating. My own job was quite tedious. But the environment was interesting.

I came out as transsexual when I was 27 in 2008. I asked my GP for a referral to the gender identity clinic at Charing Cross. I had an initial psychiatric assessment at an outpatient clinic in Brighton with a very nice psychiatrist. It was basic screening to make sure that you don't declare yourself gender dysphoric [distress caused by a mismatch between gender identity and biological sex] because of another mental health condition that's not been properly dealt with. I had a first appointment where the psychiatrist said, 'Yeah, I think you're fine, but you'll need to have a second one just to make sure. Come back in two months.' I was like, 'Two months?' The process was incredibly slow. I got the referral to the gender identity clinic. There was a process over a couple of years – late 2009 through to summer 2011 – which included psychiatrist and gender identity clinic appointments and getting a hormone prescription for oestrogen. Once I was on the hormones, I had anti-androgen injections at a GP surgery.

One thing that really stood out was how good my GP was. It was a lot easier in 2008 to have your personal GP who you struck up a relationship with. I vividly remember when I'd made the decision to transition. I thought to myself, 'I'm going to throw myself off this cliff. I have to come out to my family, friends and colleagues.' I had a good idea of how most people were going to react, but not all of them. I went to my GP and steeled myself to say these words, 'I want to go through this gender reassignment process.' My GP very calmly and casually in his unflappable way said, 'Oh, yeah, we talked about this before.' I had no memory of it. I was really quite startled when he said that, but I'd been dealing with various mental health problems. In hindsight, I think these had a lot to do with being trans in a transphobic society more specifically. But the GP was very good.

I had speech and language therapy through Hove Polyclinic. A really lovely therapist gave me an individual assessment where he measured the range of my voice, and also the way I talked. My voice came out in a fairly androgynous range. It wasn't definitively *male*, but it certainly wouldn't be read as female either. I had the option of individual or group sessions, so I went to a group session. As well as doing exercises to feminise our voices, we had lots of interesting conversations. What does it mean to have a female voice? Can you retrain yourself to speak a different way as an adult? How much do we even want to? You know, far more than my body changing, or the clothes I wore changing, or even changing my name, there was something about changing the way I spoke that felt jarring and unnatural. With the help of the therapist and the group, I decided that I would work out how to affect a voice that was going to help me to pass as a woman in certain social situations where it was just easier or safer to do so. Otherwise, not to worry too much. Most people who spent much time with me would know that I was trans. And it's something I've written about an awful lot, so I'm not in the closet about it. I had friends who supported me and I had to work out how much I wanted to have trans friends.

In autumn 2011, I started consultations with the surgical team. Late July 2012, I checked in to Charing Cross Hospital the night before surgery and got up at 5.30 the next morning. Having an enema was pretty unpleasant. I was in surgery for, I think, four and a half hours.

Nearly everyone else in the ward was also there for gender confirmation surgery. One woman in particular I struck up a really nice friendship with. I'd sit and watch football with her in the waiting room. The solidarity and comradeship that I got from some of the people on the ward was really nice. It was a really intense, strange and deeply personal once-in-a-lifetime experience.

It felt like an old-fashioned hospital. The food was very bad. I remember asking myself, 'How have you fucked up a cheese roll?' I really wanted it to be good because I believe in the NHS, so I don't want to come away criticising any aspects of it. There was a moment of great liberation on my penultimate night at the hospital where I was able to get myself over the road to Pizza Express with my friend who'd come to visit.

I was in hospital for a week and was in great pain. After a night at home, I went to see my parents to recover. I got an infection, which was incredibly painful, and had to get antibiotics. It was a couple of months before I could walk. After about 10 days, my mother tried to walk me to the top of my street – about a minute's walk. I was in absolute agony. It was really hard for me to do it and for her to watch. Mum used to be a nurse, so she was good at looking after me. I remember going to a football match maybe three weeks after my surgery, and I was able to walk the 15 minutes to the pub, and meet my friend and go to this game together. It took me about nine months to play football again, I think.

The recovery was slow and painful. I was able to eat, to read, to watch films. I also had to dilate. They gave me these really unpleasant Perspex dilators. The body interprets the new vagina that's been created as a wound that it tries to close, so you have to dilate for a long time. You started off doing it three times a day for half an hour. Then tapered it down to twice, then once and then less regularly. I did it for years.

There were certain bureaucratic frustrations. At one point I moved house, but the information didn't get to where it needed to get to and I missed an appointment. 'Why did you miss this appointment?' You know, if you miss two appointments, they can throw you off the pathway. And little things like them refusing to use my female name until I provided them with a deed poll. I wrote about that in *The Guardian*. That protocol has probably changed now. So little things like that stuck out.

I did a blog for *The Guardian* called 'Transgender Journey', fortnightly before the surgery then every couple of months afterwards. Then I turned the columns into a memoir with the title of *Trans: A Memoir* in 2015, which built on the columns, but talked a lot more about the media environment in which I understood and wrote about trans issues. That book was as much about the media as about being transsexual.

If health professionals aren't aware of the power dynamics or, worse, if they are given that kind of medical gatekeeping over something that, to the transsexual person, feels like a matter of life and death – you know, that's a very loaded relationship. I was very conscious of that when I was doing my own writing. The way that the writing changed the power dynamic again. Because if I wasn't careful about what I wrote, then I might get kicked off the pathway. But if they kicked me off the pathway, then I would write a high-profile piece about it. So my writing added an extra-complicated layer to an already pretty loaded power dynamic. The impact gender reassignment has had on my life has been pretty huge. I mean, I'd be dead without it; there's no way I could have carried on living as a man.

Now a writer and filmmaker, Juliet continues to advocate for LGBTQ+ issues.

ANDY BURNHAM

Andy was born in Liverpool in 1970. He went to school in Newton-le-Willows, a mining area, and his experience of the miners' strike in the mid 1980s was vivid. 'I became quite political.' After Andy graduated from Cambridge, the 1992 general election happened. 'A feeling of utter despondency after the election made me, at that point, resolve that I wanted to work permanently in politics.' Andy served as health secretary between 2009 and 2010, and was elected mayor of Greater Manchester in 2017. He was interviewed in the run-up to the NHS seventieth anniversary celebrations in 2018.

It's funny having this conversation with you because I was quite involved in NHS 50 – which makes me feel very old now! As parliamentary officer for the NHS Confederation, one of the first big things that we did in the newly unified organisation was plan for 1998, which was the fiftieth celebration. I remember going up and down the country doing a lot of work, talking to people about exactly what you're doing now.

I was the first frontbencher ever to call for the full integration of health and social care in that speech, and I remain utterly convinced that that is the only way the NHS makes the transition from a twentieth-century treatment service towards a twenty-first-century, person-centred health and well-being service. I remember quoting, in a speech at the King's Fund in 2013, the World Health Organization definition of health – it being a state of complete physical, mental and social well-being, not the absence of disease or infirmity. That is what good health should be. The NHS should be a vehicle to achieve that. At present it is only a vehicle that seeks to remove disease and infirmity. The NHS will only be twenty-first-century ready when we can say that it supports people with dementia as well as it treats cancer today.

That's what we're aiming for in Greater Manchester. The vision is very much around full integration of the system. Complete breaking down of the silos. Commissioning with one budget for physical, mental and social well-being. I would say at the moment we're in the foothills of that journey. There's different ways of describing it. A 'National Health and Care Service', you could say, or an 'NHS for the whole person', I think is the way

I would describe it. In primary care, I talk a lot about social prescribing. I think the notion of social prescribing needs to be a core offer in every GP surgery. It's about mental health being much more centre stage in the NHS. That's a work in progress. It would be a completely different way of supporting older people with ongoing needs, and the home not the hospital being the default setting for their care.

As we hit NHS 70, I think more than ever before, there's a consensus about it. There really wasn't in NHS 50. Then, there was a lot of voices out there saying that the model was not fit for the modern age. I like to think that the government of which I was a part disproved that and showed that if you invest in it, it can provide a good service to everybody. When I left the Department of Health in 2010, the NHS had record patient satisfaction, and the lowest-ever waiting lists. The Commonwealth Fund said it was brilliant in terms of health services across the world. So that's why the Lansley reorganisation in 2013 was such a frustration. The NHS was performing well. It was settled. It needed to focus on the efficiency challenge ahead, not have a reorganisation that distracted it.

I think there is now a set consensus, on the left and on the right of politics that the NHS model is the right model. It's the most efficient model. It's not something that people used to say, but free at the point of use is the most efficient way of providing healthcare. The debate about privatisation has almost gone now. I was the first secretary of state to talk about the NHS as the preferred provider and I did become estranged myself from some of the more aggressive Blairite policies around the market. If I look back at that, I was a bit of a pariah at that time. It's amazing how that debate's moved on in the last decade. I think people have completely come around to the idea that privatisation and healthcare don't mix at all, like oil and water, really. So in terms of NHS at 70, I think there is a consensus. The question comes – 'Well, it needs more money, where's it coming from?' I think the public are ready to pay more tax for it. All the polls suggest that.

The big change I keep coming back to is changing the way social care is funded. We need a solution for social care that aligns it with the NHS principle. Everyone contributes and then everyone is covered. When I was secretary of state, I proposed a compulsory levy on all estates to pay for social care. I remain of the view that that is the right policy. You can't pay for everything from general taxation because it wouldn't be fair on the working-age population. You have to find a way of making the baby-boomer generation pay something towards the cost of their social care. If it was done in an equitable way, by taking some value from the housing assets that they've built up, you could have then a fully-free-at-the-point-of-use National Health and Care Service. That is such a powerful vision. It's only when social care is free at the point of use that the NHS can move into the home and become much more focused around health promotion and independence.

In 2012 the NHS featured in the Olympics opening ceremony.

I got invited to the dress rehearsal by Tessa Jowell, shadow minister for the Olympics, who was heavily involved. I sat next to Frank Cottrell-Boyce, who'd helped Danny Boyle with the opening ceremony. When that NHS thing came up, I confess to a small tear creeping up. There was all the stuff, dancing staff and hospital beds. I knew what was coming when I was watching it on the TV. I thought, 'What other country would celebrate its health services at the Olympic Games?' That said everything, didn't it? The pride everybody felt. In terms of its history, I think you could look at that moment and say, 'That is the moment when the NHS truly was as entrenched as the BBC or any other institution you could think of.' It's absolutely part of the fabric of the country, and I think will always be so.

Andy shares his reflections on the future of the NHS in Chapter 10.

ETHEL ARMSTRONG

After retirement Ethel continued her deep involvement with the NHS through the HS Retirement Fellowship and serving as governor to trusts in the north-east. She was awarded an MBE in 2018 for seven decades of service, and attended many of the NHS's birthday celebrations.

In 2018 I shared the platform for the very first time with Simon Stevens, then chief executive of the NHS. He said to Antony Tiernan, then director of NHS communications, 'Antony, I want Ethel for one or two more things.' I'd only done this 20-minute session question-and-answer thing. It literally went ballistic. I was on the platform and Jeremy Hunt, then minister of health, was there. Well, he was as good as a chocolate teapot. He said, 'Well, we're not going to have to worry, Ethel, because in a year's time we're going to unroll this app that you can attach to your phone. And it only costs £10 and anybody that can't pay it, I'm sure we'll find some means of getting it to them for free. The app will tell you who their doctor is and what their symptoms are and what their prescriptions are and whether they need this and that.' I looked at him and said, 'For £10 – but you have to put it onto a smartphone that costs you £95, so we'll get the numbers right.' 'Well, yes, it has to be attached to one of those.' 'I'm going to ask you one question. Can you think of anything that you can attach to a smartphone that will replace care and compassion? I would like to think that when I was snuffing my last, I'd got a nice, warm, compassionate hand just to hold my hand and say, "It's alright, you can shut your eyes, I will make sure that you're not in any discomfort."' There's no app ever will replace that. You still will always need people. (An app in my day was something that, if you were good, your mother gave you and you ate it. You gave half of it to your best friend, she would have the middle and you could have the outside bit.)

The NHS has been my whole life, but until 2018, people would see me on the street and have no idea. Now, I go into the village and they say, 'I heard you on the radio this morning.' I said, 'Then you've done more than me, I was on the train.' 'Oh, you were being interviewed.' 'Oh, saw you on the television. You were with some lovely men!' The one thing that has literally knocked them all for six in the village – oh, I'm a real star in my hairdressers' – was the fact that I had the four celebrity chefs who came up to Newcastle to do my interview and then they all cooked for me. I was the special guest at the *Great British Menu* show on the NHS and stayed at the London Hilton. Who were my escorts for the whole of the evening? Nick Knowles and Peter Andre. That really got them buzzing. Peter Andre, all to myself, holding my little hand. He said, 'I can't believe, Ethel, that you don't have a speaking note.' I said, 'No, I don't need a note, I tell you as it is.' (I've never had a problem with words. Never. It comes from the two essential organs. It comes from your head and your heart.) He and Nick Knowles were both absolute gentlemen, attentive and courteous.

I am always optimistic. I'm an eternal optimist. Every one of the people I've worked with has enriched my life. If somebody said, 'Would you do it all again?' 'Yes, I would do it all again. Every bit of it.' The day that I drop off the perch, just say, 'Here goes Ethel, who worked and enjoyed every day.'

My autobiography will be called *Shiny Shoes and Half a Crown*.

Ethel died in August 2020, aged 90.

GRAINNE TEGGART

Grainne was born in Belfast in 1985 and is Amnesty International's Northern Ireland deputy director. She campaigned for the decriminalisation of abortion and, in October 2019, MPs in the UK Parliament in Westminster voted overwhelmingly in favour of the changes. Although healthcare is devolved to the Northern Ireland Assembly at Stormont, the assembly was still suspended following a breakdown in power-sharing arrangements between Sinn Fein and the Democratic Unionist Party in 2017, and in that case, a law can pass without involvement from Stormont. 'It was probably one of a very few good things that came out of the collapse of Stormont.'

For the best part of 50 years, women in Northern Ireland have been treated and have endured treatment as second-class citizens. Women have received very different treatment on the NHS compared to their counterparts in other parts of the UK.

I've been with Amnesty International for 10 years and my background is as a lobbyist. It's my job to change legislation, to change policy, and lobby – whether that's at Westminster or here in the devolved administrations. I have always been very passionate about rights. I grew up in a household where it was impressed upon us very early on. My mother works in children's rights. At Amnesty I was doing a lot of work on different domestic issues and it struck me that abortion is the most pressing rights issue. It's one of those issues, for good or ill, where you have two people on opposite sides of the table. There wasn't anything in the middle. I approached this campaign to throw light on the fact that there's a big spectrum. It wasn't about reinforcing the notion of good abortion versus bad abortion, but rather, we need to have this conversation through the lens of women's lived NHS experiences.

It is a human rights issue as well as a healthcare issue. The United Nations had been very clear to the UK government that this was something that needed to change. They had been ignoring that. For me, it was about, 'How do we get this on the agenda?' It was the combination of Amnesty, with our rights expertise, together with women's lived experiences. That combination makes for a very compelling argument. It is very difficult for politicians who, historically, had deliberately washed their hands of the issue or ignored it, to sit across the table from a woman who had had to travel to England for an abortion and been through that trauma and tell her, 'No, we're not going to talk about this issue.' I was aware that we were operating in a very hostile political environment and that there were different ways we would need to bring our politicians to the table, and part of that was through the courts.

In 2013, under a Democratic Unionist Party health minister, draft guidance had been published which did nothing to clarify the law for healthcare professionals about when they could provide terminations, and reinforced the threat of prosecution if they made a wrong decision. Healthcare professionals pushed back. 'If you're not going to tell us when we can legally provide this, then we can't provide it.' Our healthcare professionals felt like they were failing women, and were quite open about that. But their hands were tied, and they couldn't do much different. That's when we've seen a big difference. Not necessarily in the number of women travelling, but particularly with abortion pills.

When we think about the women who are going online and buying abortion pills, who are those women? They are women in domestic violence situations – perhaps spousal rape. Women who have other children, but don't have childcare and can't travel. Women who don't have confirmed immigration status, etc. So we're talking about women who are already marginalised and were going online, buying abortion pills and risking prosecution. Whilst we were pushing through the legislative change at Westminster, we were able to secure a moratorium on prosecutions. Otherwise, you would have had a woman in this part of the UK facing a jail sentence for accessing healthcare that was freely available in England and Wales and Scotland.

The Northern Ireland public have long favoured change, and that includes decriminalisation. People recognise that this is a healthcare, not a criminal justice, issue. We're now the only part of the UK where that's the case. Doctors in other parts of the UK could still be prosecuted if they are deemed to be outside of the exceptions under the 1967 Abortion Act. We went from this position of being 160 years behind to leading the way, which is a wonderful position, but we want the rest of the UK and NHS to catch up.

How did it feel when the law did go through in October 2019?

It was a significant moment in the fight for women's rights here, because it was the first time there had been the acknowledgement in law that we are equal. That our bodies are our own, and we should have a say on what happens with them. We can't undo everything that has happened in the past, but we can now safeguard future generations from facing the same discrimination. I cried. I still get emotional about it. Such a fight, even through the courts. We had an attorney general and others coming out in force against what we were trying to do. When it passed in the UK Parliament with such a landslide majority, it was a really important moment. One that I'll always remember. I cared very deeply about this issue because I care very deeply about what happens to women.

For me, the NHS is one of our greatest gifts. It's such a model of how to do things that it's something that we should share, particularly with other countries where people don't have the same access to health. They neglected this healthcare for women here for a long time, and they've got it wrong in other parts of the UK as well, because we need to see better improvement of abortion services in England. I think history will show the politicians got this wrong and that, eventually, in the Northern Ireland context, they got it right. Women's rights and women's healthcare have to be a priority of any government.

Grainne was interviewed in November 2019. By April 2023 abortion services have still not been fully established by the power-sharing executive at Stormont, and women continue to struggle to access services.

ALFRED SAMUELS

Alfred grew up in London in the 1960s. The NHS was part and parcel of his life. 'I watched my father take ill and be nursed by the NHS back to good health. My mother was an auxiliary nurse. We've been exposed to the NHS from birth, so to speak. We've never really got into private care. That was never a thing that we could look at, probably not afford.'

In 2011, aged 53, I started to feel some funny pains in my lower back. I was jogging, as I used to keep fairly fit. I stopped jogging. I thought I was maybe overtraining and I left it for a couple of weeks. One day, probably about 1 a.m. in the morning, the most excruciating pain radiated from my spine, right across my back, down the right side of my leg. I didn't deem it a 999 call. I called my brother, 'Look, can you take me to the A & E?' Long story short – they thought at first it was sciatica. They could not do an MRI because it was something that they said that my doctor had to suggest. So they filled me with drugs – codeine, morphine, etc. Eventually, things started to subside. I left the hospital a few days later. I was back to normal.

Alfred visited his GP on several occasions and eventually was referred for an MRI.

Two weeks later, appointment with my doctor. That's when the news came through. It was awful in many ways, because it was the worst kind of news that you can expect. But for me also, it showed a human side to my doctor. Because my doctor had tears in his eyes when he gave me the diagnosis. Something I've never seen. You could just see the humane aspect of this doctor: 'I'm sorry to tell you, Mr Samuels. It's cancer.' And I didn't cry.

So with that, I was referred to St George's Hospital. Within weeks, I was there with them. I was given the hormone treatment as the introductory aspects of treating the disease. It was then that we found out that it was advanced because, obviously, initially we didn't know. Once we found out that it was advanced, the option for surgery had been removed because they realised it was stage four. The oncologists suggested, 'There is a possibility that you could go on the STAMPEDE trials.'

In 2012 Alfred joined Arm G of the STAMPEDE (Systemic Therapy in Advancing or Metastatic Prostate Cancer: Evaluation of Drug Efficacy) trial, which included a new drug, abiraterone, and injections of Prostap.

The fight started, and the comeback – it's not been easy. It's been a real rocky, hard road. I've never spent the amount of time I spent in hospitals like I've done in the last six years. I was not somebody that complained about illness. Prior to going to my doctor, I had not been to my doctor in four years, which also suggested to me that on my side of things, that was probably a big mistake. I knew the history of our family. I always say this to people, I was so busy making a living, I forgot how to live, and my whole health suffered as a result of that. I lost my mother to breast cancer in 1983. Six months later, her sister died of cancer. Five years later, their brother, my uncle, died of prostate cancer. I was definitely at risk, without a doubt. Here I am now, luckily. There is no remission for me, that's been made plain and clear. I accept that. However, it's managed. But it's baffling them. It's baffling them because I'm still on the same drug. So, we shall see. Watch this space, as they say!

I kept a diary of what I was going through on a daily basis just for my own purposes. I thought to myself, 'Why don't I write a book?' Because when I looked out there, there was nothing written from a personal perspective. The book was called *Invincibility in the Face of Prostate Cancer*. It was about my journey. How I felt, the medication I was taking, how my life was panning out, the side effects, the pain that was still going on. A couple of years later, I wrote another book, *Motivated to Inspire*. Everybody who's read it have said, 'Spot on. You said what we couldn't say.'

I'm educating myself as I go along. I'm starting now to see the real issues that are out there. Right now, we do not have a national screening programme for prostate cancer. But the issues are that the PSA [prostate-specific antigen] test is flawed. The finger test [physical examination of prostate] is flawed. So if those are flawed, you can't have a national screening test. Until we get those sorted out, we can't have a national screening programme. The big issue is that, unfortunately, I fall into an ethnicity that are at higher risk. When you look at the statistics, one in four Black men,

Afro-Caribbean men, will fall prey to prostate cancer at some stage in their life, as opposed to one in eight in the general population. That is a ratio of two to one. That is not satisfactory at all.

We have a wonderful organisation in the NHS. We have something the world basically sits back in awe at. It's 'going down the Swanee', as they say, and we – the government and Joe Public – have got to get together and get this sorted. Once you've gone through my diagnosis, or a life-threatening illness, you will start to understand that if we go another route and that route is private, there are going to be a lot more dead people out there. Because how are you going to afford it? When I look at the cost of my medication – you'd be astounded at what it costs. I thought to myself, 'If I was anywhere else in this world, I'd be dead.' So what does that tell you? We've got a wonderful system. The nurses, the doctors, they don't have to do this job. Because it's not a thankful job, for sure. We have a group of people who, day in, day out, try to and help people. I think they need to sit down all political parties, all the people involved and sort this out. Because we have something that is the envy of the world. There is no 'ifs'. There is no 'buts'. But if we do not sort this out, there is going to be a bigger problem. I'll tell you that now.

Since his interview in March 2018, Alfred has continued to advocate. In 2019 he was ambassador of the year at the Cancer Research UK Flame of Hope Awards and, in April 2022, won an Outstanding Achievement Award from the World Film Carnival in Singapore for his film, A Survivor Amongst Survivors, *which is available on YouTube.*

MAXINE BALL

Maxine grew up with her family in Glasgow. She had issues with alcohol and drugs through her twenties and things became progressively worse.

I had a normal upbringing for growing up in Partick, Glasgow, in the seventies. Both my parents were alcoholics, which at that time made no difference because everybody else's mum and dad did the same thing. We left Glasgow and relocated back to Ayrshire. That was good, but it was a complete change of lifestyle. Coming from the tenement flats in Partick to Saltcoats, the town by the sea, was like a different world. People said good morning to you, people had gardens.

In my twenties I was seeing a CPN [Community Psychiatric Nurse] in my doctor's surgery regularly because there was so much bad happening with my mental health, with my alcohol addiction. Being involved in fights, all that kind of stuff. I had my daughter and my son and didn't see any reason in changing my behaviour because all through this, I still worked. I still paid my taxes. I still felt as if I was a pillar of society because I was still putting in to society. I wasn't your average drunk sitting in the end of the street tying my jacket with laces, so in my head, I thought I was a wee bit better. I had been seeing doctors, nurses, psychiatrists who could not help me remove the void that I felt. There was always something missing, and no medication they gave me, no therapies, no groups, no activities was going to remove this.

When I reached 31, I had a friend who had stopped drinking the year before and her life had changed dramatically. I thought, 'How has she done that? Where has that change come from?' On questioning her, she had stopped drinking. I told myself, 'I am going to try this.' I stayed with her for three months and I got sober. I didn't do it the correct way. I just stopped drinking completely and that is not recognised as doing it in the proper manner. I was practically ill for that three months. I went to AA [Alcoholics Anonymous] meetings. Got myself healthy, got myself back on track. Went back to my doctor and made them aware of what had been going on for the past years. The doctor said, 'That explains so much that has been happening.' She offered me different medications. I thought, 'No, I want to do this with a clear head; I want to be aware of what I am doing.' I have got a fear of being allergic to stuff as well. While my brain was functioning normally, I didn't want to take anything, in case it put me into anaphylactic shock. I carried on seeing my therapist. We went through the CBT, the cognitive behavioural therapy. They took the time with me. We got a lot of stuff out and worked through. In 2008 after a year of remaining sober and drug-free, I enrolled in college. I did social care, then moved to biomedical science. It gave me more awareness of how your body worked, and I sucked that up. I loved it.

Maxine had a traumatic experience having her third child in 2012 because the baby's shoulder became stuck and Maxine didn't want to take pain relief. After the birth the staff noticed that Maxine 'panicked' when she was changing the baby's nappy, and they contacted her CPN.

They kept me in for five days, which nowadays doesn't happen when you are in giving birth. I thought, 'They don't need to do that.' I felt humbled that they took the time to be so nice. It was me who couldn't cope with changing a nappy. For these ladies to recognise that straight away, and be on the phone, and get my CPN and get me involved with the maternity mental health team – that kind of treatment, you don't get that everywhere. I was very grateful to the staff when that happened.

Maxine fell pregnant again, but tragically, Georgia, the baby, was stillborn at 22 weeks.

During her next pregnancy, Maxine was monitored intensively.

They made such a big deal. They sent me to hypnobirthing classes, they put me forward for reflexology. They did anything they could do maintain my calm and to make me worry-free, as such. They put me in the birthing pool. Everything was just so calm and reassuring, and it was textbook. It went to plan from beginning to end. It was such an enjoyable experience, that is my wee George. I kept thinking, 'I want to do something like that, I want to give back. The way these ladies looked after me.' I kept thinking, 'I want to go back and study. I want to do midwifery. I want to do nursing. I want to be able to do something positive.'

It came up by accident. I saw a job advertised on the NHS website for a peer addiction worker, which specified 'lived experience necessary'. I was like, 'Are they talking about lived experience of me? My lived experience?' Then, I am thinking, 'No, nobody wants anybody that has had an addiction issue to work for them.' I read through the application and thought 'I'm going to try this.' In the summary statement, I skirted over the fact that I have got the lived experience and elaborated more on experience with family members.

There were three on the interview panel. 'Tell us a bit about yourself, tell us how you came to be free of your addiction.' I thought, 'Holy shit, they really want me to talk about my addiction. They want somebody with an addiction to work for them.' It blew my mind. I rushed through my life, what had happened and how I had got sober. I went home. They called, 'You were the best applicant, and we wish to offer you the job.' The only thing which is bad about the NHS is the time period. I got the job on 25th May 2017, and I started work on 9th September 2017 as a peer recovery worker.

I knew my co-worker from our AA meetings. The peer worker role was a new role, so he and I made this job our own. We had a job guidance summary, but it was, 'Let's see how it works, let's try this, let's try that.' Nobody really knew how peer workers would work. I now work the Kilmarnock and Cumnock areas. Most of my clients are in active recovery. My job role is to assist and support them. I will accommodate them however they choose to pursue their journey of recovery. If they want to meet me twice a week and have a coffee and talk over how they are feeling, that is fine. I can be there. I will help them if they wish to attend college but don't know where to start because their whole life has been consumed by alcohol or drugs. I will accompany them to appointments, courses and groups.

My clients include people who live in a tent to people who live in quarter-of-a-million-pound houses. I have a great relationship with all my clients. Nothing is off limits. I have a better relationship than most staff because I am not a threat to my clients. I don't have any role with their methadone or cutting medication. I love my job role. I feel I am giving something back. I am able to help. Even though I didn't go down the route of heavy drugs, addiction is addiction. I had that feeling of what they are feeling, and now I don't have that feeling of having to fill a void. I feel that my void is filled and I don't need to actively use to get that feeling. I come to work to get peace from my children nowadays!

Addiction has not got a class. It will affect anybody. It makes no difference who you are or how much money you have got. If addiction is going to take you, it will take you. I have thoroughly enjoyed the interview. I could talk for Scotland.

Maxine would advise anyone thinking of having a career in the NHS to go for it: 'I love my job.'

LISA PETRYSZYN-EDWARDS

Lisa joined the NHS aged 19, working in the Business Service Centre in Swansea at a time of big changes in IT.

I was working on a project, 2DRx, which is for 2D barcodes for prescriptions and rolling that out across Wales. We were looking to go to automatically printing a 2D barcode where you take it to the pharmacist, they scan it, and then you've got all the information there on the computer. It takes away all the risks involved in typing those medications, particularly with the volume of prescriptions that the pharmacists get. That change was very exciting to me.

In 2017 there was a ransomware attack, 'WannaCry', on some NHS England Trusts.

I was senior product specialist for the LIMS [laboratory information management system] at the time. I was accountable for the system across Wales. We had over 100 servers just for that system across a number of environments, all of which are connected to the NHS Wales network. We were very well aware that a number of NHS Trusts in England had instances of this ransomware getting on the machines. We needed to ensure the same didn't happen with us. There was a huge amount of patching, rebooting, keeping record of what had been done, what hadn't been done. If you think 100 servers within one system for LIMS and about 80 national systems, that's a lot of servers. There was a lot of pizza. There was a lot of coffee. It was a lot of pressure because, as the day was going on, we're hearing more and more stories on the news about more organisations that were at risk. It was a massive piece of work to identify which machines needed the patch against WannaCry to prevent a ransomware attack.

Lisa moved into cybersecurity in 2018.

I've always been excited, a bit geeky about cybersecurity. I thought it'd be a really good opportunity to enhance and develop some of my technical skills in this relatively new role as a senior cybersecurity designer. It allowed me to do more consultant-type work, which helped with the work-life balance with my children. There was a new team set up, and there's a lot of investment going into the team. It was an exciting change to work with the health boards in Wales, because I think it's extremely important that we have strong links and networks in there.

I look at any new projects or any new or existing IT services where there's a big change. I work with a product specialist, the developers or the technical architects to really understand what is being delivered, what they're looking to achieve, how it's been hosted, whether the IT system is being hosted within one of our [NHS Wales] data centres, whether it's going to be hosted by a third-party supplier, or in the cloud. I work with them to define the security controls to ensure that the patient data, staff data, is kept secure, whilst balancing usability.

It's always a balance between security against usability, so that you have good controls in place, but not to the point where things are locked down, where you can't access information or it's so slow that you're not going to be able to use the system.

It can be very challenging because I think a lot of the time as a security person, you want to lock things down. You can't do that because systems won't be used. You can't exchange data from one system to another. You've constantly got to think about how we can mitigate the risk.

It takes a lot of money to invest in cybersecurity, particularly when you have things like security incident and event management [SIEM] systems – they're very expensive. Again, it's balance. We look at what the risk is as opposed to the cost. But I'm a taxpayer. I think if this was my money, how would I spend it? You have to think wisely in all of the decisions that you make because we're working in a public-sector organisation. You think about, 'If I waste this money here, how many nurses would that be?' I'm very mindful of that at all times.

The challenges are keeping up with the level of threat. Every day, there are new cybersecurity vulnerabilities all over the World Wide Web. You're getting more groups developing viruses and enjoying putting these out on the internet. Patient data has to be secure. There has to be confidence that data isn't going to be accessible by anybody else, isn't going to be stolen and sold. It's very sensitive data that's being held, so it's a massive challenge to keep up and understand what threats are out there. Because of the amount of infrastructure and applications we've got, being able to respond to patching those machines in a timely manner to prevent breakdowns in data security is always difficult to manage, and I think that will become greater as time moves on.

I've seen huge improvements. Personally, I've gone to an out-of-hours setting, seen clinicians log in, see my children's data and then be able to prescribe the right medications. I've gone into a secondary-care setting and seen clinicians log in to the Welsh Clinical Portal, view all of my tests and results, view my images. Ten years ago, that wasn't available. They'd be logging into multiple systems, pulling paper from drawers. I went to see a locum who was new in the area. I was able to say, 'Oh, if you log in here …' and he viewed the scan immediately.

I feel like I've been given masses of opportunity. I still wish I was a dancer [*laughs*], if I'm completely honest. But I would never have been able to perceive that this is what I'd be doing, particularly in cybersecurity. I'm very happy to be doing what I'm doing. I dance in the evenings instead. The relationships that I've built working here have been fantastic. And it's given me that sense of pride so I can say to my children, 'Mummy helped with that.'

Lisa now works in cybersecurity outside the NHS.

COLIN ANDERSON

'My actual name is Keith but I'm always called Colin. It's a pet name, but many of us from the West Indies, especially from Jamaica, have these names that we're known by.' Colin joined the Blood Transfusion Service in South London in 1982 after leaving school.

I joined as a medical laboratory scientific officer and, over the years, qualified as a biomedical scientist. In those days you rotated through different disciplines within the Blood Service. We had the blood products laboratory, where you make the products from the blood that came in, through to the viral testing and the group testing of those blood donations. Then there was specialist areas that we called the 'reference laboratory' back then. If the hospital blood banks had difficulties cross-matching the donor blood with the patient's blood, they'd send it back to our reference laboratory. The laboratory would investigate what the problem was, what the antibodies were, what the serological issues were, and then provide compatible blood for people who had antibodies, etc. The antenatal side of it was when mothers with unborn babies would make antibodies which could impact the development of the baby. We would measure the level of the antibodies and give advice about what was best to do to safeguard the baby.

In the 1990s I worked in the Red Cell Immunohaematology services. That involved identifying very rare antibodies and going up and down the country to find compatible donors. In South London we had one of the most diverse set of blood donors. We'd be sending very rare units of blood across the country and also take part in international exchanges of blood. Looking back on it, I fitted in with the culture, fitted in with how things were done. The first 25 years of my working life were laboratory-focused in the testing of blood. That gave me the foundation of investigating and doing things thoroughly because any mistake in your transcription, or writing it down wrong, could have severe impact. The analytical side of my brain was really boosted.

In 1999 Colin took on an unpaid role in the union.

I said, 'I could do it.' I was involved in church life. I was aware of how committees worked, and procedure was what I knew. I'm a person who has a sense of equity: that every person has a right to be heard. For me it was a matter of two parties meeting and coming to an understanding. I was never the type of rep that banged the table. I was very much into people being heard and finding a resolution. I avoided conflict. There may be a difference of opinion, but it doesn't have to descend into conflict.

Agenda for Change was an NHS policy introduced in 2004 to harmonise grading and pay across the NHS, with the exception of doctors, dentists and some senior managers. Pay had previously been determined for each occupation.

In 2004/5 we had the big issue of Agenda for Change. The NHS Blood and Transfusion service [NHSBT] had become a national body by then. It was decided that all biomedical scientists across the board would go over to the same terms and conditions and, more importantly, the same broad reach of job descriptions. You can imagine 6,500 to 7,000 people across the country – trying to get them into the same sweep of job descriptions was very difficult. Every region, every centre did things very differently. NHSBT set up a team and I was elected to the staff side. I became full-time in 2005/6. We were undergoing a massive period of organisational change. Essentially, reconfigurations. What reconfigurations means is that there would be closures and reconsolidation of services. So that was going to be a difficult time. Because we worked so well during Agenda for Change, they wanted to use the same working model for the reorganisation. So I went from being a part-time rep in 1999 to working full-time as a senior rep and a national rep, working alongside the executive. I learnt that change was constant. But change is one thing, as human beings, we don't like. So how we introduce change is important, and often more important than the change itself.

In 2014 Colin decided he needed to move on, and became the diversity engagement manager in NHS Blood and Transplant, managing a team across England.

Development courses encouraged him to think differently about the role he could play as a Black leader.

I learnt so much about my currency as a Black man and recognising I was in leadership roles. I had done what I had because I enjoyed it. But now I was viewing myself through a different lens, as a leader with currency, and thinking about how those coming up behind me can maximise their potential. I'd seen a lot of African Caribbean colleagues not developing in the way I knew they could. They were still stuck in lower-paid roles, whether as a scientist or non-professional. It became apparent: if you can help people unlock their potential, it can deliver vast improvements in the work environment and have significant impact on patients.

Colin had always been deeply involved with the church through music – his parents had insisted the children learnt to read and write music. Colin had run community choirs since the early 2000s, including Birmingham Town Hall Gospel Choir which had won the BBC's Songs of Praise *competition. But he'd always kept work and music separate, even though his colleagues had encouraged him to develop a choir at work.*

In 2017 they came back to me. 'We want you on board. We've teamed up with MOBOs [Music Of Black Origin music awards] and we want a choir to sing at the awards in November and then make a single for the Christmas charts.' I realised this is a calling I can't run from. The choir would give a platform to attract young Black people to be blood donors.

We got the choir together, chose the name – B Positive – and delivered. In November we sang for the MOBOs. We invited a great gospel singer to be our lead vocalist. It went off really well. Carting around 50 to 60 people was a logistical nightmare. But people started talking about sickle cell and about blood donation. I worked my butt off to get the single recorded and produced: 'Rise Up', featuring Lurine Cato. As far as I was concerned, that was it. But in December, whilst I was in Birmingham, the B Positive choir sang carols in St Pancras station. Somebody said, 'Have you thought about doing *Britain's Got Talent?*'

Long story short, one of the managers said to me, 'If we get to the first televised stage, the message goes out to millions of viewers ...' 'Fair enough, guv.', I thought. So we started *Britain's Got Talent* in 2018, and that was an absolute whirlwind eight months. It was pressure. It was fun. We got through to the semi-finals and our website crashed. It was a good problem to have.

It meant the message was getting out there. We were blessed to get through into the finals. The message carried all the way through. At the end of 2018, I was like, 'Breathe ...'

I never thought in a million years I'd be working with NHSBT and doing something called marketing. B Positive is the standout moment because it brought all the sides of my life together. Before that, I compartmentalised my life. As a young Black man growing up, as a Jamaican growing up, as a churchman growing up. All those different parts of me, I compartmentalised. I never brought them into the workplace. It was never the thing to do. It was too much hassle. It all came to a head in 2017/18, where I was able to live my best life because I was bringing my whole life into the workplace.

The main challenges have been me not fulfilling my full potential as a biomedical scientist in terms of studying and moving up. That was down to a lack of confidence in myself. And to me acquiescing to the culture that exists. NHS is so hierarchical. In your laboratories, your biomedical sciences, it is so hierarchical, and it continues to this day. It's really shocking. It's one of the things that saddens me the most about the NHS, not just BTS. We refer to each other, not by our roles, not by what we do, but by our pay bands. That is awful. It continues to this day. It really saddens me. As a Black man, you know, when I look back, I see how I just had my eyes 'closed wide shut', as they say, to seeing how that impacted me. How I just went along with things. I allowed that to happen. Part of my legacy is to open up people's eyes, especially my BAME colleagues, through coaching. It's opening up people to the idea that they don't have to stay; they can think bigger, and it's systems and people that are making them suppressed. I should have stood up and spoken out loud.

But that's where this compartmentalising, for me, worked. I didn't get the full satisfaction from work. But I was enjoying myself outside. Playing squash. Doing music. Coaching and mentoring is key for me. Now the narrative is out there. We don't talk about diversity engagement anymore. We talk about inclusion. Too often, we've allowed ourselves to be trodden on and never challenged it. I wish I had started challenging a lot sooner in my career because it saves and improves lives. I encourage my NHS colleagues to be brave. To have those uncomfortable conversations. There's no blaming. Just acknowledgement that what was done before needs to change. If we don't, then the youngsters coming into the NHS now will not stand for it. They won't necessarily shout. They'll just walk away and we won't have the right people to deliver the service. One of my mottos is based on the mythical Sankofa bird from Ghana. The bird that's flying into the future bringing the pearls of the past with them. We have to learn from the past and bring ourselves into the future.

Colin retired in 2021. 'I absolutely am looking forward to the future. But I'm giving myself time and space to breathe.'

JOANNE HARDING

Joanne's first experience of Trafford Park Hospital was helping take newspapers and sweets round to patients on the wards. In 2004 she gave birth to her daughter there.

My midwife who facilitated all the antenatal classes, Greta Young, was just brilliant. I remember saying to my husband, 'I really hope Greta is my midwife when I go into labour.' She inspired confidence and assurance. When I did start in labour, they had to induce me, which was something I didn't want to happen, but anyway, it did. It was a nice, personal little maternity ward. Really clean, comfortable. The staff were great. I started in labour and it was pretty awful. Next thing, this midwife popped her head around the curtain and it was Greta. I thought to myself, 'Wow, I feel really lucky that it's her.' She said, 'Oh, I recognise you, you're the little one that's always smiling.' I was thinking, 'I'm not smiling now.' She was absolutely brilliant. I had a horrible, horrible labour that culminated in me having to have an emergency caesarean section. They said, 'We've got five minutes to get this baby out.' That's when panic set in, in me. I remember saying to the anaesthetist, 'Oh, I'm not going to see my baby.' He said, 'You'll be fine but we have to knock you out.' Then waking up in recovery. Seeing my baby wrapped up in a Trafford General towel, like orphan Annie. Really fantastic treatment from the maternity services.

The campaign I was involved in 2010/11 was called 'Save Trafford General' and that was around the A & E. There was lots of rumours flying around that Trafford was no longer financially viable. It had a huge deficit and, as a trust on its own, it wasn't sustainable. I started doing lots of delving and reading and researching and looking about how the deficit had come about. And of course, when you lose things like paediatrics and maternity services, the income goes, then the hospital starts to struggle. So there were issues as to why deficits built up. At that time, I was a member of the Labour Party, and I got more involved in local politics. When I got elected as a local councillor in May 2011, I set the hares running. I thought, 'I'm going to use my position as an elected member to get answers to questions. This is a public service. And I want to know and understand what the future of this hospital is.'

I was known for doing a bit of questioning, and there'd been some press activity, as the *Manchester Evening News* ran a story: 'Newly elected councillor starts campaign'. I had staff approaching me with leaked documents that evidenced there was going to be significant changes and that A & E wasn't part of it. It was going to be an Urgent Care Centre, which is very different to an A & E. I leaked that document as well. I thought, 'Well we need to know what's going on.' I went on record and said, 'I've no regrets about doing that at all.' I then got a position on the Health Scrutiny Committee. I think they probably thought, 'Oh, God.'

Health Scrutiny is a body that scrutinises all the health provision across Trafford, and it does have constitutional rights. It's part of the council function. I used both roles as a way of saying what's happening.

I was actually a Labour councillor leading the Save Trafford General campaign, but it wasn't a Labour campaign. It was a community campaign. As things progressed, both Wythenshawe university teaching hospital and Central Manchester Foundation Trust put in a bid to acquire Trafford. I went to public meetings and again, it was a case of, 'Well, if you get the hospital, are you going to guarantee to keep services?' Both of them fudged it. 'Well, we'd need to review... blah, blah, blah'. Anyway, Central Manchester University Hospitals NHS Foundation Trust acquired the hospital and they held a public meeting in a local church. That was very busy. Lots of staff came along expressing concerns and, at that point, UNISON, the union, was involved, but there were some contentious issues with that, really.

The detail started to come out, that yes, they were going to close A & E. But they presented all the statistics, and decided 'We're going to close it from midnight till eight in the morning.' So those were the first changes, because 'The footfall shows that people just aren't using this facility. There's no point having these consultants, you know, if nobody's going to use it.' It wasn't just A & E that went, though. A brand-new intensive care unit that had had a million-pound investment – that was closing too, and the paediatric observation assessment unit closed too, because they are all interdependent with an A & E. There's all these co-dependencies within the hospital setting, and you can't have one without the other. It meant that if we lost one, the others have to go too. It's a significant chunk of services, the acute care that went from Trafford, so we just played merry hell.

I thought to myself, 'So what happens to a Trafford resident who has a heart attack?' 'What happens if there's a match on and you've got to get an ambulance through traffic, if Manchester United are playing at home?' You know, we're close to the airport, we're close to the Trafford Centre, the M60 services, all of that. Why would you remove an A & E from this? We were told that we're in a luxurious position because where we are positioned geographically, we had A & Es at Wythenshawe, Salford and Manchester, so we don't need Trafford. We went to every one of the public meetings and asked lots of questions. We started a petition in 2012. People were queuing to sign this petition. We had a website, we did little vox pops and videos of people telling their stories. Because everybody's got a story to tell about the hospital, about how the A & E has been there for them. The community were really engaged by this campaign. We did a lot and then we had a march. The march was amazing. I don't think any of us in the campaign imagined it would be this big. It was the birthday of the NHS, 5 July, and, of course, Trafford General is where it all began. It started at Golden Hill Park in Trafford and we passed the hospital, we walked through the hospital grounds and the staff came out cheering as we did that. Then we went back to Golden Hill Park for a rally. We easily had 1,000 people marching through Urmston. It was incredible. It's a boiling-hot day, absolutely boiling. Since then, I do a party every year for the NHS on Golden Hill Park.

Well, of course, they closed those services. We put up a really good fight, but they did concede some ground in that the out of hours became an urgent care centre. I've used the urgent care centre a couple of times since and it's a fantastic facility. They've got the walk-in centre and the urgent care centre. You go in one door, you're triaged and you'll go one way to the GP and all the way to urgent care. Brilliant treatment when I've used that facility, but I think now the pressure is on just to absolutely make sure that we don't lose anything else.

Joanne is now chair of the Age Well Board in Trafford, leading a campaign to raise awareness of benefits available to older people suffering from the cost-of-living crisis.

PUNAM KRISHAN

Punam grew up in a Glasgow tenement flat with her extended family.

There were about 12 of us living in our two-bedroom flat. The moment that really struck, and still sits deep inside, is when my grandfather had a heart attack and passed after that. It was our GP, Dr Cossor, that picked the pieces up. My family fell apart. My grandfather was a really important head of our family, our community. My GP did a home visit and he sat with my gran, my parents. It felt like hours. I haven't really thought about that moment until talking to you right now, but it was that sense that your doctor is there for life and they do care.

I wanted to be a neonatologist. I absolutely looked up to this consultant neonatologist who had the ability to wear scrubs and six-inch heels to absolutely every situation – cardiac arrest, you name it, she was always there looking fabulous. Brains and beauty. I did a placement in paediatrics. I loved working with children and families, but the first death of a baby on the unit was just far too much for me to handle. 'Okay, this isn't really for me, but how else can I still make a big difference to children and families?', I thought to myself. General practice was the perfect answer. At the back of me was always Dr Cossor, and a feeling that I wanted to be part of people's stories from birth to the end.

A typical day in general practice is crazy. And I love it because it's crazy. No two days are ever the same, no two patients are ever the same, no two scenarios will ever be the same, and that is just exciting as it can be. I will have a surgery in the morning, and that usually starts somewhere between half eight and nine, depending on days that I can coordinate getting my son to school. It will be 15 to 20 patients that I will see face to face. In between that, you have special requests, so that's repeat prescriptions to sign, you have referrals, so if somebody needs a further assessment in hospital you need to do the referral for that, so that's letters that we would be dictating after our consultations have finished. We get correspondences from the hospital, so you can have anything up to 100 and 120 letters from the hospital that you need to action. You have your blood results for all the times you've told your patients that they need to go get their bloods done, and then they arrive in your inbox. So you have multiple inboxes open in front of you. And once surgery finishes there may be one or two or more home visits for the frail and elderly, housebound patients. Usually you get an hour between the two surgeries. Some practices differ – sometimes you can get two hours between a morning clinic and an afternoon clinic, but that time is often spent doing home visits or all the other paperwork. Then you do the same in the afternoon, and you pray every day that you'll finish on time and every day you're not surprised that you did not even come close to it. But I absolutely love everything that happens in general practice. I firmly believe that you, the doctor, can also be the medicine – and I'm a big believer of social prescribing, which is not every patient needs a pill. What we need to be doing is empowering people to take a step back and start looking at the root cause of their problems.

Nine times out of ten, it's down to the way that they're living their lives or the lifestyle choices that they're making. Or 90 per cent of the time it's stress because of the pace of lifestyle. As a GP you have this overview of not just the patient, but sometimes you're fortunate to have the rest of their family as your patients. You can plant a seed somewhere to really help inspire them to want to change. I think that magic never leaves, and you get to do that every 10 minutes. Yeah, that's right, we do get only 10 minutes per patient, which I never stick to. I think that when you know that you've just lit a light bulb in somebody's head and you know that you've helped them make a change or make a choice to change the progression of their lifestyle in a way that can actually prevent them from being ill one day, I don't think anything comes close to the exhilaration that you feel.

All of these interests led me to join in the British Society of Lifestyle Medicine, of which I am now a director and trustee. We are a charity but our mission is to help empower the public and healthcare professionals to look at lifestyle medicine in a greater context and to start focusing more on prevention of disease rather than simply curing disease. I came across NLP, neurolinguistic programming, which was the study of the mind. I was never taught about the mind at medical school. Not about understanding the way that the mind works, both on a conscious and subconscious level.

Neurolinguistic programming taught me, over a seven-day course, about understanding the parallels of the subconscious and conscious mind and how can we use certain techniques to break habits. To help people stop smoking or stop fearing certain things, and really empowering them to go forward and take their life into their own hands, for the better.

I've had patients who have really healed themselves, and they've not required countless drugs. I've had patients where we've managed to get them off long-term drugs. I've had patients where we've managed to put their Type 2 diabetes into remission through diet and exercise. When you get that thrill at the end of every day, there's no wonder that you want to go back the next day. Maybe I'm addicted to general practice; I might need to see an NLP practitioner for this.

One of my personal big moments was that I hit a burnout point two years ago. So after I had my son five years ago, I took up a partnership, and I joined a practice where there was just the two of us and we were responsible for three and a half thousand patients. At the time, I guess I was fairly newly qualified as a GP and I thought that the only option was to be a partner, where you were in charge of the business and it was your responsibility: the premises, the staff, the business side of it, as well as the patient care. I think what happened was it was far too much to juggle all of that and we didn't have a practice manager. We were two GPs running a 3,500-patient practice.

There came this pivotal moment where I was on holiday in Turkey, on a beach, sitting down, trying to engage in a conversation with my family and friends, and I was ordering toilet paper for the practice. I thought, 'This is not why I became a doctor.' That was a huge moment where I realised, 'I want to be a GP. All I want to do is help my patients. I do not wish to negotiate and fight over contracts. I do not have the headspace or, actually, the knowledge and skill to manage businesses on such a scale.'

I left my partnership and now I'm what we call a portfolio GP, which means I locum [provide temporary assistance]. I locum four days a week and I work predominantly between three practices, because continuity of care is really important to me. It means that I turn up, I see my patients, I do all the jobs in and round my patients and I get to leave at the end of the day not worrying about what will happen if the alarm goes off in the building tonight, because I can just about manage that in my own home.

I was really moved by the exhibition put on by the Royal College of General Practitioners on the immigrant doctors that made the NHS in 2018. It still makes me emotional. I walked through the exhibition and looked at these incredible immigrant doctors. The amount of challenges they must have faced in order to keep slogging away and believing in the National Health Service, because this wasn't something that was available to them back in their own countries. I saw a picture of Dr Cossor, can you believe it? 'Oh my God, that's my doctor.' He definitely was somebody who made the NHS because he made me and my little sister, who is also a GP in Glasgow, want to grow up to work the way that he worked.

I'm really proud to be a Scottish-Indian. To all those that asked me to get the boat back home, I say, 'Can you tell me how I get a boat back to the west end of Glasgow? Because that's where I live.' Recently, I had a case where a patient refused to register with our practice because they didn't want 'that Asian doctor'. Thankfully, my badass receptionist, who – you just don't mess with her – turned round and said, 'But she's Scottish.' The patient went, 'She doesn't look Scottish,' and my receptionist went, 'Well, what do Scottish people look like?' I have never been more proud of somebody as I was in that moment. Not just because it was my receptionist standing shoulder to shoulder with me, but also showing me that we are a team. That patient did register with us, did come and see me, was delighted with the outcome, and apologised profusely for having that judgement.

In 2022 Punam published her first children's book, How to Be a Doctor and Other Life-Saving Jobs.

At the end of the 2010s

The NHS enjoyed two extraordinary high points during the 2010s. It was showcased in the opening ceremony for the London 2012 Olympic Games, created by Danny Boyle. Featured alongside other iconic aspects of British history, NHS staff participated in the extravaganza, which attracted huge interest from a global audience. It was an emotional and compelling visualisation of the depth of public feeling for the NHS. In 2018, the NHS seventieth anniversary was commemorated with a year-long programme of events ranging from fun runs to tea parties to thanksgiving services in Westminster and York Abbeys. Ethel Armstrong, with her lifetime of work and support for the NHS, became the face of the celebrations, challenging politicians and leaders alike with her quick wit and common sense.

But the high public satisfaction with the NHS that resulted from the New Labour reforms during the late 1990s and early 2000s did not protect it from yet another reorganisation. One of the most disruptive factors during the decade was further reform of NHS structures and processes. Andrew Lansley was appointed health secretary in the 2010 Conservative-Liberal Democrat coalition government. Since the 2000s he had been working on a major reorganisation of the NHS. Huge efforts were made by the NHS and the professions to resist these changes, and they seemed particularly unnecessary at a time when there had been measurable improvements reflected in the public ratings. The Health and Social Care Act 2012 has been described as 'the messiest reorganisation the NHS had ever undergone'.[15] In short, the reforms intensified commercialisation and competition within the NHS and, by 2014, Conservative MPs were going on record saying the reforms were 'our worst mistake'. Before the decade was out, further reforms introduced the idea of integrated care systems in England, which created new partnerships of NHS organisations, local government and the voluntary sector. It was a further attempt to address some of the weaknesses inherent in the NHS since 1948, especially the connection between health and social care.

The decade drew to a close with reports of a new coronavirus emerging in China. Few could have anticipated that the NHS would be brought into the eye of the storm as never before.

Chapter 9: 2020s

'... I did webinars with the guys from Wuhan and the guys from Italy. That was really important to understand the scale of this.'

NICK HART

'... we are at our best when we care for others.'

KLARISSA VELASCO

'That was the first patient I intubated
and he subsequently went on to die.'

AMIT PAWA

'... I'm actually in the hotel across the road. I took myself
away from my family a week before the lockdown.'

ARCHIE FINDLAY

"... this morning I got up, expecting to do some dentistry,
and suddenly, I'm standing in a theatre and a
baby's being delivered in front of me."

PRITI ACHARYA

'There was a feeling of huge responsibility to present honestly, and with integrity, the results of the studies in as transparent way as possible.'

ANDREW POLLARD

'I always want to be humble, becuse I'm doing it for the nurses, the paramedics, the doctors, the dentists, the people that are actually on the frontline.'

CLAIRE GOODWIN-FEE

'… it was good that we had that long prayer session because that's what the family needed.'

YUNUS DUDHWALA

'Thank God for the NHS. I'm proud of being part of the NHS.'

RACHEL LEWIS

'The care bit is much more important than delivering the treatment. That will stay with me for the rest of my life.'

GRANT MCINTYRE

'I've been involved in pandemic planning for years, and we always thought of it being a gradual build-up. But for us, it was like a storm hit.'

KATIE TOMKINS

'There is no point in us being amazing at vaccination in the UK if we then don't vaccinate the poorer countries across the world that don't have the resources that we have.'

ALICE WISEMAN

*'I want to be someone who champions the things
that patients really care about.'*

GEORGINA BOND

'So, yes, I'm getting better. But it feels glacial in its speed.'

PETER JULIAN

*"... we could have predicted – based on what we already
know about disease trends – that Covid would have a
disproportionate impact on minority communities.'*

PATRICIA MILLER

*'I keep saying to everybody, "I've got the easy part.
I'm at home, I'm safe.'"*

NATALIE PARR

*'... if we're going to have any data-gathering on this catastrophic
event, and a massive change to patient experience ...
it needs to be as widespread and as diverse as it possibly can be.'*

DEB TROOPS

*'The energy and intelligence and determination that goes about
bringing our healthcare system together is miraculous.'*

JONNY EMMS

NICK HART

Director of respiratory and critical care medicine at Guy's and St Thomas', Nick was in no doubt about the contribution of NHS staff: 'The talent of this institution is beyond a shadow of a doubt, from senior leadership to people working on the ground – that includes all our housekeeping and domestic staff, who have been phenomenal. Everyone has taken a view that we'll get through this.'

On January 8th, 2020, I was in Beijing lecturing. That is when the story broke about the isolation of a novel coronavirus which was identified from the Chinese government by the World Health Organization [WHO] on 31st December 2019. Being in Beijing at that time, it struck a very big chord straightaway.

I followed all the data coming out of China at that stage, really to try and understand what this was and what it was going to potentially do. We've been told by our infectious diseases and virology doctors constantly that Armageddon is coming. We'd seen SARS CoV-1 [Severe acute respiratory syndrome], we'd seen MERS [Middle East Respiratory Syndrome]. Guy's and St Thomas' was under significant pressure with H1N1 swine flu 2009. The interesting part of that is I remember the working together. The idea of everybody working as a team, and everybody with a 'can-do' attitude to looking after patients. That lasted quite a short period of time – three to four weeks. But it was a period of time with significant numbers of patients coming to the ICU, significant numbers of serious decisions being made in the ED [emergency department] about whether patients should be escalated or not.

I flew back on the 10th January, and I was following the high-impact journals. They did a good job. They just got data out. In late February I did webinars with the guys from Wuhan and the guys from Italy. That was really important to understand the scale of this. Stefano Nava, professor of respiratory and critical care, University of Bologna, who's based in Northern Italy, was really helpful. I could see in his face how difficult this was, and I've known him for 15, 20 years. They were just about holding in there. That's when we started discussion about the disease. What it was, what it was doing and how you were going to treat it. So you're trying to interpret this in terms of physiology. At that stage it was a viral pneumonia. The older folk were coming in and would have a relatively slow deterioration and become increasingly unwell and require ventilatory support. The younger folk coming through, 55 years or even younger, had a condition where they could be sitting reading the paper in the morning, and the afternoon, they needed intubating. Stefano said, 'It's a very rapid condition.' He goes, 'Nick, we've run out of intensive care beds. We don't have them. We've moved to using CPAP [continuous positive airway pressure] machines.' He said, 'The reason we went to using CPAP is because you can't use anything more than that outside of the ICU or HDU [high dependency unit]. We're doing it on neurology ward, we're doing it on gastroenterology ward, we're doing it everywhere.'

That was really powerful and striking to me. We had an intervention in a condition we didn't really know that produced acute respiratory failure, that seemed to give a one in two chance of being successful. This is observational data, and you've got to be really careful. Probably the second week in March I said, 'Guys, I'm coming off Twitter. Everything's a bit too busy at the moment.' I was trying to get as much information out there in terms of what this disease process was.

The first Covid patient was early on and I bagged them. I went, 'This isn't ARDS [acute respiratory distress syndrome]. This is a nasty inflamed lung that we've got to treat with kid gloves.' It was that understanding, and also the patients were so hot. Nobody had said, 'Oh, by the way, they're all going to be 41 degrees.' Incredible this part of it had got lost in translation.

I posted on Twitter on the 29th March 2020. I said, 'Covid-19 was this generation's polio.' What I meant by that is we need to make sure we look after the folk who survive, because the polio survivors were not looked-after. I've looked after polio survivors for 16 years and people were not looked-after well. It's our responsibility to make sure we do better, and we look after their cognitive, psychological and physical issues as they arise or they have arisen. I'm really keen that we see that we've got through this part, and the next part is going to be equally as tough.

Nick is now part of a research initiative to follow up with Covid-19 patients for 25 years.

KLARISSA VELASCO

Klarissa arrived from the Philippines in October 2019 and began work in Southend University Hospital, Essex, as a theatre recovery nurse. Her father had died shortly before she left: 'The grieving process was cut, and then when I was here, it was almost winter and everything was dark and gloomy.' She was fascinated by the NHS and its system of providing healthcare to everybody. 'It was very different from healthcare in the Philippines, and thank God that the work environment I had to walk into was very warm and loving. It was all so supportive, it made it easier for me to adjust.' She was redeployed to the ICU at the start of the pandemic, choosing to do night shifts so she could talk to her family back home during the day. She poured out her experiences in writing and shared it with the project.

'Brave' by Klarissa Velasco

'You have to fight, Andy. Your family's waiting for you outside, love,' I whispered to my patient as clearly as I could muster under the tight protective mask I was wearing while I checked on his temperature for the nth time tonight. Andy is just one of the six intubated patients in our bay inside the ICU, just one of the 100-plus (and counting) Covid-19 positives admitted in our hospital at present. As I was checking his observations, I overheard that they were intubating five more in the Recovery Room – which, ironically, is now part of the Covid-19 'hot area'. Elective surgeries have been cancelled. The OR theatre, once a sterile area, now harbours one of the most treacherous viruses known to man.

I'm an overseas Filipino nurse, one of the thousands who took that gigantic and harrowing leap of faith in search of greener pastures. 'You're such a brave girl,' my British colleagues would often say. And even now, I'm still stumped as to how to respond to that. Because I don't think I'm brave. It was merely a decision born out of necessity. If you're a nurse in the Philippines, I'm sure you'd understand. So here I am, far away from everything I'd ever known – barely navigating my way through this foreign country, its people, and the dreams I set out to fulfil – and now, inevitably, caught in the deadliest line of fire.

It's been two months since our superiors told us we ought to get ready to be uncomfortable. What an understatement that was. Fast forward to today, with me writing this note during my 30-minute break (10 of which I would have to use in donning and doffing a gown and PPE, washing my hands with soap, extra hand gelling – being every bit as careful as I possibly can to ensure I'm not contaminated). These days, the dents of the N-95 mask feel as if they've already become a permanent feature on my face, with the bridge of my nose and the backs of my ears in perpetual agony. It really isn't the most ideal feeling, but how could I dare complain about such trivial inconveniences?

I have to admit I'm scared to die. Petrified. I'm only 28. Haven't made something out of myself yet. Haven't seen enough of the world. Haven't even found the love of my life. I didn't sign up for this. But I know I don't have it in me to give up this particular battle either. Because lying on those beds are someone else's mothers, fathers, brothers, children. And I could only think of my mum, whom I left back home just a week after we buried my dad, how heartbroken she'd be were I to end up dead just because there wasn't anyone brave enough to try to nurse me back to health. She would always be in anguish over the fact that I had died alone. Alone. With nobody there beside me. Because this is what this virus means – that you die in the saddest way possible, leaving a wound in your loved ones' hearts so big it wouldn't ever heal.

So I won't turn my back on these people.

Maybe this is why this profession chose me. It was for this moment in history. It was for one person's life. Maybe I was meant to save Andy. Or maybe I'm meant to just stay beside him and not let him die alone. Either way, after all is said and done, as countless tragedies have consistently proven, we are at our best when we care for others.

Klarissa continues to work in the NHS.

AMIT PAWA

Amit's family moved to the UK from Bangkok, Thailand, a few months after his birth in 1976. His grandfather was a GP in North-West London, so medicine seemed a natural career. His grandfather was keen for Amit to specialise in cardiology but Amit was attracted to anaesthesia because he liked the concept of intensive care. Amit was 'really excited' to secure his first three-year training post in anaesthesia, but his grandfather, who had practised in the days before anaesthesia was fully developed as a speciality, was 'distraught' – he saw anaesthesia as a lower-status speciality. 'The anaesthetist I am today is a culmination of all the skills and techniques I've been exposed to during my training. Anaesthesia is an art.'

It was the anaesthetic department who raised the flag and said, 'We need to stop elective surgery, we need to plan, we need to have increased provisions.' It was a Herculean task to mobilise the workforce and change the working patterns. I knew something was coming, but I didn't realise how much of a change to consultant life it was going to be. Elective lists were scaled down. Outpatients were scaled down. We got new terms introduced into our vocabulary. Donning, doffing, aerosol generating procedures or AGPs, which initially was a little bit scary because I had no idea what they were talking about. But we had a crack team of people who were designing action cards. These involved breaking down every step of procedures that we do every day and also procedures that we were going to start doing into a stepwise manner. Even things as simple as cannulating a patient with full personal protective equipment on was going to be different. I discovered that it's quite difficult to listen to a patient's heart with the stethoscope when you're wearing a full visor and a face mask.

Somebody sat there and watched me put on a gown, gloves and mask. That bit was easy, but removing all of the items in a way that didn't contaminate yourself was actually much harder than I thought. It seemed a little bit surreal. At various points in my life, I thought, 'Someone's having me on here. Is this real?'

I had a choice: working on delivering care in theatres or being part of a specialised team who were going to be putting patients on ventilators, the mobile emergency rapid intubation team (MERIT). I volunteered to be part of the intubation team.

The academic literature supports the idea that the risks of infection are higher for staff involved in those procedures. Why did you step up to something that put you at greater personal risk?

You're asking the same question that my wife asked me when I volunteered. It's difficult to answer. Part of me felt that I was relatively young, fit and healthy. I had a skill set and I could utilise it. I would have hated for there to be a situation where there weren't enough volunteers and so people had to be coerced. It was my choice to do it, but it felt appropriate. I appreciate of all of the jobs, potentially it was one of the higher risks.

It's come to light subsequently that people who come from the Black and Asian minority ethnic groups, which I fall into, are disproportionately affected by Covid-19. So maybe I would have not wanted be included. But if I'm being entirely honest, I think ironically, we were very well protected by virtue of being on the MERIT team. We were given high-quality personal protective equipment. We had short, sharp, albeit high-risk exposures, but then we were able to remove ourselves from the situation. My colleagues who were in intensive care, certainly the nursing staff, who had long periods of time exposed to these patients, had as high, if not a higher, risk.

Our hospital strategy was to intubate patients relatively early. What I mean by that is these patients weren't absolutely on their last legs, for want of a better phrase. These were patients who were critically unwell, who were hypoxic, who had low oxygen levels, but they were still talking. You wouldn't think they were unwell until you looked at their physiological parameters. My first recollection of an intubation was a gentleman who was from Africa. As we walked into the room, he was on the phone to his bank trying to sort out releasing money to deal with his affairs. Seemed a bit odd. I thought, 'Why is he doing this, it's fine, we're going to intubate him, he'll be okay.' But he insisted that we wait for five minutes whilst he made telephone calls. He got his credit card out, he gave a PIN number. Just before we put him off to sleep, he spoke to his nephew. It was on speakerphone and he told his nephew that he loved him. It was bizarre because it almost seems overkill. I thought, 'Why is he doing this, he's going to be okay.' But the fact that he had the presence of mind to think, 'I want to sort my personal affairs out.' That was the first patient I intubated and he subsequently went on to die.

Amit became upset at some points during the interview. 'I think it was important for me to share some of the things that were deep down there. If I hadn't had a chance to talk about that, I might have walked away without getting tearful. But it's felt very good to do this.'

ARCHIE FINDLAY

Archie came to the UK from Jamaica at the end of the 1960s. He joined Guy's and St Thomas' NHS Foundation Trust in 2019 as a porter after working in the decorating and building trades. 'I wished I actually was in this maybe 10 years ago, because I just love it.'

In the beginning I thought, 'It's just portering.' But actually doing it, I realise it's more than being a porter. Every day to day we have to interact with patients. Sometimes you go and pick up a patient you're taking to theatre. You can see that they're stressed and worried. I just communicate with them. There are a few patients that I've handled and they come in for their check-up and they go, 'Oh, you pushed me to theatre, I remembered you.' You meet so much different cultures and nationalities. It's just amazing to work in there.

I'm based in operating theatres Monday to Fridays, 10 till six. If I'm doing bank, covering gaps, I could end up anywhere. In theatre, even though you work all over the place, you interact with patients. It's more intimate. We could move up to 20 different patients and you've got basically 20 different conversations. Some patients might not converse with you, but you still converse with the nurse and it's always different.

At the moment, I'm actually in the hotel across the road. I took myself away from my family a week before the lockdown, maybe two weeks before lockdown. Basically about 20-odd miles away from my family. The accommodation in the hotel across the road – I've been in it for nearly six weeks. I've got a three-year-old granddaughter who's got asthma. My mum will be 93 in October. So, for their health, I took myself away from them before they put the lockdown on, and I've been away from them ever since.

I'm out of the hotel by nine o'clock – not that I need to be here at nine, because my shift hasn't started. Once I wake up and have breakfast, I come over here because over the last seven weeks this has been my family, you know. If I have to do an early shift, that's when I find a problem. It's from six till two in the afternoon, and then I've got the whole day. The lockdown, you can't go nowhere, and you're in this room all by yourself. My daughter, my granddaughter, that is the most heartbreaking thing. I go there, my three-year-old granddaughter and my seven-year-old grandson, they want to run and come and hug me, and I have to stop them, 'No, you can't.' I walk away with tears in my eye. When I used to go home from work, I'd be in the room watching TV, my grandson would run, come jump on the bed, and sit and say, 'Oh, Grandad, can I watch TV?' All them things that you miss, even though it's for a short while, but you do miss them. Because that was an everyday part of my life. And right now it's, to be honest, like I'm homeless. I really feel homeless. That's that.

Archie was interviewed in May 2020 at the height of the first wave of the pandemic.

PRITI ACHARYA

Priti grew up in Mombasa, Kenya, and came to the UK aged 16 to study for her A levels. Her father was a doctor and advised Priti to become a dentist so that she could control her working hours. But Priti disliked the thought of dentistry until she did work experience.

I fell in love with dentistry within half an afternoon! I realised the things that I associate with dentistry are not true. What I saw was people coming in and letting a virtual stranger into a very personal space and handing over immediate trust, which is such a privilege in itself. I realised that it's so artistic and it's a long-term relationship you build with people. Nowadays, we don't use harsh products and chemicals at the dentist so it doesn't smell half as bad as it used to.

Since 2013 Priti has worked as a specialist orthodontist at the Eastman Dental Hospital, part of University College London Hospitals NHS Foundation Trust.

I look at the NHS and I think we are so blessed to have it in this country. I think you work exceptionally hard as an NHS general dentist and you have to be very efficient at what you do. You're doing so much good for so many people. Most people do a mixture of NHS and private dentistry because they want to be able to offer more than they can do on the NHS, and they want to be able to give their patients more time and do excellent-quality dentistry as opposed to good-quality basic dentistry.

I'm an NHS consultant, so I work within the hospital services in orthodontics for the NHS and I'm in private practice outside that, so I think I have the best of both worlds. In the hospital I do all sorts of things that you would rarely get the opportunity to do in practice. You work with so many different specialists in a big teaching hospital such as Eastman Dental Hospital, and every day is different. Your mind is challenged every day. Sometimes you come home and your brain actually hurts. I love my job.

I always ask every patient, 'Was it worth it?' That's the phrase I will use. 'Was it worth it?' Because they have very long courses of treatment, some of them spanning eight years, sometimes longer, because of the complexity of what they have done. Every single patient has looked me in the eye and said, 'Yes.' So that's extremely rewarding. It's that effort that patients put in to get there. We are a team. I'd say that's the most rewarding thing when it comes to patients.

In most hospitals, by the time patients come to see an orthodontist, it's because no one else out there can give them the sort of care that they need because of their complexities. You really are the last stop in their line, and when you look at them and say, 'Don't worry, we will look after you, we will make sure that we can give you the nicest smile possible and the best bite possible,' you can see that immediate relief.

On a professional level, my colleagues keep me sane. We're all different people with different personalities, but we really look after each other. I am very fortunate for that. You get very attached to your registrars [junior trainees] because so many of them are amazing and you nurture them, you see them qualify and then they move on. That's always a bit sad because you wish you could keep some people forever, but then it's lovely to see them grow and develop in their careers. The core of consultants stay around you. It's knowing that when I go to work I have colleagues with this kindred spirit who have got your back when you need it.

During the first wave of the pandemic, Priti was redeployed to obstetrics and gynaecology. Her consultant colleagues had elderly parents and were anxious about contracting Covid-19 and passing it on to them. Priti's parents were in Kenya, so she didn't have the same sort of worries. She set up a rota so that all the junior dentistry staff could be redeployed to obstetrics and gynaecology.

They said, 'We do 12-hour shifts day and night.' I said, 'I have never stayed awake at night my entire life, not even when I was a student. Can I please do days, because I don't think I will survive a night shift? I would be useless to you.' So I did 12-hour day shifts, which means, in reality, much longer – so you have breakfast, lunch and dinner at work.'

The team that we joined was extraordinary. If you put me in their shoes and said, 'Right, I'm taking all your junior orthodontists away and

I'm giving you dentists [not trained in orthodontistry],' I think I'd probably have had a meltdown, but we were greeted with exceptional kindness and patience. The teams turned it into something that was fun. They really tried to incorporate you into everything. There's three layers to maternity work. There are general labour wards. Then there are the planned C-sections for the day. And then postnatal care and covering anything for women who are expecting and having issues. The first day I went across with a colleague of mine who is an oral medicine consultant. He is a dual-qualified dentist and medic. We met this lovely consultant. 'Right, I'm doing C-sections today, why don't you guys come and join me?' We went into theatre and I remember thinking, 'Oh my God, this morning I got up, expecting to do some dentistry, and suddenly, I'm standing in a theatre and a baby's being delivered in front of me.' The consultant was extremely competent and very relaxed. The mother is awake and the father is in the room. It's like an everyday outpatient conversation, except the patient's body's is open, as opposed to her mouth. I stood there and held the doyen – the instrument that keeps the bladder protected – and that was as helpful as a pair of hands. Dentists are good at suctioning and we're good at infection control and zoning areas, so I think that was helpful. We would start cutting sutures or following the stitch. That was easy. Some consultants were happy for you to stand in the background, others wanted you to get stuck in. The postnatal floor was very different to usual because normally, all the fathers are allowed in. There are lots of balloons and cards. Suddenly, fathers were only allowed one hour with their baby and then they are evicted from the building, so the mothers are on their own. The staff had to work much harder.

We had to prescribe for these mothers. The first doctor I met was reeling off all these medications to me and telling me what to do. I looked at her and said, 'I don't even know what the drug does.' I could see her eyes go, 'Oh my God, who is this person that you've sent to me?' I said, 'Look, I'm a consultant, I get things, just explain to me what this drug does and what your pathway is in terms of deciding when you prescribe and when you don't.' The drug was enoxaparin, which is like a clot-buster. It thins your blood and there are very specific reasons for which you would prescribe it or not prescribe it. We also had the pharmacists who would double-check everything in the background. So I got a flow chart and I was happy to just plug away.

They had some amazing junior staff because these doctors realised that post-delivery, most mothers will go to their GP to get contraception. But with Covid-19 there is no contraception via GP. They devised a Q & A flow chart for people to go through with the mothers so they could prescribe emergency contraception in the hospital. Every mother, we had to go through and tick them all off to make sure that they either have their contraception, or they don't want their contraception and that's recorded somewhere.

Orthodontic services were re-established and Priti returned to her usual post.

Dentistry did shut down for at least six to eight weeks across the country, but my hospital took on a contract for Covid-19 'hot patients' – patients who were Covid-19 positive who had raging toothache. They set up a service for how these patients could come into the building, have treatment and flow out without infecting others.

In orthodontics we used to have a walk-in emergency service and, because we're a really large department, we treat a lot of patients. We created a flow chart of every potential emergency that patients have, with advice that you can give over the phone and a very few things that they'd physically have to come in for. We were posting out elastics and wax to patients. Telling them how to cut bits of wire if they needed to. We sign-posted them to videos – the British Orthodontic Society was very active putting up videos and advice.

Once dentistry started to come back online, we had to contact the entire cohort of patients to get them booked in with the right people. A lot of our registrars were overseas registrars who had gone home and then couldn't get flights back to the UK. Our clinical leader set up extra services for evenings and Saturdays for these patients to be seen by a group of staff who would get paid for the extra hours. That's how we got through it.

The leaders I met in maternity and labour wards were extraordinary. They got the job done and they were kind in the face of a lot of stress – when they're losing all their junior staff. I encountered some beautiful examples of leadership, which I would hope to be able to draw on if I was ever put in that situation. Leadership in the dental hospital where we completely lost services and had to put them back online and create services to see Covid-19 positive patients – that was also extraordinary. University College Hospital London is an amazing hospital for teams coming together, getting things done and being innovative.

Whilst working on maternity I remember meeting this lovely Indian girl. She was about to become a consultant obstetrician. We suddenly realised that she was from Kenya too and her father was also an obstetrician-gynae-cologist. I said to my father, 'Do you know so-and-so?' 'Yes, I do. He was a couple of years older than me. We worked in the same hospital in Nairobi.' The next day the girl brings in a picture of her with my older sister and her parents and my parents. She remembers, as a little child, coming to our home town, Mombasa. She was standing with her arm around my sister. I was a tiny baby in that picture. I suddenly realised, 'How small the world is!' I met someone who knew my father, knew my sister. Her dad was in the same profession as my dad, and I met her as a baby. Until that moment I didn't know who she was, or where she came from. You realise how small the world is. It gave us such joy in those moments. That sense of camaraderie.

'Why are you giving up a couple of hours of your time to share your experiences?' Priti's other half asked her before the interview. 'I think it's a privilege to be able to share your story, so I feel blessed. Thank you very much for asking me and including me.'

ANDREW POLLARD

Andrew is a paediatrician who specialises in infectious diseases of children and has an academic role as director of the Oxford Vaccine Group at the University of Oxford. The group had expertise in developing vaccines for coronaviruses and they worked with AstraZeneca to develop a vaccine for Covid-19.

I've worked in the NHS for the whole of my career. I think the last few years have been enormously important for the NHS and vaccines have been central to getting us to this point in the pandemic. And it's only been possible through the testing of them that was done in the NHS and then the rollout through the vaccination programme.

I was certainly very aware of coronaviruses that have this potential to cause large outbreaks over the previous 20 years, because of previous coronavirus outbreaks in 2002, and then in 2012, which didn't go anywhere, but they were very frightening because they killed between 10 and 30 per cent of people infected. Fortunately, those viruses didn't transmit very well.

During February, looking with the mathematical modellers at their predictions of spread and mortality from this virus, it became very obvious that this was an extremely worrying situation. Like most people, I woke up to that fact, with a bit of a shock, as we started to realise that this was a virus which will change all of our lives forever.

My colleagues Sarah Gilbert and Teresa Lambe, with this interesting problem of a new virus in China, had been working on developing a vaccine. More as a follow-on to work they were already doing with a previous coronavirus vaccine, and to see whether they can make a vaccine against this new interesting virus. It wasn't until February that we all became aware that this was much bigger than the one research interest. We took the decision, collectively, to come together to form a team across Oxford, to try and respond to the emerging pandemic threat. I work particularly on bacterial vaccines. I do some research and development in the lab; we do very large-scale trials. Sarah and her team are very focused on early-phase studies, developing new vaccines and testing technologies, various forms of manufacturing. So we brought together lots of different skills that we had across the university, realising that you need multiple skills to be working in parallel in order to move quickly in the pandemic. And also that we needed the capacity that it takes to do development rapidly. We came together as a big consortium to work out how we could tackle this problem.

There were meetings almost every day as a result of the huge amount of work to be done. I led the clinical part of the development. My colleague Teresa Lambe worked on the animal studies and also setting up the laboratory, ready to measure the immune responses to the vaccine. And Sarah Gilbert focused on some of the coordination, particularly coordinating manufacturing with sites in Europe, as well as here in the UK, to make sure we have enough vaccine doses available.

We got our first results towards the end of November 2020. The results arrived on a Saturday evening. They were presented to me by our data-safety monitoring board because the results met the criteria for sharing the data publicly. We then had to verify all of the information over the next 24 hours before Monday morning, when AstraZeneca had to release the data to the market. I found myself Monday evening in Number 10 Downing Street at the press conference, announcing the results, having had very little sleep over the course of the weekend, with all of the work to do to prepare everything for that first media release.

It was a very surreal experience. There was a feeling of huge responsibility to present honestly, and with integrity, the results of the studies in as transparent way as possible. Also, I think, some anxiety because everything was very fast in the way that the information was released, because Astra-Zeneca wanted to release early because of the insider-trading rules and their concern that they couldn't hold back the information from the markets once they opened on Monday morning. I think our natural instinct as scientists was to have more time to assess the data and to do the further analyses to understand subgroups and so on. The recognition that communication was extremely challenging to do at such a pace when we only just got the results, and the importance of getting it right. Because we knew we had a vaccine that has the potential to save many lives around the world. And so, a big responsibility. So I'm not sure I felt satisfaction at that moment. But certainly a feeling of considerable pressure. And I don't think travelling down to do a Downing Street press conference is something that gives you satisfaction – it was more stress.

The AstraZeneca vaccine was licenced on 30 December 2020 and Andrew received the vaccine on 4 January 2021. 'Our thinking was that it was a very positive message for someone involved in leading its clinical development to demonstrate I was very comfortable with receiving the third ever dose of the vaccine we'd developed.' He was knighted in 2021 for services to public health.

CLAIRE GOODWIN-FEE

Claire's experience of the care received by her father when he was critically ill in 2018 led to her setting up Frontline-19, a psychological support service for frontline workers, in March 2020.

I'd not had much contact with intensive care units prior to this episode with my dad. But it's amazing. The NHS is at its finest in those moments. My dad had an intensive care nurse, highly trained, at the foot of his bed, filling in charts. If my dad had a sniffle, they knew what it was, how much it was, and they'd tested it. If he had a bowel movement, they'd measured it, tested it, they knew what it was. Scientifically, intensive care units are cutting edge. World-leading for what they do, but psychologically, which is my background, I realise that staff don't always have the psychological support to look after themselves, or even have the time to know what that entails.

Fast forward to when the pandemic started. I kept thinking back to these people. I remember Dr Lucy (I don't even know her surname), a lovely young doctor who spent three hours after her shift ended in a tiny, scrappy room in King's College Hospital, explaining some quite complicated brain scans of my dad's, when my mum and I were absolutely petrified that my dad was going to die. She took time to talk through them, to share the gravity of the situation, but did it with such openness and compassion and patience, and she must have been incredibly tired. So, she and the team there were a massive inspiration for me to want to try and give something back, at a time which I just thought would be unlike anything else. I wanted to try and support them the way that they'd supported my family.

Frontline-19 was an organisation that I founded and set up. I had the idea on March 22nd, 2020. I was sitting on my sofa in my front room, thinking about these staff, and how could I support them. I knew that psychological support would be key. I've worked in counselling/psychotherapy for around 16, 17 years, and I know quite a lot of people within the industry. I also work as a clinical supervisor for other therapists. So I've built up a network of people that work in the same industry as me. I set up to offer frontline staff free counselling sessions. They get up to 12 counselling sessions as standard. It's done via FaceTime, Zoom, Teams, on the internet, so like a virtual meeting. We do some telephone counselling too. Anybody that works for the NHS or frontline services, and care home staff are included in that, and paramedics, fire brigade, police and some teachers. They come along, they register via our website, they put in a request, and we match them with a qualified therapist. The therapists that we work with all belong to membership bodies, so they have to have insurance and they have to have clinical supervision, and be qualified in what they do. The idea is that we support the NHS and frontline workers to be able to continue to do the work that they do.

I'm incredibly proud to say that the quickest match we've done is 25 minutes. We had a suicidal NHS worker who needed support, who'd got in touch after I'd been on the radio. In 25 minutes we matched them. Generally speaking, we match within a couple of days. It's not long at all. We work incredibly hard, and the volunteers that we have are very focused.

There's probably three cases that will always be upper in my mind. One is the person that worked in the care home where around 60 per cent of the residents died. They were elderly. The carers would wash their face, feed them their lunch, tell them their stories, tuck them into bed at night, stroke their face and say, 'I'll see you in the morning.' That person had to wash all of those bodies and dress them for the undertaker, and then go home and have their dinner. I don't know how you're supposed to manage that without any support, and even with support, how you're supposed to manage that. The doctor that, I think in one shift, in the space of perhaps six or seven hours, lost around 20 people, and put his head on the desk and sobbed, because he didn't know how to tell another person that their loved one had died. The nurse at my local hospital that had to phone up all the local undertakers to see if they had any space to put these people, 'cause they'd lost 60 people in one night to Covid, and they'd run out of refrigeration space.

I always want to be humble, because I'm doing it for the nurses, the paramedics, the doctors, the dentists, the people that are actually on the frontline. It's intense at times, but I snuggle up with my little chihuahua, Bella, and I'll read fantasy books about stuff 'cause I need that distance.

That's what keeps me sane. I want to keep clear-headed and healthy, so that I can help as many people as possible.

The pandemic is this generation's shell shock. This generation's Vietnam War, which sounds incredibly dramatic, but that's how I feel about it. I believe in oral history, I believe in leaving a legacy for people that come after me, to understand how we lived our lives and what we can learn from that.

Frontline-19 is continuing to offer psychological support to people working at the frontline of care.

YUNUS DUDHWALA

Yunus had been working for over 20 years as a chaplain at the time of the pandemic and was seconded to the Nightingale Hospital London, the first of the temporary hospitals set up by the NHS in 2020 to deal with Covid-19 patients.

I work in chaplaincy at a large NHS trust in London and I was at the forefront of the pandemic response, especially in caring for families, caring for patients, being a bridge for families who couldn't come into the hospital because of the pandemic. As head of chaplains I am looking after a team of about 11 paid chaplains and a team of 30-plus volunteers. My role is to make sure that there's enough chaplains to cover the need for the hospital, whether it's patients, staff or relatives, to receive spiritual, pastoral or religious care whenever they requested. And to ensure that there are spaces within the hospitals for people to pray, or to reflect and be in a quiet space.

It's a total honour, you know. How many people in the world are invited to a space where somebody's leaving the world? There are three events in life which are usually the most important: birth, marriage and death. The chaplain is so privileged that they are invited to these. I can't remember the number of times I've cried with a family. We're praying at the end of life so that the person who's in front of me is forgiven and the family are given patience at that particular time.

Pre-pandemic, the team was much smaller. We had about eight chaplains at a time. We cover five different hospitals. My job was to make sure that we've got enough chaplains and to make sure that we had the right mix of faith within the hospitals. Our majority communities are Christian and Muslim. But we also get requests from Jewish and Hindu communities.

One of the hardest things that happened during the pandemic is that loved ones could not be with their loved ones when they were dying. I think that was huge. We can't express that in words. I can't imagine how families have dealt with that over the past few years, and whether they have overcome that grief or not. I think that that will live with them for many years.

On the Saturday, the patient deteriorated quite rapidly. We set up a video call and one of the daughters was allowed to go in. She was given the full PPE. She was holding the iPad and it was connected to my iPad. Then I had connected the rest of the family. There was a daughter in Manchester, wife and daughter here in London and a few families joined into the call. We started around five to two in the afternoon on the Saturday, and we finished five to three. For one hour I did prayers with the family. Usually I take between 10 minutes and half an hour depending on family members, etc. This one was very unusual. I was doing prayers for about one hour. We finished around 2.55 and he died around 3.20. We knew that he was going to die. The prayers are for the person who's dying, that they are forgiven, that their journey becomes easy. But also, the prayers are for the family, that God makes it easy for them to cope with what's going to happen. I'm trying to prepare them mentally for what's going to happen. It was very emotional, but it was good that we had that long prayer session because that's what the family needed.

Within Islam, we have to do the funeral as soon as possible. I wanted to know from the family whether they wanted to do it on the same day or the next day. At 4.05 they rang: 'We'd like to do it today.' 'Let's see if we can do it.' I made a few phone calls to the funeral directors, to the mosque and to the cemetery. Everything kind of fell in place. We got the doctor to write the death certificate 4.20, I got the registrar to issue the burial form. I got the funeral director to collect the body around 5.30. The body was taken to the mosque for six, washing, and shrouding. He was in the cemetery by seven o'clock and buried by half seven.

My thoughts are we did exactly what the family wanted. And that's what we are here for. It was the quickest I've ever turned it around. Everyone came together. I was just coordinating the funeral directors, the cemetery, the mosque, the staff in the hospital, the registrar's office. Everyone worked in sync to ensure that the family received the best care that they felt they needed at that particular time.

Emotionally, my colleagues and I were looking after each other. That was really important. Every day, we used to speak to each other at the end of the day. That phone call used to be a half an hour, one hour. Just to offload.

And although we don't remember most of those conversations, that offloading was key to keeping us emotionally set for the next day.

My perspective has always been, as part of my faith, that death is a reality and death will come at any time. I've seen that throughout my life within the hospitals. I remember a death of a two-year-old. I remember a death of a 12-year-old. I remember a death of a 20-year-old. I've seen deaths at different stages in life. My philosophy has always been that death can come at any time, at any place, to anyone. The pandemic was just cementing that personal belief that I've had for years. Yes, it was traumatic. Yes, it was emotional. But I've always believed that we are not in control of our destiny. God is in control of who dies, when they die, whether they die. And I saw that during the pandemic.

Yunus believes that the pandemic has made people value the work of the chaplaincy more. 'I'm really looking forward to how the chaplaincy will develop in our hospitals.'

RACHEL LEWIS

Rachel was among the first women in Wales to be ordained in the Church of England and she spent 30 years working in rural communities in England, Wales and Ireland. 'A very rich life and a very privileged life, inasmuch as you have access and opportunity to be alongside people at every moment of their life. So in hard times as well as times of celebration, which was very satisfying in terms of vocation.' In 2016, after 30 years' service, she returned to Wales.

I was fortunate enough to get a post with the NHS in the chaplaincy Cardiff and Vale University Health Boards, where I am part of a team – multifaith and multi-denominational. We're available for patients and staff and their families. At a late stage in my ministry, it has given me the sense of being liberated to engage in the aspects of care and response that took me into the church in the first place.

During the pandemic the role changed inasmuch as everybody's roles changed in hospitals. It was constant in that we were caring for people who are very poorly, but it shifted inasmuch as we are talking and listening through masks and visors. That was a very big physical change in how we looked and how we dressed to be available to people and to care for them. It makes it different physically. You'd have to speak louder. You'd have to move differently. Your face isn't seen the same. So lots of people learned how to do the most extraordinary, fabulous caring with eyes, and smiling with eyes. It's hard work, and heavy and hot. I've been lucky enough not to have to work in full PPE for long when we were called in. It wouldn't be a 12-hour shift like other staff.

The other important thing that we do is we pray. I don't mean that in a noble sense, but that there is time spent in intention and holding people in positive thought for good, which somehow bears witness to the tragedy we're all living through in a way that honours people's lives. It seems important in respecting what strength people are having to show to get through their day-to-day existence. We wake up with a pulse and a choice. In terms of practical prayers, we have people who are at home, praying and remembering us and lighting a candle or sending good energies out into the universe. It doesn't matter how people do it; we appreciate it very much. My Catholic colleague, Peter, says mass every day in the chapel. People leave prayers in the various books that we have, for folk who've died that they want to be remembered or for folk who are very poorly, or in thanksgiving that somebody's recovered and gone home. Confronted with the adversity of disasters, political scandals and all sorts of other things that are paralysing the planet, I think a very real recourse becomes faith.

How do you support people with other faiths?

The bottom line is about human connection and I think it's about mutual respect. I will often sit prayerfully, with my Muslim colleague Amina, and we will be keeping each other company in the presence of the divine. She understands it in practice in one way; I do it differently. Nobody has a monopoly on God.

Thank God for the NHS. I'm proud of being part of the NHS. I'm very fortunate. To have the chance to say it out loud is great. And I hope that people who listen to this in the future still have a wonderful NHS that looks after them as well as ours.

'It's an extraordinary opportunity to have a voice from a hospital chaplaincy as part of this research,' reflected Rachel at the end of the interview. 'We live in extraordinary times, where to be able to give voice to anything is both a challenge and a great opportunity.'

GRANT MCINTYRE

Grant grew up in the west of Scotland in the 1970s. His uncle was a dentist, which gave Grant a role model for a career. 'He's got a good lifestyle, has a good living and is in control of his own day-to-day work and so forth.' For the past 25 years, Grant has worked in Dundee. 'As a consultant orthodontist, I say to people, "It's the best job in the world."'

It takes me back to why I wanted to get into dentistry in the first place, and that's to have a degree of autonomy and a degree of responsibility that naturally go hand in hand. As a consultant, my job, ultimately, is to care for the patients that are under my name, but I'm given the freedom to be able to decide how best to care for them. In addition to that, I've got a management role which allows me to do a bit of shaping of my own and, indeed, the sister services within hospital dentistry. I really enjoy the mixture of what I do day-to-day, clinically as well as the management. I'm also an active researcher, and being able to answer some of the questions that have dogged my specialty for many years is also an intellectually stimulating opportunity.

In the third week of March 2020, I felt dreadfully unwell and, for the first time in my career, I couldn't go to work. My breathing worsened, my wife phoned for an ambulance and paramedics took me off to the hospital in which I have worked for 25 years. I turned from professional to patient instantly. I was discharged the next day and was given the news that I was positive for Covid. I had two further admissions back to hospital over the following few days. The third admission I don't have any memory of whatsoever, and that third admission was to prove one of the big turning points in my life. That night, my breathing had worsened significantly and overnight, I had had an out-of-body experience and by the time the morning doctor's ward round came to my bedside, I had to say to the medical team around me that I felt that I was dying – and I actually asked them to save my life. There wasn't a huge conversation at that point. I guess they probably weren't having much conversation with patients who were all positive for Covid, but I suspect everybody realised that I was a deteriorating patient at that point.

I was taken around to the second intensive care unit that had been set up in the hospital and within a matter of minutes, I was anaesthetised. I'd asked to be put onto a CPAP machine to help me with my breathing, but there wasn't any discussion and I was put onto a conventional ventilator. I was in intensive care for a week and, whilst my family were given the news that I was reasonably stable for a few days, by the end of the first week, I crashed into critical illness and multi-organ failure. Then the decision had to be taken as to whether or not I would survive the condition that I was in at that point. I was fortunate that a bed was available for me in the ECMO [extracorporeal membrane oxygenation unit]. In Scotland, it's based in Aberdeen, and I spent the next seven weeks on, effectively, life support.

Despite the doctors' best efforts, day in, day out, and the rest of the team, I showed very little signs of improvement until day 42 on the ECMO life support machine. The doctors had had a conversation with my family that there was one last roll of the dice, as it was put. That a fairly significant dose of steroids would either give me the kickstart that I needed, or it may, sadly, hasten my demise. To my luck, the steroids did work and I started at that point, apparently, to show signs of improvement.

I was transferred from ECMO life support onto a tracheostomy and the life support machine was eventually turned off, which was good news. Then we had to start making the long journey towards rehabilitation and recovery. I was transferred back to Dundee and I spent a further 36 days in intensive care, starting the initial rehabilitation phase of care. Some of the highlights of that were learning to speak again, learning to stand, learning to feed myself and, eventually, on day 96, taking my first fledgling steps again, naturally, with the help of a whole team of allied health professionals. We recorded that moment on camera for Facebook and beyond, of course. After several more weeks, on day 128, I was finally discharged from hospital to start the long journey back to the life that I knew at home. It took the next eight months for me to get back to being relatively healthy and able to survive independently, on my own.

At this point in the interview, Grant says, 'This was a story you probably didn't expect to get this morning!' to Jane, his interviewer.

Whilst nobody has ever said to me that patients had to be prioritised at either wave one or wave two of the worst of the pandemic, I know that some decisions had to be made as to who would be likely to survive on the basis that ECMO's not a panacea by any means. It's only giving the heart and/ or lungs a break to allow them to recover. I fully understand that if there's disease and pathology that are not really compatible with life, then it was only going to postpone death in many ways. I'm very grateful for the fact that the medical team looking after me thought long and hard as to whether I would have a chance of survival. Indeed, I'm glad that they did think I did have a chance of survival, because the stats for ECMO, as far as I understand, are not really that good. It's a 50/50 chance of survival across the board, and for the 50 per cent that survive, only 50 per cent of the survivors really ever return to a functional lifestyle afterwards. I'm very much aware of the very narrow, little channels that I've passed through on this journey and how fortunate I have been in many ways.

It did take some quite considerable time for me to start to get the normal cognitive functions coming back together. I was aware that I wanted to get back to work. It had been such an important part of my life until being struck down by Covid. When I was trying to have a look at some emails on either a phone or laptop, one of the intensive care doctors told me that I was there to get better, not to work, and if he saw me doing that again, I'd be evicted. I knew they were just being very kind. When I did eventually get back to work, nine months after leaving, there were 17,000 emails.

The one abiding memory that I have of everybody that I met as a patient and still continue to meet as a patient, is that nobody can do enough to help me as a patient. That's something that is absolutely crucial to the NHS. It's that level of care that the professionals show towards patients as well as undertaking the actual treatment, so to speak. The care bit is much more important than delivering the treatment. That will stay with me for the rest of my life. I've been in absolute awe of what everybody has done for me in this whole journey as a patient. At one point, I tried to count up the number of people involved and lost count. Over 200 people had been involved in my own journey.

Grant recovered and returned to work in winter 2021. Interviewed in August 2022, he has been left with some permanent symptoms of chronic pain and post-viral arthritis. 'I look at them in relation to the fact that I have survived an illness that should really have killed me outright.'

KATIE TOMKINS

Katie is the mortuary and post-mortem services manager at West Hertfordshire Teaching Hospitals NHS Trust.

I remember it so clearly. It was about January 13th 2020, and my manager came to me. 'We need to have a conversation like, what if this coronavirus comes here?' Stupidly, I shrugged my shoulders. 'But we've got the most capacity in the whole of the county, like we've got 175 fridge spaces. How many more do we need?' If I could go back and kick myself, I would, but so many of us were naïve as to how it would pan out.

In West Hertfordshire we have three hospital sites. Two have mortuaries. We've got a small team, five of us, and I'm equally split across the two sites, managing the Watford mortuary and the Hemel mortuary. I also manage the post-mortem service. We work with the Hertfordshire coroner and provide post-mortem services for the coroner to establish the cause of death for people whose death has been sudden, unexpected, or unexplained. We also meet with families, and we conduct viewings. But we are here to care for the deceased patients and all of their families that we come in contact with.

March 17th was the first phone call. 'Katie, we've got our first Covid death, what do you want us to do?' I contacted all my staff, let them know we've got our first Covid-19 case. 'Nobody touch it. I will handle this person. I will book them in. I will check them out. I will release them.' I remember giving myself a massive pep talk as I was getting kitted up, 'You've got to do this properly, Kate, you know, if you make a mistake, you could catch it, you could pass it onto everybody, you know, people could die.' We didn't know then how infectious it was after death. Seven days later we got our second one. The moment lockdown happened – that was the tidal wave.

I've been involved in pandemic planning for years and we always thought of it being a gradual build-up. But for us, it was like a storm hit. It hit so quickly, and we were caught off guard, we really were. One day things were relatively normal. The next day it was suddenly just like a tidal wave and the deaths were coming quicker than we could physically deal with. It engulfed us so quickly. It was really difficult to respond because by the time we needed help, we were already overwhelmed. Our trust were really good. 'Look, Kate, what do you need? How can we help?' In terms of making sure we had enough cold storage for our deceased, that was arranged relatively quickly. In terms of my team, we literally just pulled together. We worked seven days a week, 14, 15 hours a day, nonstop, just doing what we could to maintain the service.

The only saving grace for us in the first wave is that the number of people who required a post-mortem dropped because we were swabbing people. If the swab came back positive for Covid-19, the consultant would do an external examination and the coroner and the families were content with the cause of death being Covid-19. We were able to concentrate on making sure that we had space for our deceased and we were getting our deceased out to the funeral directors for funerals.

We were doing a lot of keepsakes for families. Taking locks of hair and disinfecting them and putting them in nice little packages that could be handed to the undertaker to give to the family. Or taking off jewellery, again packaging it up nice, because a lot of the undertakers stopped doing that during the first wave. They literally just collected the deceased, and if they were Covid, or suspected of being Covid, they were just put in a coffin and sealed. The family didn't get to see them, and if there was property or jewellery, the family didn't get it back. We tried really hard to do as much as we could. Handprints, footprints, taking off jewellery, locks of hair. Anything to give families that little something, because they couldn't come and say their goodbyes. So, that's where a lot of our resources went, managing the admissions, managing the releases and then trying to give families some kind of comfort and support.

Every mortuary in the whole of the United Kingdom was in exactly the same position. We were all struggling. Traditionally, mortuaries are staffed to the bare minimum. We're not overstaffed and people were getting sick, or there were people that had to shield. We were all struggling to work our way through the kind of guidance that was coming out quite regularly about what we should be doing, shouldn't be doing.

In the early days families weren't allowed to view their relatives who had Covid, because we didn't know how infectious it would be, or how infectious they might be if they'd been in contact with them. Two years down the line, we're understanding a lot more. There is a risk, but with proper handling of the deceased, gloves, masks, the risk is luckily minimal to staff. Covid-19 is still deemed as a category-three infection, so similar to that of HIV, hepatitis, and tuberculosis. The risk comes more at post-mortem because we are then inside the chest cavity and handling the lungs of the deceased, so we take extra precautions, like we would with any high-risk category-three examination.

West Hertfordshire Teaching Hospitals NHS Trust nominated Katie to have her portrait painted by Roxana Halls in recognition of her outstanding leadership and celebration of her extraordinary courage. The portrait has been acquired by the Science Museum. 'I'm so proud to represent mortuaries and anatomical pathology technologists forever in that portrait, that it will be seen by people and they'll remember that mortuaries are here, and that we care and we are professionals. We shouldn't be forgotten.'

ALICE WISEMAN

In 2016 Alice became director of public health in Gateshead in the north-east of England.

Covid has impacted on everybody across the whole spectrum of our communities. However, I do think that the people it has affected most are people who are from more disadvantaged circumstances. People who are from particular groups that were potentially restricted more than others. I worry a lot about young people who have been at home, in houses where they've had additional stresses from job loss, or from furlough on 80 per cent of the national living wage. I spoke with teachers about them worrying about their kids being fed. That's an ongoing issue with the cost-of-living crisis.

So if you've got additional stresses at the home, those adverse childhood experiences impact on the way that our kids develop and grow. I was worried about the inequalities of home learning for some families, where maybe there wasn't a quiet space for the kids to sit and study or, you know, maybe they didn't have access to IT. I worry about the long-term implications for those young people, you know, because unless we do something really robust in our recovery, which is challenging because of austerity and other financial pressures, then there's a whole generation of kids that are going to be adversely affected in an ongoing way.

I looked back at some data in the 1980s. The kids who were teenagers in the 1980s, when there was all of the difficulties in the north-east, and the mines were shutting and the shipyards and all the rest of it, and there was loads of poverty around then. If you map drug- and alcohol-related deaths, there's a direct correlation with that age group. So in the 1990s, there was a spike of drug-related deaths of people in their twenties. And 2000s to 2010 it was people in their thirties. And 2010s to 2020 it was people in their forties. Now, that's only one example of a long-term poor outcome, but we've got kids who have gone through 10 years of austerity, plus the Covid pandemic and now cost of living. I genuinely do think that there is a real concern.

In Covid the demand for our children's services has gone through the roof. I've never seen there being need in Gateshead like that. And they're just the kids who are ending up in statutory services. What about all of the other kids on the edge of care? What about the kids who are leaving school, who would be going into apprenticeships, and there just aren't the opportunities out there that there were previously? Children and young people are a massive concern for me.

I worry about people who have lost work during the pandemic, or maybe they've had their own business and it's folded. The sort of stresses that come from that and the impact that that's had on health. We have seen a massive increase in the number of people who are drinking at higher, and harmful, levels of alcohol. So there was a 21 per cent increase in liver disease in the first year of the pandemic and a massive increase in alcohol-related hospital admissions and deaths. That came as a consequence of people feeling so anxious and stressed at home that they were self-medicating. You know, cheap supermarket prices, availability of alcohol all over the place. It's interesting because hospitality was closed – and we often blame hospitality because that's where you can physically see the harm from alcohol, of people having fights or getting really drunk. Whereas the hidden harm is much more concerning, from a health perspective.

I'm the addiction lead for the Association of Directors of Public Health, so I'm lobbying on minimum unit pricing, looking at whether we can restrict promotions in the way that other countries, like Scotland and Wales, have done. And particularly thinking about how children are protected from alcohol being as normalised as it is in our society. People often jump straight to the individual who's using alcohol as an addiction substance. But the reality is it's harmful in much broader ways, as it's linked to seven types of cancer. We're doing media work at the moment around making sure that people have that understanding around the link between alcohol and cancer.

My little brother said to me a few years ago, 'How big is your "us"? And is your "us" just about me and my immediate family? Or is your "us" about me and my community, me and my region, me and my country, me and the world?' With infectious disease, there's no point in having a small 'us'. No point in me sitting and worrying about me and my teenager, because the only way that I can protect me and my teenager is by caring about my community. And the only way I can protect my community is by caring about my region and my country and then, ultimately, the world. So for me, infectious disease teaches us a lot about how we do have to care. We do have to recognise that we need to meet each other's needs in different ways. Vaccination's a great example of that. There is no point in us being amazing at vaccination in the UK if we then don't vaccinate the poorer countries across the world that don't have the resources that we have. What will happen is we'll end up with a new variant that will evade the vaccine and we'll all be back at square one.

Alice shares her broader reflections on the NHS in Chapter 10.

GEORGINA BOND

Georgina is a medical student on the combined University of Manchester / St Andrews School of Medicine programme. At the beginning of the pandemic, the students were removed from ongoing hospital placements.

Suddenly to be pulled out of a placement felt like we were abandoning everyone that we'd known in hospitals. I wanted to go back and help if I could. Luckily, I was already on a bank healthcare system roster, so I could begin working as a healthcare assistant. I worked basically anywhere where they were short-staffed, which was everywhere at that point. I was so struck by the amazing generosity of the people. I saw so many instances where staff stayed late, long past their hours, or they did things that their job descriptions wouldn't normally suggest that they should do, or even put themselves in situations that were higher risk than they were really required to, just because it was what the patients needed. Instances where we didn't have any FFP3 masks. But there were patients who were on aerosol-generating procedures with Covid, who needed changing or their medication. Everyone was like, 'Well, if I don't do it, a patient's going to suffer. So it's happening.' It's like the Blitz spirit. This sense of duty. I was so struck by the generosity of the people around me, and the nursing teams particularly.

The gowns when we were in proper, full PPE were supposed to be fluid-resistant, but often they weren't. I remember some of the nurses coming in and wrapping themselves in bin bags and duct-taping themselves in before they put the non-fluid-resistant gowns on. Most starkly, I remember the cleaning crew coming up to clean one of the ward bays that a patient had just been moved out of, and there being no masks, no gowns for them. I remember watching one of the team wrap plastic aprons around their arms and tape them on with that paper tape that we use for dressings. We wore the same gowns for whole shifts regularly, even though they were they weren't supposed to be used for so long, but we only had so many. There was definitely shortages. I do get a bit frustrated sometimes when I hear politicians saying now that there weren't shortages, that the reports were exaggerated and things. I think that's a bit disrespectful to the people who persevered.

I was looking at emails in a Manchester hospital and one mentioned the Nightingale. I went online and filled in the application form. I never thought I'd get a response from it. I got a phone call: 'Can you be in Manchester tomorrow morning? And we'll do an induction.' It all happened very quickly. My family were furious with me. They really didn't want me to be any more exposed to Covid than I already was. My mum came around eventually, but at the time, she was very upset that I was going to be in an entirely Covid-positive environment. My brother and my mum moved into an Airbnb for a few months because they didn't want to be living with me while I was so exposed. I started only a day or two after it first opened. I worked there until the last Covid patient was discharged.

It was an amazing thing to be part of that first day when I had the induction. We saw photos of them turning the convention centre into the hospital. The army did just such an amazing job setting up, I would say, a world-class, excellent facility in such a ridiculously limited time. The first time I walked in to the temporary hospital setup, I was sort of expecting it to be like that old show, *M*A*S*H*. Like temporary beds and green army tents. But it was excellent. It really did look like a proper hospital – except when you looked up, and then you could see the roof of the convention centre.

There's one patient I remember, who was really struggling with the CPAP [continuous positive airway pressure] mask, but also persevering. I was helping wash and change him one morning; he was very weak. He had this big beard. I said something about his beard and just tried to make him laugh. He said, 'Oh, actually, I'm always clean-shaven. I've never had facial hair in my life.' I could sense from his voice that he really didn't like it. I said, 'We could try and shave you around your mask.' He said, 'I'd love that.' But there wasn't time on my shift. So at the end of the shift, I went back and sat with some of those really terrible NHS razors and a load of the shaving cream sachets and for three hours we put him on and off the CPAP mask, and on and off the oxygen mask, keeping him hooked up to a SAT machine [for checking oxygen levels] and slowly gave him a shave. It was a real labour. It took a long time. We talked while we did it. I spent hours with him. I felt like I had a connection. You come away and think, 'Gosh, I hope things go well.' I didn't work on that ward again for a while. When I went back as a medical student, I saw a member of staff and I said, 'Do you remember that day?' She said, 'It's so sad.' He passed away, not so long after that. He was one of the first patients on that ward to pass away. It still makes me sad to think about, but I don't want to forget it because it was something that I'm really proud I did. It was a day that I felt like something small made a big difference. It was why I became a medical student and want to be a doctor. I want to be someone who champions the things that patients really care about.

What does the NHS mean to you?

Gosh, I'm gonna sound really pretentious. But it's my raison d'être. Caring for people is such a huge part of why I do anything. I really want to spend my life doing something that genuinely helps as many people as I can. I'm really lucky, because being a doctor is something that's going to be rewarding in so many ways. But honestly, any role within the NHS has the same end result of being so good for so many people. What does it mean to me? I couldn't even begin to answer that question, really.

Georgina qualified in medicine in 2022.

PETER JULIAN

Peter started feeling poorly at the end of March 2020 and, after five days, was so ill he was admitted to hospital. He was interviewed in October 2020 by Christina Jones, a retired ICU nurse who works with the ICUsteps patient support charity. 'I think a historic archive of the people, as opposed to filtered through journalists or politicians or novelists, is a really important historical archive for the future. Covid and its effects on the UK, the NHS and society is one of the biggest things of the last 70 years. That's why I chose to get involved.'

I got progressively worse, which culminated on 2 April 2020, where I couldn't really talk. I couldn't stand. I couldn't walk. My wife had to call an ambulance. I had 25 per cent oxygen levels at that point. I remember part of the ambulance journey. I remember getting to ICU and being told I was gonna go on a ventilator. I had enough wherewithal to send texts to my family and to my kids. I distinctly remember being on a trolley, and an anaesthetist putting the mask over my face, and saying he would knock me out, or words to that effect. That image of being on a trolley with three pretty burly blokes around me, from the viewpoint of a trolley, stuck with me.

I was in intensive care for 11 days. They tried bringing me off the ventilator at day five. I remember coming off the ventilator the second time about nine days in. It's very hazy, because I had delirium at that point. So it's very hard to know what was real and what wasn't. You got this sense of the staff being really focused on saving the life of everybody there. I think pretty much anything else was stripped back. At the hospital I was at, they'd had to grab other wards and places to extend ICU capability.

Knowing I was leaving ICU was an exciting experience. I remember leaving on a trolley with a person from ICU and two ladies from what I'm calling the 'recovery ward' and just thinking, 'Oh, crikey, I've made it.' I remember being clapped by the staff as I went out. When you've been in such a dark place, it was so uplifting. The sensation was one of overwhelming kindness from the staff there. I felt a sense of relief. I felt I was on a road to recovery – that turned out not to be necessarily true – but that was what it felt like at the time.

I went into this recovery ward on 11 April and I left on 18 April. Looking back, I was on pretty heavy drugs. I was in a ward with three or four other people. I was largely out of it a lot of the time. But the delirium got progressively more unpleasant. So it started off in a fairly nice way. It was pleasant delirium. Thoughts about fireworks going off at night, Christmas lights being around one of the other patients. Then the delirium took a really bad twist. My memory of it was shrunken heads around the ward. I thought people were coming to kill me. As a junior doctor's coming to talk to me, I could see a samurai assassin with a sword over his shoulder coming for me. Anyone would be upset by believing that to be true. It was deeply terrifying.

What do you think could have been done to help you?

Everybody in that recovery ward had their phones mislaid. That meant we weren't in contact with our families. Had we had our phones, that would have helped us. We couldn't move, we were not able to walk, we were on catheters, we've lost muscle. The idea that you can use the TV screens, which act as a phone above your bed, is really not likely. Losing our phones and, in my case, losing my glasses, when I'm deeply short-sighted, really made my recovery and probably my delirium much harder. On my wife's birthday I had one nurse who told me that I couldn't ring my wife. That was that and maybe that's fair enough in the circumstances. I had another nurse who gave me her private phone on another day and allowed me to contact my wife. That humanity was much appreciated. I understand later on, the ward invested in some iPads to allow people to communicate with their families. You have to see in the context of the time. We had people on the wards who had not been on a ward for 10 years, or had no experience of ICU. They didn't all understand what delirium and hallucinations were. I had one very good nurse who said she knew all about delirium, and it just put my mind at rest.

When I came home, my wife and my neighbours did a lovely clapping thing, which was just lovely. I was told when I left hospital that my GP would take responsibility for my care. Physically, I was very lucky. I could walk up the stairs on day one, which wasn't a universally shared experience of other people in the same situation. I was very weak, but just delighted to be home.

About a week later, I was just in bits, I was really upset and in a really bad place. I had my first contact with my GP. 'Don't worry. What you're experiencing is common for people that have been in ICU. And you're not going mad.' About three weeks after I came back, I was getting concerned because I was having worries around my physical recovery and about my ability to process conversations and understand. I rang up my GP and explained I was really struggling. I couldn't negotiate websites. I couldn't do any planning. 'What Covid support will I be having?' 'There is no Covid support.' I was told I would have to phone up for an appointment in a month's time. At which point, I said, 'Given that I've told you I can't negotiate websites or do any planning, this really isn't helpful.' And that was that.

Physically, I was well and fit before Covid, I had no pre-existing conditions and cycled about 30 miles a week. I'm now six months out of hospital. I'm grateful to be cycling. I can do about 15 to 20 minutes once a week. In terms of walking, on a very good day my record is 22 minutes. My average is probably 16 minutes. I do that three times a day.

Before Covid, I was a director and then a business consultant. The work involved a lot of thinking, constructing things, a lot of emails, processing numbers in Excel. I really can't do any of that. Let's take using Excel spreadsheets as an example. What would have taken me five minutes takes me an hour – except that I can't do an hour, I can probably do 25 minutes. So my short-term memory is affected. I used to be very good at spelling; now I make spelling errors. I can do this stuff to a much lower level than I used to. But if I overdo it, I get fatigue. In fact, I get fatigue anyway, because I wake up with it every day. I can see I'm getting better. But I guess it's about how long it takes. The biggest problem was I had no benchmark. I now reckon it would take me a year to 18 months. Initially, I was hoping for three to six months. So, yes, I'm getting better. But it feels glacial in its speed.

Peter joined the ICUsteps charity's Chester group and went on to set up a similar group in Manchester.

Whilst there's a lot of talk about the provision getting better for people out in the community, the truth is that people like me aren't really seeing it. ICU staff and outreach services are really stretched. But there's a real need for this kind of informal support. One of my aggravations initially was it took me about 20 weeks for the ICU team to reach out to me. Only when I speak to them do I find out that there's just two of them and any reach-out services are in addition to their day job of saving lives.

What I'd like to end on is the kindness and compassion shown to me by nurses and doctors at the hospital was fantastic. Many healthcare professionals have just massively supported me beyond and outside of their normal work. Finding the ICUsteps charity has been a godsend. I've gone from feeling utterly alone and out of my depth to feeling I have a team of people that care. Psychologically, that's a massive support.

Peter continues to support other ICU survivors.

PATRICIA MILLER

Patricia is the third generation of her family to work in the NHS. They came from Barbados in the 1960s, 'part of the last tranche of the Windrush generation'. Even though the NHS wasn't an initial career choice, 'If somebody opened me up, they'd probably find the NHS running through my DNA, because I really believe in the principles under which Bevan founded the NHS and the values that it has.' She joined the NHS in the late 1980s, working in the information department, providing statistics to the then District Health Authority. To get more responsibility and the scope to make decisions that impacted on communities, she took time out to do a business degree. She joined Dorset County Hospital NHS Foundation Trust in 2011, becoming chief executive in 2014 and leading a 'turnaround' of the organisation that had been placed in special measures by the regulators.

As we started to have some discussions in the NHS about what we would do if the situation in Italy was replicated here, I was diagnosed with breast cancer. I had to very quickly put some plans in place for the organisation to manage that, knowing that I was going to be away from work for anything up to six months. I ended up being away for four months. For me, that was very challenging whilst I was at home – keeping in touch with my team and different parts of the organisation who I knew would be struggling. I was also dealing with my own dilemma. The thing that I found the most difficult was that a big part of being a chief executive, in the public sector, is your pastoral role for your staff. Making sure that they are looked-after and cared for. For me, the biggest challenge I had was – being the person that usually has their arms around the organisation – that I wasn't there at that moment when they were absolutely terrified. I found that very difficult.

The thing I am most proud of my staff for is that they rose to the challenge. They did whatever was asked of them, no matter how difficult it was. Especially at times when we were actually putting them in harm's way. When they were looking after people who were incredibly ill, in circumstances where even with the best PPE in the world, they could have contracted coronavirus themselves.

I was really fortunate in that I didn't need to have chemotherapy, but I did have surgery and radiotherapy, and I chose to be treated at my hospital by the teams that I trust. So that was interesting and challenging. Arriving regularly at the organisation when it's going through a lot of turmoil, to receive treatment for a condition that is really worrying. But even though the staff were going through their own difficulties, their own fears, I always felt cared for, I always felt cared about. I don't think a single week went past at home without a bunch of flowers, or a card, or a gift arriving from someone at the organisation. One afternoon, having been at the hospital in the morning to have some radiotherapy, a delivery man turned up with an afternoon tea. There was a note from one of the clinicians, 'I hope this brightens your day.' They're just fantastic human beings. They had their own stuff to deal with. I felt really privileged that I was never far from their minds.

I think my patient experience changed my view about how the NHS delivers cancer services and what is important to people. As professionals, we think we know what our patients want. We think we know what's in their best interest, but actually, there's nothing can beat being in their shoes. You see the world through a different lens, and you see the Service through a different lens. It has made me think very carefully about what the NHS does really well, in terms of support for individuals with that diagnosis, but also what it needs to do differently.

We've always known that health inequalities existed. Successive governments have been clear about that. The NHS has always known that there is inequality of outcome within the services that it offers. I think there hasn't been enough focus on that. So when governments say that a pandemic has shone a light on something, I don't accept that. I think they've always known it. I think what it has done is uncovered the fact that nothing has been done to change that. So we could have predicted – based on what we already know about disease trends – that Covid would have a disproportionate impact on minority communities. We could have predicted that it would have a disproportionate impact on deprived communities. We could have predicted that it has a disproportionate impact on those with learning disabilities. Because we already know that these communities are disaffected by the services that we offer. We need to make a fundamental shift to do something about it.

If not, we will have missed a golden opportunity to focus on the things that are really important. If you're an adult with learning disabilities, your life expectancy is significantly shorter than someone without disabilities. If you are from a BAME community, you are between 80 and 240 per cent more likely to live in a deprived area, which means that your life expectancy is considerably shorter, you don't have access to the same employment opportunities, you don't have a right to have a decent education. All that plays into health inequalities.

We've got an opportunity now, where the public start to realise where those inequalities are, to really change the dial on the conversation and do the right thing. But health can't do that on its own. It needs local government to work with it. And it needs the ministerial support of the secretary of state for health, and the secretary of state for local government and communities to be joined up in that agenda to make sure that the right plans are put in place to really reduce the level of debt provision that we have in this country and make a real difference to the communities that we're responsible for. Because it feels at times as if we're letting them down.

When I'm having a stressful week, spending time with and talking to staff and patients is what gets me back to, 'This is what it's all about.' The other thing is remembering that I'm not a superhero. That none of us in the NHS are superheroes. We're just human beings. And it's okay to have an off day. It's okay to feel emotional about a situation we're in. It's okay to be vulnerable. Even when you're the leader of the organisation, it is okay to feel like that and it's okay to tell people you feel like that. It shows that you're human. It gives everyone else the signal that it's okay not to be okay at times. And that when you're not okay, there is support out there to help you. We can get into this mindset that we're here to serve. That we're required to be superheroes and that we're not allowed to be human beings. And we are.

Fifty years from now, is there one thing you would like people to know about the pandemic?

That 15 years ago, a professor and epidemiologist, Sir Michael Marmot, wrote a White Paper. He said, if this country doesn't fundamentally change the way that it not just offers health services but deals with the wider determinants of health, that health inequalities in this country will increase massively. And we'll have one of the highest child poverty rates in Western world. We ignored that report. And we ignored it to our peril. The fact that we ignored that report is one of the principal reasons why these communities were most affected by Covid in terms of death rates. The fact that we didn't do the work that Michael Marmot said we should do is one of the single reasons why those people died of Covid. So the one thing I would want us to remember in 50 years' time is not to get into the same place. Marmot has just written a follow-up to that report, after Covid. And this is the moment where we need to listen to him.

Patricia is now CEO of Dorset integrated care system.

NATALIE PARR

Natalie trained as a teacher in the 1990s and worked with children with severe disabilities. But in 2002 she was diagnosed with Guillain-Barré syndrome, a rare condition in which the body's immune system attacks the nerve cells, leading to weakness and paralysis across the body.

I was 25. I was very fit and healthy. I woke up one morning, had a shower and then I collapsed. Guillain-Barré paralysed me from the chest down. Basically, it stops the messages from getting down to the nerves. So you need a lot of hospital support, and then a lot of rehabilitation. For me, it's caused permanent damage. I'm tube fed, I have oxygen, I have a lot of lung problems and things and I'm in a wheelchair permanently. So I rely on people for 24-hour care.

At the beginning of the pandemic, Natalie had to adjust to having her care delivered in different ways, as she was asked to shield at home.

It was announced that people needed to be shielded. I had a text and about four letters. Then I've had my consultants phoning me at home, which is really helpful because I've got so much responsibility. All of a sudden, you think, 'Wow, we've been left to deal with this.' There are people at the end of the phone but you know that they're busy, so you don't like to bother them. I also came down with shingles. I got the matron at the end of the phone, she's the advanced nurse practitioner. She spoke to my GP, got me some meds that they delivered to me. So that was sorted really quickly. So all of these phone numbers that you've got for an emergency suddenly come into practice. I was given a big bag of PPE stuff for nurses to wear here. All my medicines got delivered. So I was shielded, Mum was shielded and Dad's over 70, so he was asked to stay in as well. None of us can leave the house.

The equipment required for Natalie's ongoing care, including oxygen cylinders and the food for tube feeding, was delivered to the house.

I did get a bit excited. It was near my birthday and I had a huge box delivered. I thought it was a great big birthday present, but then it had got a big sticker, 'urgent medical supplies'. It was catheters and things like that – it's exciting, but not as exciting as a birthday present!

I keep saying to everybody, 'I've got the easy part. I'm at home, I'm safe. I just have to stay here.' All you want is for us all to still be alive at the end of it. So I'm quite happy. And I feel that I'm being well looked-after in a way that is appropriate.

Natalie reflected on the ways in which adjusting to the pandemic were similar to the changes she experienced when she first had her diagnosis.

I had my feeding tube changed last Thursday. The nurse comes out from the ward and she is still wearing a mask and PPE. That feels normal. You hear so many people saying, 'Oh, we just got to get on with it now.' But this is how we're getting on with it. Life has changed massively. But life changed massively when I was ill. I went from walking, eating, working. I had to change overnight and I had to adapt to the new life. Like not be able to walk in the sea. I think that really helped me with all this. Some of the change, it's really good. I'm really quite independent with everything that I do now. Mum had surgery last week on her knee. She had a PCR test and did the isolation, then went to Rugby hospital, which is seen as the green non-Covid hospital [the green pathway was the term given to hospitals with Covid-free areas]. I've got bladder surgery next week and I'll be having a PCR for that. It does make you feel a bit better that people are still taking it seriously. We have the FFP2 and the FFP3 masks, which are the ones that protect you. I think it's a case of, 'This is what we need to do.' As much as you feel quite abandoned by any governments, we've learned that this is what we need to do. We've had a canopy fitted in the garden and set our own rules. We'll live like this as long as we need to and, yeah, at one point we might catch Covid. But the more time that's going past, more treatments are coming out. So it has become a new way of living, really.

The NHS means everything to me. You can't take it for granted. In the last couple of years, it's made me feel so proud of everyone in the NHS.

These people are holding us up, these people are carrying us, and we cannot live without everybody in the NHS. They've carried us, every single one of us, for two years. These are humans, these people, and they've given up everything for us. I'm just so grateful.

Between April 2020 and May 2022, Natalie contributed 27 interviews to the collection.

DEB TROOPS

Deb worked at the BBC for most of her career. She has several long-term conditions, including the rare disorder Dercum's disease. She became involved in health advocacy after her son suffered a brain injury. 'I learned very quickly that people don't get what they need when they're sick, or injured, or suddenly disabled, and that it's a fight every day. The best way of me dealing with what had happened to me personally was to reach out to others, and to join forces and work together to improve things. I am a doer, I'm not a talker.' Deb is now campaigning for support for people suffering from long Covid.

Being a journalist, you can take the girl out of the BBC, but you can't take the BBC out of the girl. I first started to hear stories about Covid-19 around July, August 2019. There were little threads about this new virus that was making people very sick and had started to kill people. But it was confined to China. And it was something that we shouldn't really be too worried about. By September, October, that had changed and there were reports that Covid had arrived in Europe and in the UK, though it wasn't being taken very seriously.

As a journalist, you think to yourself, it's either a story or it's not. It's not getting any traction. There could be two reasons for that. It could be because we don't want to create a story from it. Or it could be that there's no story there at all. I just kept an eye on it. But it didn't affect the choices I made, or the places I travelled to, or the way I lived my life. We went to Spain for a few days in December 2019. There was much more conversation in the Spanish media, in the bars, in the cafés. That was my first immersion into conversations about Covid-19. I thought, 'I really need to do some digging.' Towards the end of that four days, I didn't feel well and I couldn't put my finger on what it was. I felt weird for a few weeks. I never made any association between that and Covid. We went to Lanzarote in January 2020. The Spanish media again were taking this very much more seriously. I was still feeling out of sorts. I was getting a lot of pain in my left side. I put it down to an old back injury. I literally could not stay awake on the flight home and was unwell for a few days. About the third week of March, I got Covid properly. I believe I caught it in Malaga and it hit me in March.

I'm chair of the Greater Manchester Neuro Alliance [GMNA]. I'm very proud of the fact that we're always about the patient. We support all people living with neuro [neurological diseases], including health professionals, because they live with it too. The one thing about the smaller organisations was that, during the lockdowns, we didn't shut. The traffic to our website went up by 400 per cent. I know it's because when people come to our website, they only get official information and advice. People trust us.

The experience of working with the neuro community – that is used to having a lack of support and services, particularly around rehab, and a lack of understanding about the conditions and disabilities and illnesses, of which there are 600-plus – prepared me for the sudden influx of long Covid patients now coming to the GMNA. 70 per cent of long Covid patients are presenting with neuro now, much more than they are with respiratory or anything else. It means that our experience as a neurological group is that we understand their frustrations. And it's hugely disappointing that we now have a whole new group of patients who are fighting every day to be understood, listened to and get help. They're now in the same boat as the neuro community. I would have hoped that through the pandemic we would have learned that we can't treat an entire group of patients in such a casual way, but it's meant that for me, you know, I understand where they're coming from. Most importantly, I fully understand because I have long Covid – 28 months now.

My experience of the long Covid clinics is rubbish. As chair of the GMNA, I also sit on the Tier 4 stakeholder group for Greater Manchester. I know what we agreed the long Covid clinics would do. Out of nine clinics, there's only one actually doing it. Now that's not acceptable. I am incredibly frustrated that nationally, many of the long Covid clinics are still offering graded exercise therapy and talking therapies. NICE [National Institute for Health and Care Excellence] have said these should not be prescribed for people with ME/CFS [myalgic encephalomyelitis/chronic fatigue syndrome] and long Covid. It is too dangerous for those patients, yet it is still being pushed as a cure, mainly by the private sector. That shouldn't be allowed to happen. The long Covid clinics are predominantly modelled on respiratory and pulmonary services. Well, not many of the long Covid patients that I come into contact with have those issues. There's a phrase for people who just bounce around the NHS, being passed from one specialty to another – it's 'patient tennis'. We haven't got patient tennis anymore; it is literally patient ping-pong. Some clinics only provide a service for six weeks. Well, I'm 28 months. So where do I fit in? Some services will only do a triage. If you don't tick enough of their boxes, they don't offer a service at all. That's not acceptable. It is alarming to me that when we know how dangerous Covid is, and how debilitating long Covid is, we are not taking seriously a huge number of people who now can't work, can't look after their families, can't care for others and can't play an active role in society. Covid is non-discriminatory. It doesn't care if you're a hedge-fund manager, or someone who cleans toilets for a living. Why are we not taking this seriously and doing everything we can to get these people rehabilitated and as fit and well as they can be? I don't know.

The NHS was moving in the right direction before Covid. There was much more engagement with smaller organisations like GMNA who represent patient groups that are enormous, but underrepresented. Aside from A & E, we are the biggest group of people who will depend on the NHS long term, yet we have no national clinical director, and we have no strategic clinical networks. That is a nonsense. That means an entire group of people who use the NHS most have no voice and no representation. So the NHS was talking to groups like ours. Since Covid, there seems to have been a return to the bad old days of talking about patients, not to [them]. And a lot of short-term, quick-fix solutions to a problem which is going to be with us forever.

Is there anything further that you'd like to add?

That I hope I'm wrong. I feel a bit emotional, tearful. I hope with all my heart that I am wrong. And that somewhere in the next few months, someone gets a grip. And says, 'No, we have to do this. We have to go forward in a totally different way to what we've done thus far. Because I fear for my grandchildren. I really do. And I fear for the people in the Ukraine, and Lithuania and Estonia and Poland and Hungary, because if this is not gotten a grip of, then there is nothing to stop despots using viruses like Covid to control populations. That's my fear. I hope I'm wrong. I want to be wrong. I want you to come back to me in 12 months' time and say, 'Crikey, Deb, you were so wrong.' And I'd say, 'Patrick, I'm so glad!' [*laughs*] What we need is a Jacinda Ardern [former prime minister of New Zealand].

How has it felt to be interviewed?

I've been able to say things that needed to be said.

Deb wanted to contribute her experiences, 'Because I don't believe that the real voices of Covid-19 and long Covid particularly are being heard. They're certainly not being listened to. I feel very strongly that if we're going to have any data-gathering on this catastrophic event, and a massive change to patient experience, it needs to be as wide-spread and as diverse as it possibly can be. And that's not my experience of the patient engagement groups I've experienced so far.'

JONNY EMMS

Jonny graduated in medicine from Newcastle University in the summer of 2012, just as the London Olympics was beginning and the NHS took centre stage at the opening ceremony. 'That was quite memorable because my first job working surgical nights was a couple of days after the opening ceremony in London, and that seemed quite a momentous time in August 2012.' Jonny graduated as a GP in 2017 and did locum work around South London until early 2020, when the birth of his son prompted a move back to Harrogate, North Yorkshire, to be close to family.

As a GP, when somebody sits down in front of you, or you pick up a phone and start speaking to them, you literally could be talking about anything. You're in a privileged role to have people talking to you and share things with you that they wouldn't tell anybody else. As a GP, you get to form really close relationships because you see these patients again and again.

The biggest thing has been the change from working face to face to working phone to phone. Because that changes the dynamics of a relationship. You can have spoken to a patient four, five, six times and not know what they look like, walk past them in the street without realising that's the person you've spent six hours with on the phone. That's a big difference. It's often harder to form a rapport over the phone than it is in person, and so that's changed the dynamics of the job and how we work. You might have anywhere between 25 and 50 phone calls to make during a day. Some of those patients we will need to see in person, in which case we arrange for them to come down and see us. But it might only be a few a day that we'd see face to face. Like much of medicine, it's experience. So, for example, if somebody has tummy pain and told me that they were in quite a bit of pain, it's difficult to get a sense of that without putting a hand on their tummy and feeling it. Something like that, I'm quick to invite patients to come into the surgery so I can assess them in a bit more depth. Other things, you can comfortably consult about over the phone. You don't necessarily need the person there if they've got a blood-pressure machine and tell you what their blood-pressure readings are. Other things are a halfway house. If somebody has a rash you can't discern what that is just from a telephone consultation, but you can invite them to take a picture of it and send it to you. It might be that, from that picture, you've got your diagnosis right and you can call them back and, with confidence, tell them how to manage the problem.

There's days that are really tough and I come back and need to sit down in a dark room for 10 minutes. There's days when you feel that you've started very compassionate and empathetic and as the day's gone on, you're more hectic and more stressed and you feel that compassion and empathy start to dwindle a little bit. I think most GPs would acknowledge that that, unfortunately, is the way. Other days, everything seems to work out nicely. You've got a nice pace to your day. You're not too rushed. You manage to get through it feeling that you've done a good job, given everybody as much as they wanted or needed, and everything feels more calm and relaxed. You have to make sure that you're doing your best, but also that you're practising safely. Sometimes that means you're going to be finishing an hour or two later. It means that you miss getting home to put your son to bed. But, ultimately, it means that, actually, you can enjoy your evening when you do get home, because you know that you've done your best, and you've tied up all the loose ends and you've not cut any corners or taken risks just to get through the day.

It's easy to say this now. I always thought and hoped that the vaccines were going to be the only way out of this situation. But I have to hold my hands up and say I didn't think that they'd be able to get them rolled out as quickly as they have done. That's a miracle of modern technology. Certainly, the end of November 2020, when we started to hear the results from the trials, gave everybody a huge spring in their step that the trial was so positive. It meant that the vaccinations were just around the corner. That did lift the spirit, especially amongst the healthcare professionals. We gave our first vaccinations on Saturday 19 December 2020. That felt like a game changer.

The mood was fantastic, as good as I've ever seen it in everybody. It was a big privilege to be one of the first people giving out the vaccinations to these elderly patients who had been sat in their house, many of them for months and months on end, just waiting for something to happen so that they would be able to get back to some normality. We did something like 160 vaccinations that first morning. The patients were thrilled to be there. We've never had more generous feedback and warmth from the patients that we were helping. It felt a really positive experience and something that we'll look back on and cherish.

We had to keep them, the patients, in for 15 minutes while we monitored the after-effects of the vaccinations. They were sat, socially distanced, in a big waiting room. These elderly people chatting away to each other, having a mince pie and a cup of tea while we kept an eye on them. It was a really happy experience. A lot of these patients hadn't left their house for months on end, so you can imagine what they felt like at seeing the outside world again.

People have started to distrust the people at the top and the way they go about doing things. I didn't think I'd end up mentioning Dominic Cummings in this interview, but that at the time was very important in respect of how patients saw the government. It lost a lot of trust, and once you've lost that trust, then you go and look for reasons to disbelieve them. It saddens me that the government hasn't managed this better and hasn't been able to come across as a trustworthy and believable source of information. That has made our job more difficult over the last 12 months. If the government had stuck to the rules that they were trying to implement, that would have made it easier for everybody to enforce. That would be number one. Number two, they should have listened to their health advisers a lot more. Listening to the press briefings, it was like you had to listen to two different stories. Chris Whitty and Patrick Vallance would be urging extreme caution and then the government saying, 'Oh, things by Christmas will be a load better' and so on. Those of us with any sort of medical background were well aware that this was absolute nonsense. I found it hard to stomach, the fact that the government were seen to say things that the medical experts were going completely against.

Big strengths of the NHS are the diversity of it, the public love for it, and the pride that the people that work within the NHS have for the Service. The energy and intelligence and determination that goes about bringing our healthcare system together is miraculous, and everybody that's a part of it can be proud of what they've been able to do. As for the weaknesses, because it's a big beast it can be hard to mould into what we need it to be. But we've seen that we can be quite adaptable and creative, and things have changed at a very fast pace over this last 12 months. It shows what we can do if we've got that determination and drive, and that's still a challenge moving forward.

Covid will be the defining event of our generation. For me, it will be bittersweet, in terms of the birth of my son but then the absolute decimation that the virus has had on us as a society at the same time. It's a massive, life-changing event, and who knows quite how we'll reflect on it in years to come?

Jonny reflected at the end of the interview: 'While we've not been, as GPs, centre stage of the whole operation, we've certainly been on the stage to do what we can to help.'

The 2020s

In the longer history of the NHS, the 2020s will be coloured by the Covid-19 pandemic and the remarkable performance of the NHS during the darkest of times. The NHS showcased the incredible response of science and medicine with new treatments, diagnostics and vaccines and the technological revolutions around education and work. The Service's ability to rise to the need to treat huge numbers of patients suffering from Covid-19, a previously unknown disease, was underpinned by the strength of its human capital. NHS staff proved themselves to be willing and able to cope with the most challenging and unprecedented of circumstances. Public donations to NHS Charities Together hit new records during the spring of 2020 and the public showed their high support for NHS staff with weekly clapping sessions.

On the NHS's seventy-third anniversary in 2021, the NHS was awarded the George Cross by Queen Elizabeth II. It was in recognition of 73 years of dedicated service by NHS staff, especially their courage in responding to the pandemic. But these extraordinary contributions of NHS staff were not made without cost. Many staff have suffered illness and the deaths of family members and colleagues during the pandemic. Inequalities in health have been starkly exposed through the pandemic, as has the continuing racism experienced by NHS staff from ethnically diverse communities. Work has been enormously challenging, with long shifts, limited resources, and uncertainties about the longer-term impacts on the NHS, such as growing waiting lists and unmet needs. Public acclaim of the NHS has given way to frustration with the difficulties in getting treatment. Many health workers are taking industrial action in protest over pay and working conditions.

It is too soon to fully evaluate what the long-term consequences of Covid-19 will be on our lives, communities and the NHS. But what is certain is that 75 years on from its creation, the NHS is much more than a healthcare system for people in the UK. It is part of UK culture, intrinsic to national identity and a unifying force across political, social and spiritual divides. The previous chapters have shown how the NHS has both shaped our history since 1948 and been a site on which the broader historical changes have played out. As the final chapter will show, there is no shortage of critical and thoughtful reflection on the NHS's strengths and weaknesses, and the ways in which it can be better moulded to fit the health needs of 2023 and beyond.

Chapter 10: Reflections

What is the meaning of the NHS?

What are its strengths and weaknesses?

And how does the future look?

Some of our narrators offer their reflections.

JUNE ROSEN

Bevan was a man with a vision. He was a real left-winger, but he was a pragmatist. If you remember, he said about the consultants, 'I've stuffed their mouths with gold.' He didn't think much of them, but he knew he had to work with them. It was the pragmatism that got things moving. What would he think now? I think he'd be very proud that it was still going and very proud of the amazing developments. He might have a little nostalgia, because we all do, don't we? You look back with rose-coloured spectacles, but you forget that you were a different person then than you are now, with a lifetime of experience. I think he'd be very pleased that the sort of people he grew up with, who had nothing, now could have pretty well everything. We all, as patients, need to appreciate that. Because nothing's for nothing, is it? And although we say it's free, it's not actually free.

NORMAN SHARP

Without the NHS, nothing would have been possible. I could never have paid for the treatment that I've had and the attention. Father could never have paid for it when he had to contribute. It was a marvellous thing, the NHS. It included everybody.

I wouldn't be very popular, but I would say they should look at the contributions. I foresee that the youngsters today may not have pensions and the sick pay. National Health won't be so good to them as it was for me. Because everything is money-oriented today and they're more conscious of what everything costs. I can see the time coming when they won't be able to afford it. Of course, prices have increased, and wages have increased, and now it's so big. I couldn't get my head round it today. Such a big thing, financially, especially.

The NHS is like Stanmore (see page 43 for Norman's interview). Stanmore got into me – I couldn't get it out my system. Stanmore was my home. I was brought up there as a kid. Spent 18 months there. I can imagine anybody that works for the NHS must get the same feeling. That it's the most wonderful thing and it is part of them. And I feel like that about the NHS. I think it's definitely part of me.

GILL WAKELY

Gill has had rheumatoid arthritis since the late 1970s and reflects on her care as a retired GP with medical knowledge.

I think it becomes very obvious that I have knowledge very quickly when I say, 'Why do you want to do that? So-and-so's study says something else.' Then the consultant will turn to the trainee, 'You can see how difficult it can be sometimes …' I'm aware that I'm not the easiest patient to manage because I argue. The thing I find is that there's still this attitude in hospitals that you should be really grateful for being seen. And I don't really like that very much. I think it should be a more equal interaction. There has been a shift in attitudes, particularly amongst the young, who tend to have this attitude – we pay for the health service so, you know, we've got a right to expect a service from it. I think some of their expectations are unrealistic. I think a lot of older people have still got the sort of attitude that they should be really grateful that they're being seen at all. And they are very undemanding, when they should be more assertive. There's still an awful lot of patients who don't say, 'Why are you doing that?' or 'What's wrong with me?' I'm still amazed by the number of people I come across who haven't been told the diagnosis, or if they have, they haven't understood it. There's still a big power imbalance there. I think, with some of the younger people, they are perhaps too demanding and less prepared to look after themselves. I don't know how you balance that out. Because I think it should be more equal. But on the other hand, equality means that patients have got to take responsibility for their own health as well. I don't think that's happening enough.

GEOFF ADAMS-SPINK

A lot of people like me were born into a world that doesn't remember what it was like to live without the NHS. The fact that you couldn't afford to go to the doctor, you couldn't afford to go to hospital. You will die quite young of things that could quite easily be treated. I think in our quest for ever-improved healthcare at the frontier of longevity, we tend to forget why the NHS was created in the first place. And the whole welfare state, come to that. The Attlee government in '45 to '51 really laid a lot of the foundations in education in and in welfare provision that govern how we see ourselves now. Six years. But what a difference those six years made.

If you want a vision for how the UK would look without the NHS, just go to America. Just try and get treated. Look at the opioid scandal that's going on there. Why are people being prescribed opioids? Because they can't afford proper treatment for a lot of the ailments. So an opioid drug is a bit of a sticking plaster. It's horrendous and it's scary. I know the NHS has been criticised over the years for dishing out treatments to people who haven't contributed, or people who've just landed on a plane from somewhere. But I'd rather live in a society that treats somebody and worries about their ability to pay second, rather than somewhere that says, 'Yeah, just before we load you into the ambulance, what's your insurance? Where's your credit card?' I don't want to live in that kind of society. I'm sure we can do a lot more to recover costs. But the NHS historically doesn't have mechanisms for taking money in because it was always set up as a free-at-the-point-of-use healthcare system rather than a reimbursement system.

I've been thinking a lot recently about older age. I'm thinking about my thalidomide cohort as we move from middle to older age. And as our care needs increase, for me, I have to have a self-determined future. I do not want to have my life bookended by institutionalisation. A lot of us feel very much along those same lines that, okay, we know we're going to need more care. But it has to be care that we've negotiated and participated in. Rather than one-size-fits-all. You will go and live in this place. You will lose all autonomy and dignity. I want to have a riotous, joyful old age. Partying.

Going on holiday. Taking recreational drugs, if you fancy it. Perhaps a glass too many of Champagne. Just doing stuff that you want to do. All too few people get that amount of autonomy once they get sucked into the system. Only their basic needs are taken care of. That's very sad.

I would like to see more formal mechanisms for making the patient voice heard and included in decision-making. I think it's great to have committees where people give voice to their concerns. But unless they've got any executive authority to change things, it's almost like a release valve. Let them vent a bit over there. Then we can just carry on doing what we're doing. No, that's not good enough. You've got to include people in decision-making. From the lowest to the highest levels. A certain element of patient empowerment rather than just the voice of the patient needs to be there. We both know that the demographics of this country, as with most developed countries, are changing. You're going to have a lot of people in their sixties and seventies and early eighties, who may well be retired or semi-retired, but will have time and, crucially, have experience to be a part of that kind of decision-making process. So instead of them being just passive recipients of healthcare, they should be consulted, and have a say in shaping that healthcare. That's what I would say.

I consider the NHS to be a much-loved but slightly dysfunctional aunt. You have to make allowances for the fact that she sometimes puts a cardigan on inside out or she turns up in her slippers or whatever. But she's still much loved.

ETHEL ARMSTRONG

There was an NHS at 60 celebration, but it wasn't a big event like 70 was. The history of what was before 1948, and what is now, is something that we should preserve. We've got to stop taking it for granted. It does mean that Joe Public has got to become a little bit more self-sufficient. I know from the girls in A & E. Someone was going to an evening do, all dressed, all posh, and her nail had caught and lifted it out of the nail bed. Why the hell didn't they just use a bit of Sellotape to stick it back down? Then she complained that they were having to wait. As a hospital governor, you say, 'Oh, was it really worthwhile waiting three hours?' 'Oh, well, we've paid for it.' I think, 'God, you haven't lived long enough, you haven't been on the planet long enough to pay for what you've just received today.' I'm hoping that all the work that has gone into commemorating 70 years of the NHS in front of Joe Public isn't going to be done today and forgotten tomorrow.

Technology has advanced so much, and IT is becoming your master and not your servant. The balance has got to be right. You can't instil enthusiasm and total commitment into something that you press two buttons with. It's not rocket science, is it? I roll it out every time I've got the podium and nine times out of 10, it will get people standing up in the audience, you know. I'm passionate about getting all of our retired NHS [Retirement] Fellowship members to become members of an NHS foundation trust. Because who better than somebody who's been at the sharp end? At a governors' meeting, they will know what they're talking about. Everything now is abbreviated. Half of the letters, if you're not from an NHS background, you wouldn't know what they meant.

I went to Bristol and 100-year-old Sophie said, 'I can't believe, Ethel, that you've come all the way from Durham.' I said, 'I'm so pleased that you've asked me to have some of your birthday lunch and your birthday cake.' The fellowship president's collar is royal blue and gold, and I had got a jacket on in a yellowy gold colour. Sophie had got a yellow hat on. I said, 'Sophie, I'm so pleased you wore a hat for your birthday party.' She said, 'We just look like two canaries, Ethel!' I have no idea what she did in the NHS and I couldn't care tuppence. She's a member of the NHS fellowship and that made her day. That was a 17-hour travelling day for me to get there, to do the lunch and then get back again. But it was worth every minute. Every member of the NHS workforce, present and past, refuels me and tops up my batteries every day. Otherwise, if it didn't do that, I may as well just go and have a cup of coffee in the village and come back and think, 'What am I going to do today?'

STEPHEN LIGHTBOWN

The NHS doesn't always get it right because it is made up of human beings. Human beings make mistakes. It's about how you deal with those mistakes. Unfortunately, they can sometimes lead to catastrophic events. When those happen, it's really important to rebuild faith as quickly as you can do in that organisation, in that area of the NHS that might have been impacted. There's no question that if somebody reads that headline and they're going in to have an appointment in that place, they will feel more anxious. We have a really important job to make sure that we build faith as quickly as we can. The part about being humble is to recognise that we don't know all of the answers.

The NHS is always changing. It's always going through a period of evolution. Every government that comes in thinks that they know how to run the NHS better than the last government. Every health secretary wants to stamp their authority. So there's always change. We can't ever forget that we need to involve the people that use the NHS and benefit from the NHS in that decision-making. It's irrelevant that they haven't had X years of medical training, or they have not worked in a management position for 30 years. They use the NHS. They know what they want to experience and how they want to receive care. They've had good experiences and bad experiences, and know how those bad experiences could be made into good experiences for the next person. We should involve people in the design of what happens next, from the outset.

LINDA LAMONT

The NHS is the one issue where it goes across the political divide, doesn't it? Having spent the last five years paying for a nursing home for my husband who had dementia, it seems to me that an illness of the brain should be an illness. Not something which you have to pay for if you're lucky enough to be able to afford to pay for it. Or if you aren't, then the council pays. I think social care should be funded in the same way as the NHS. On the basis of shared risk. We support the NHS. Everybody practically does. And the idea that if you're lucky enough not to need it, you're happy to pay for the people who do. That should apply to social care as well, I think. I don't think there should be a clear distinction between them. People interestingly say they're prepared to pay more taxes until it comes to an election. Then they don't vote for a party which says, 'You'll have to pay more tax.' I'm afraid it's hard not to be political about this.

The NHS has always been a compromise. Well, any big institution is. We keep saying we're the best in the world. We aren't at the moment. Not until we pull our finger out and get on with it. We've wasted billions on different IT systems that haven't worked. We've got electronic communication, so it should be possible to pass reports from a consultant to the GP and not lose it on the way. It's ridiculous, isn't it, in this day and age, that we can't get it better.

I've seen with my husband's care there was some excellent people from Bulgaria, Romania, Italy, all over. What got me going on a campaign I'm involved in with others is to get a real living wage. It was because I saw the carers looking after my husband doing 12-hour shifts of really difficult work. On minimum pay. They often had families to look after as well, and they were really not earning enough. Some were employed by agencies and that, of course, takes a lot of NHS money. It seems to me that we have to pay more and train people more so that it's a respected profession, instead of being treated as not important. We've got to make it respected enough by having good training and by paying people decently to do such an important job.

KATIE TOMKINS

I'm at the hidden end of the NHS for work, but then as a human being and a patient, I'm trying to access services. So I have two different views of it. I understand processes and I understand the way in which referrals happen and the pathways that people have to take. But then from a patient point of view, I understand the frustration of not getting where you want to get as quickly as you want to.

We are so lucky in this country to have the National Health Service and to be able just to get those services through phone calls or seeing your GP. But I don't think it was built for what it is now. I love it but I'm also frustrated by it. We are so lucky. When I speak to friends who live in other countries, what healthcare costs them is just astronomical. It is something to be very proud of. I'm proud as an NHS worker and I'm also proud as a British person to have the NHS. When it works, it works amazingly, but we've got some problems and some tough times ahead of us.

JULIET JACQUES

The NHS means security. It means knowing that whatever happens to me, there's a baseline. I talk to Americans about their healthcare and it really influences their life decisions. I was speaking to an American friend who was talking about how she spent $300 a month on health insurance. There's no way I could have pursued my writing career if I was having, on top of rent, on top of living costs and everything else, to find £200 a month for health insurance. I couldn't do it.

There's all sorts of ways in which the NHS lets me live the life I want to live, beyond the most obvious one. It's the baseline of care for the public and, to me, it's what a government should be doing: taking care of its citizens. The most fundamental principle of government is embodied in the NHS and that's beyond the practicalities of it. That's ideologically. That's why, more than anything else, it's the thing we should be fighting for.

GRANT MCINTYRE

The NHS hasn't stayed still since 1948. The biggest change I've noticed is the fragmentation of what we call the NHS. It's actually different in Scotland, Northern Ireland, England and Wales. In some ways, 'N', the national bit, is a bit of a misnomer because it's such a different service in each of the different four nations in the UK. We've gone through various models of providing and delivering primary and secondary care, and so on. At the end of the day, we're all still here to treat patients. That's the reason why I think so many people stay in the NHS and make it a successful career. We shouldn't forget that patient care is at the heart of everything that we should do.

The challenge that I've confronted for most of my career is the fact that waiting times are always far greater than anybody would want them to be. I think that's a bit unfair for most of our patients. To have to wait for care that they either want or, indeed, need. Having been a patient myself in recent years, I have experienced how efficient the NHS can be when things have to be done. But I'm also aware that my own service is dogged by much longer waiting times than anybody would want. Whilst we've gone through various processes of change to improve that, we still have the fundamental issue that the demands are greater than the supply in terms of the NHS.

I think we have to have a conversation with the UK public to say, 'Here's what the NHS can and can't deliver.' Or indeed, if we are going to provide everything for everybody, we have to be a bit more honest about the waiting times and the fact that the change management processes we've gone through in recent years haven't really addressed those.

Before Covid, the major strength of the NHS was all about teamwork and responding to individual patients' needs. I think that's remained the same through the pandemic and into this post-Covid era that we're now entering into. The biggest single weakness of the NHS has been the issue of chronic underfunding in order to deliver the services that are needed to be delivered and, in doing so, patients having perhaps a slightly disjointed or lengthy care pathway compared to what they could achieve if they were to pay for it privately.

We need to be better at making sure that patients have not only equity, but also equality of care in services across the UK. Part of that is down to workforce, but it's also partly down to resources and, indeed, patient expectations. As somebody who's worked for the NHS for my whole career, I haven't seen this improve. Indeed, I would argue that perhaps we've got worse at equity and equality in the 30 years or so that I've worked for the NHS, which doesn't fill me with good heart, I have to say.

AVERIL MANSFIELD

I'm much more on the receiving end of the NHS since I retired, so I can see its deficiencies more, which is a shame. The thing that impacts most is getting a GP appointment. I've got a wonderful GP, but they're flat-out busy; they haven't got the time. To me, the biggest defect in general practice is there isn't the room for emergencies, for the man off the street. So those patients are all ending up in A & E. It's not really necessary. I don't know how we make it that we can treat emergencies in general practice. If we could do that, I think a lot of the problems with the health service could be eased. As a child, I could see my GP's house from where I lived, and we never left home until the queue that was outside had gone inside. Then we'd go. We'd still have to wait, but we knew we'd be seen. It's very nice to have an appointment, but on the other hand if you really have got something urgent, you wouldn't mind waiting if you could be sure you would be seen. In Liverpool I ran a clinic in a cottage hospital where you were chosen by the local GPs to be their surgeon. It was an accolade, you'd feel very chuffed that you'd been offered this job. The system was that you'd turn up on a Wednesday afternoon with a letter from your GP, and you sat on a bench until your turn came. And I never heard a single grumble, because the people knew what the system was and they knew they would go home having been seen and sorted.

I went to a clinic the other day, and the nurse said, 'He's running 45 minutes late.' So I said, 'Good.' 'Why good?' 'Because he's giving the time needed to each of the patients,' I said. She went, 'Oh, nobody's ever said that before.' But I mean it doesn't matter to me. I'm retired, I can wait if I have to wait. It isn't the end of the world. We're used to going to the hairdresser's and being treated on time, aren't we? I don't think we should be making people wait unreasonable amounts of time to be seen. But I think if they understand that they will get seen even though it might mean waiting longer on the day, I think people might not be so averse to it. It's worth trying.

There is so much more that we can do than when the health service started. It's just not recognisable as the same body. Things have changed almost beyond recognition. There's so much more that can be done to cure patients' ills. But we've not coped with the expansion of it as well as we might. Is it just money? I don't know. I also feel that the hours of work have had an influence, because we are not allowed to work the hours that we used to work. Is that safer for patients? I don't think it is. In my kind of surgery, you need to be doing a lot of it. I always say to my trainees, they wouldn't go and play a piano concerto at the Royal Festival Hall without practising. You'd practise as much as you thought was necessary to get you to the standard to play at the Festival Hall. But we can't do that in surgery yet.

The NHS has been my life, really. I've never distinguished between work and life. It's just been all one for me. And a big core of that has been the National Health Service, and being proud of the fact that I'm part of it. And wanting to remain proud of it and see some of its deficiencies sorted out.

DERRICK STEVENS

The NHS is an integral part of British society. We're all very passionate and protective about the NHS. I think it's about engaging with the public, with the users of the NHS. What do the public want from the NHS? My fear is privatisation, although I believe the NHS will still be here. We can give more and better care. I think it's underutilised out of hours. It sits there in the dark and weekends. There's a major asset sitting there not being used. If you want to reduce waiting lists, then stop healthcare being a Monday to Friday, nine to five.

I'm proud of the work I did. I'm looking at it as to whether the NHS is a good employer or not. That's certainly changed over the years. It always was that if you worked in the NHS, it was a job for life. Now there is no such thing as a job for life. If you worked in mining, in shipyards, that was a job for life. Is working for the NHS any more secure? I don't think anymore. When you started working in the NHS the reason a lot of people went to work in the NHS was the security.

ANDY BURNHAM

What three things would you like to happen by the eightieth anniversary of the NHS?

The top one has got to be a funding settlement for social care. The longer it's ignored, the more damaging it becomes to the NHS, because older people are ending up trapped in the acute system. That will create a pressure that won't be able to be met adequately and isn't being met adequately, even now.

Number two on my list would be a funding package for the NHS as a whole. I think it needs to be taken out of the ebbs and flows of politics. It needs to be an agreement about what does the NHS need on an annual basis to provide a decent service rather than this 'feast and famine'-type approach. It's clear, if you look at the international comparisons, we spend less of our GDP on the NHS than France, Germany and certainly the US on their health systems. Those other systems, certainly the US system, it doesn't even look after everybody. So this thing we've got, why starve it? It works when it's funded properly. We need some sort of political consensus about that. Based on the consensus around the NHS model, there now needs to be a funding consensus.

The third would be the centrality of mental health. In my first year in this job as Mayor of Greater Manchester, I would say that that is the issue that gets raised with me more often in terms of health than any other issue. From young people who talk about the school system not looking after their mental health, homelessness, rough sleeping, which effectively is a mental health issue. I think the nature of modern living means that everyone is absorbing higher levels of stress and insecurity than certainly our parents and our grandparents did. So mental health. The demand for services is up there. But the provision is down there. That gap has to be closed, and it does mean a reprioritisation. The thing that I think it means is getting rid of the sense of separateness that often applies to mental health. Nye Bevan gave a great speech where he was talking about the NHS and what it would mean and what the general hospital would be like in the new NHS. He said this great thing that always stuck with me: It means if you walk into the doors of a new general hospital you will find it as easy to get treatment for a mental disorder as you would for the corn on your foot. That great vision never has been made a reality. Mental health has always been separate buildings, separate organisations. It's got to move away from the margins and into the mainstream.

ANDREW POLLARD

My feeling today is that we were in a situation at the beginning of the pandemic which we should stand back and reflect on. Every winter we have pressures on the system because we're trying to run the system over its capacity. That means there's no resilience for a pandemic. I think it really needs a fresh look at our provision of healthcare in the UK to make sure that the NHS is large enough that it can cope with a normal year, let alone a pandemic year, and have enough resilience in the system. That is partly about having more beds available. It's also about having a large enough workforce that is able to deliver a larger service without falling over. It takes time. Many hospitals need some refurbishment or rebuilding. There's a lot of work to do that will take more than a decade. There needs to be a vision of what actually is needed in order to do that. The investment has to take account of what staffing do you need, if we look forward to the years between now and 2050, to be able to cope with the expected increase in activity in the NHS? What numbers of doctors and nurses? What work do you need on the hospitals? And then to cost that out properly. Because it's one of the most important questions for society.

ALICE WISEMAN

I'm really concerned about the inequalities in the UK that were there before the pandemic but have also been generated by the pandemic. And subsequent events that are happening now, such as the cost-of-living crisis. Understanding some of that, I think, is really important. Thinking about, what actions could we take to reduce that level of inequality in the country? How do we get to that point, and what can we learn? Either when we've done it differently in the UK, and it's had a different impact or when they've done it in Germany, for example, when Germany was reunified. That bit is important 'cause you're learning from what's happened, but you're also thinking about what you could do into the future.

PATRICIA MILLER

The strength of the NHS is that it provides healthcare that is free at the point of need. I think the benefit bit of that is that we don't make decisions because we are financially incentivised, which is what can happen in areas where you've got insurance-funded care. I think that's a positive. I don't believe that your ability to access healthcare should depend on your ability to pay. We have got broad health inequalities in this country. I think if we move to that place where you only could access healthcare if you could afford to pay for it, then the health inequalities – gaps – would be much wider. Where I think it needs to improve, or move into a different space, is that when it was originally established in 1948, Bevan talks about it loosely being responsible for reducing health inequalities. I think, over the years, because the NHS has become quite politicised, we've lost our focus. We've lost the principle behind its role, which is around reducing health inequalities. Now that we've got a consultation document around moving to more of an integrated-care model, it's really focused on moving the NHS into an organisation that needs to develop services that are human-centred. An organisation where communities are at the heart of what we do. I think we're getting back to the original purpose of the NHS. If it does the job that it's meant to, I know that it will play a significant part not just in reducing health inequalities, but in its role as one of the largest anchor institutions in this country. It can be at the heart of social and economic regeneration post-Covid-19.

I will be the chief exec for the health system in Dorset. That means driving forward the development of an integrated-care strategy that takes the actions around supporting communities to live their best lives. It means that I will be responsible for working with local government and community partners in doing that work and putting communities in the league of developing solutions that enable them to achieve a better quality of life. It will mean working with the health organisations in Dorset in a partnership, but also a supervisory capacity, and making sure that from a commissioning perspective, we are commissioning the services that people really need because we're listening to their feedback, as opposed to commissioning services that we think they need, which is, I think, where the health service has been for a long time.

A big part of our role will be changing the relationship and the dynamic with communities so that we are listening to them in terms of their lived experience, what the barriers are for them in achieving good health and well-being. And also being prepared to listen when they tell us that some of the services that we may well be proud of, that we've been providing for a number of years, may actually be contributing towards various inequalities instead of resolving them. Then working together to design solutions to enable them to live longer, healthier lives, right from cradle to grave.

I think that it would be fantastic if, in the levelling-up conversations, the secretary of state for health and social care and the secretary of state for communities and local government recognise that to deliver on the levelling-up agenda, there needs to be common purpose between those two portfolios. Neither can do that single job by themselves. But they can achieve a significant amount together. We've got a responsibility in health and local governments to keep educating central government on what is actually required on the ground.

MASUD HOGHUGHI

I think the greatest jewel in the crown of Britain is the NHS, bar none. It is just about the most complex, enormous, personal organisation dealing with people as people. You know their race doesn't matter. We all look the same when we're laid on the table.

I was born in an environment where there wasn't an NHS. I came to one and I easily and gently slid into it. I became aware of the layer upon layer upon layer of complexity and benevolence. Sheer goodwill. People staying long after the hours that they should have gone home, in order to look after the patient. It's done as a gift. It is a gift that we give the rest of our fellow human beings. Forget about the salaries. You can get the salary anywhere else. But it is all the things that aren't part of the salary that you give to patients on a daily basis. The NHS has all the complexity that a human being has. All the complexity that a society has. But then multiple other layers added to that. There's nothing better for us.

There is a commitment which transcends the limitations of the service which are always there. When I visit my sister in a stroke unit, I talk to other stroke patients in their late seventies, eighties, nineties. I say, 'Do you know where you are?' They say, 'I'm in hospital.' I say, 'Are you paying for it?' They have paid for it during their lifetime. I say to them, 'Isn't it magnificent that you don't have to worry about how much all this is going to cost you because the rest of us pay for you to be here?' They become tearful. I become tearful, because the NHS is an act of benevolence. I think the health service commands a love, commands a sense of possessiveness, which transcends people's political beliefs.

Every generation of workers in the NHS have a loyalty. A sense of a deep knowledge of the good that it does, and the hardness that it has to go through in order to deliver the goodness that it delivers. It has become part of their identity. It is part of our national identity. We would fight for it to kingdom come. The reason why nobody else has an NHS is because they can't afford it. It is really an extraordinarily expensive kind of organisation to run. But it is, equally, the envy of the world.

It's getting better because it's getting more self-critical. People are getting less anxious about making mistakes and being ridiculed or held up. I don't mean that malpractice doesn't go on. How could it not? Because it has over 700,000 encounters every day between a member of the public and a member of NHS. Human beings aren't perfect. Neither patients, nor the people who look after them. They're not perfect. They make mistakes. They sometimes commit evil because you know, we don't select people on the basis of whether they have evil in them, or not. We hope to God that the goodness of the NHS will convert them. But we have a lot of payments to make to people who've received the wrong kind of care.

My granddaughter is the senior nurse in charge. She's only 25. She's doing brilliantly in the acute unit of the Sheffield Children's Hospital, which involves a network of six hospitals in the United Kingdom, but also includes Northern Ireland, with helipads, etc., to whom the most extraordinary cases come from all over. She's knee-high to a grasshopper. You can see how much I adore her. She's absolutely fierce about the protective care of children. She says, 'The notion of timetables goes out of the window. If you've got a child who needs care, the child needs care. Period. That's all there is to it.' It's not because of me. It's because she's picked up that baton. As a whole lot of other people have picked up that baton. This is not just about the health service. It is about life. It's about protecting life and the welfare of other people. Is there anything more important than that? I don't think so.

I am one person who's seen different sides of the NHS and who's operated in different capacities in the NHS, and continues to do so as a volunteer. My view of the NHS, my admiration for the NHS, almost bordering on adoration of the NHS, is born of very close involvement with it. It's something that we should be truly proud of because it is such a large collectivity of people.

Acknowledgements

Our Stories would not exist without the generosity and dedication of the thousands of people across the UK who have contributed in so many different ways to building the *Voices of Our National Health Service* archive. It has been a team effort in the best sense of the word which has produced a public collection of nearly two thousand hours of testimony which is accessible according to the permissions of the interviewees. I want to thank our funders, The National Lottery Heritage Fund and the Arts and Humanities Research Council, who made the work possible. Our interviewees for trusting us enough to share their lives with us. Our volunteers who worked tirelessly across the UK to record the stories. And our supporters across the NHS, and health and heritage communities. We are very appreciative of the contribution to the work from our British Library colleagues, particularly Hannah Tame who catalogued the collection, supported by Charlie Morgan, Mary Stewart and Rob Perks.

My personal thanks go to the brilliant people who worked with me to transcribe and edit the testimonies including Beck Heslop, Eleanor Shaw, and Terri Sweeney and to my fabulous project team, especially Angela Whitecross and James McSharry who have been part of the project since its beginning in 2017.

Katie Fulford, my agent at Bell Lomax Moreton, has been an unflappable support from the first day we met, and her constant encouragement that this book was an important book to pursue has been invaluable. I'm so grateful to Andrew Morley for introducing us and indeed, for his support and friendship over many years.

I am indebted to Oli Holden-Rea and his team at Welbeck who have been passionate about the book from the start, taking such care to maintain the authenticity of the testimonies in their published form. It is rare to find an editor with the sensitivity necessary to do justice to oral history and I am truly blessed.

I am hugely grateful to best-selling author, Adam Kay, whose passion for the NHS is unparalleled, for contributing the Foreword and for the support from NHS Charities Together.

At times, the process of getting this book across the line has become a family enterprise, involving hands-on help with transcripts and writing from my beautiful daughters, Evie, Verity and Gwyn, and my long-suffering husband, David. So thank you, and I'm sure you're looking forward to the next one!

April 2023

Further Reading

Every historian draws on the work of many other scholars and writers and these are the main sources used in the narrative sections.

Begley, Philip; Sheard, Sally and MacKillop, Eleanor, eds. 'The 1974 NHS Reorganisation'. Department of Public Health and Policy: University of Liverpool, 2017.

Bevan, Aneurin. *In Place of Fear*. Melbourne, London, Toronto: William Heinemann Ltd, 1952.

Bevan, Aneurin. 'NHS – Nye Bevan speaks about the National Health Service, 1959'. Accessed 30 July 2021. https://www.youtube.com/watch?v=CCAyUxY0Cm0

Bivins, Roberta. *Contagious Communities: Medicine, Migration, and the NHS in Post-War Britain*. Oxford: Oxford University Press, 2015.

Crane, Jennifer. "Save our NHS': activism, information-based expertise and the 'new times' of the 1980s." *Contemporary British History* 33, no. 1 (2019) 52-74.

Crane, Jennifer and Hand, Jane. *Posters, protests, and prescriptions: Cultural histories of the National Health Service in Britain*. Manchester University Press, 2022.

Cutler, Tony. 'Dangerous Yardstick? Early Cost Estimates and the Politics of Financial Management in the First Decade of the National Health Service.' *Medical History* 47, no. 2 (2003): 217–238. doi:10.1017/S0025727300056726.

Foot, Michael. *Aneurin Bevan (Volume 2)*. London: Paladin, 1975.

Gorsky, Martin. 'The British National Health Service 1948–2008: A Review of the Historiography.' *Social History of Medicine* 21, no. 3 (2008): 437–460. doi:10.1093/shm/hkn064.

Ham, Christopher. *Health Policy in Britain.* 6th edition. Basingstoke: Palgrave Macmillan, 2009.

Jones, Emma J. and Snow, Stephanie J. *Against the Odds: Black and Minority Ethnic Clinicians and Manchester, 1948 to 2009.* Manchester NHS Primary Care Trust and University of Manchester, 2010.

Klein, Rudolf. *The New Politics of the NHS: From Creation to Reinvention.* 6th edition. Oxford: Radcliffe, 2013.

MacKillop, Eleanor; Begley, Philip; Sheard, Sally; Lambert, Michael eds. 'The Introduction of the NHS Internal Market'. Department of Public Health and Policy: University of Liverpool, 2018.

Mold, Alex. *Making the Patient-Consumer: Patient Organisations and Health Consumerism in Britain.* Manchester: Manchester University Press, 2015.

Rivett, Geoffrey. *From Cradle to Grave: Fifty Years of the NHS.* London: King's Fund, 1998.

Rivett, Geoffrey. *The Development of the London Hospital System 1823–1982.* London: King's Fund, 1986.

Sheard, Sally. 'A Creature of Its Time: The Critical History of the Creation of the British NHS,' *Michael Quarterly* 8 (2011), 428–441.

Timmins, Nicholas. *The Five Giants: A Biography of the Welfare State.* London: Harper Collins, 2001.

Webster, Charles. *The Health Services Since the War. Vol 1: Problems of Health Care. The National Health Service before 1957.* London: HMSO, 1988.

Webster, Charles. *The Health Services Since the War, Vol II: Government and Health Care: The British National Health Service 1958–1979.* London: HMSO, 1996.

Webster, Charles. *The National Health Service: A Political History.* Oxford: Oxford University Press, 1998.

Appendix – Voices Of Our National Health Service

Voices of Our National Health Service oral history collection is deposited at the British Library. The collection reference is C1887 and you can search the Sound and Moving Image Catalogue http://sami.bl.uk to find items in the collection. Each interviewee has a unique reference number (URN). You can search the catalogue using either the full name or the URN. The URNs for the interviewees featured in this book are listed below. If no number is listed, then the cataloguing of the interview is still in process. Contact details for the British Library oral history section are:

Telephone: 020 7412 7404

Email: oralhistory@bl.uk

Website: www.bl.uk/oralhistory

Interviewee	Interviewer/s	URN	Interview date
Priti Acharya	Jane Hampson		2022-08-01
Colin Anderson	Lauren Young	C1887/730	2021-11-25
Dawn Adams	Fidelma Ruddy/ Lauren Young	C1887/623	Multiple
Geoff Adams Spink	Stephanie Snow	C1887/637	2019-10-04
Tryphena Anderson	Cathy Charles Jones	C1887/705	2020-01-23
Elizabeth Anionwu	Stephanie Snow/ Debra Hearne	C1887/1072	Multiple
Ethel Armstrong	Peter Mitchell	C1887/16	2019-03-12
John B	James McSharry		2019-03-09

Interviewee	Interviewer/s	URN	Interview date
Sonya Baksi	Peter Mitchell	C1887/309	2019-10-07
Maxine Ball	Alistair Hart	C1887/936	Multiple
Catalina Bateman	Gwen Crossley	C1887/154	2018-05-04
Margaret Batty	Maya Pieris	C1887/380	2020-01-17
Carol Baxter	Stephanie Snow	C1887/512	2019-07-17
Caroline Bedale	Angela Whitecross	C1887/153	2019-09-06
George Bentley	Peter Mitchell	C1887/250	2019-05-01
Jonathan Blake	James McSharry	C1887/820	Multiple
Georgina Bond	Jane Hampson	C1887/638	2021-09-08
Anne Brain	Sue Thomas	C1887/326	2020-01-20
Kathryn Braithwaite	Debra Hearne	C1887/375	2019-12-03
Basil Bramble	Michael Bowden	C1887/782	Multiple
Andy Burnham	Stephanie Snow	C1887/500	2018-06-12
Ed Bylina	Patrick Cornwell	C1887/1070	2022-05-16
Brian Carroll	Jane Hampson	C1887/149	2018-06-12
Pat Carroll	Jane Hampson/ James McSharry	C1887/149	Multiple
Antonette Clarke-Akalanne	Debra Hearne	C1887/328	Multiple
Ursula Clifford	Ruth Coon	C1887/492	2021-03-10
Yvonne Coghill	Angela Whitecross	C1887/596	2019-04-18
Edwina Currie Jones	Stephanie Snow	C1887/1071	2019-06-04
Jack Czauderna	Peter Mitchell	C1887/536	Multiple
Kevin Dadds	Catherine Mansfield	C1887/377	2020-02-04
Dipankar Datta	Margaret McMillan	C1887/41	2019-06-11
Diana	Hanna McAvoy	C1887/1092	2019-03-06
Robert Downes	James McSharry	C1887/303	2019-05-15
Yunus Dudhwala	Debra Hearne	C1887/1204	Multiple

Interviewee	Interviewer/s	URN	Interview date
Colin Eastwood	Gwen Crossley	C1887/86	2017-12-27
Ngozi Edi-Osagie	Lauren Massey	C1887/563	2018-03-15
Ruth Edwards	Colette Miles	C1887/20	2018-05-21
Jonny Emms	Debra Hearne	C1887/460	2021-01-29
Hughie Erskine	Stephen Rydzkowski	C1887/163	2018-01-15
Archie Findlay	Andrew Morley	C1887/507	2020-05-06
Illora Finlay	Stephanie Snow	C1887/808	2019-10-03
Lorna Finlay	Ruth Coon	C1887/462	2021-03-11
Megan Fox	James McSharry	C1887/77	2018-02-21
Claire Goodwin-Fee	James McSharry	C1887/787	2021-02-02
Joanne Harding	Stephen Rydzkowski	C1887/880	Multiple
Nick Hart	Andrew Morley	C1887/685	Multiple
Tom Heller	Peter Mitchell/ Jane Hampson	C1887/704	Multiple
June Hewett	Debra Hearne	C1887/373	2020-04-24
Eileen Hill	Lauren Massey	C1887/88	Multiple
Edmund Hoare	Jane Hampson	C1887/159	2018-07-13
Masud Hoghughi	Debra Hearne	C1887/386	2020-03-05
Gill Holden	Jane Hampson		2022-09-02
Juliet Jacques	Sarah Woolley	C1887/1122	2020-01-16
Lionel Joyce	Jill Davidson		2020-01-28
Peter Julian	Christina Jones	C1887/570	2020-10-19
Kenye Karemo	Linda Mezaks	C1887/1131	2021-04-16
Mary Keer	Diana Kuh	C1887/758	2020-06-02
Punam Krishan	Alastair Hart	C1887/53	2019-04-10
Linda Lamont	Peter Mitchell	C1887/274	2019-10-07
Brian Lascelles	Lynda Kiss	C1887/330	2020-02-10
Rachel Lewis	James McSharry	C1887/694	2021-01-22
Stephen Lightbown	Debra Hearne	C1887/700	Multiple

Interviewee	Interviewer/s	URN	Interview date
Patricia Macartney	Jane Hampson	C1887/687	2019-07-19
Averil Mansfield	Stephanie Snow	C1887/609	2019-10-03
Lauren Massey	Patrick Cornwell	C1887/828	2017-12-20
Grant McIntyre	Jane Hampson		2022-08-23
Elsie McMahon	Cathy Charles Jones /Jane Hampson	C1887/631	Multiple
Monica McWilliams	Stephanie Snow	C1887/842	2020-02-07
Rajan Madhok	Stephanie Snow	C1887/1172	Multiple
Raj Menon	Jane Hampson	C1887/1171	Multiple
Harold Mercer	Peter Mitchell	C1887/26	Multiple
Joan Meredith	Patrick Cornwell	C1887/167	2018-02-01
Patricia Miller	James McSharry	C1887/944	Multiple
Peter Moore	Louisa Peters	C1887/692	2019-08-14
David Morrison	Peter Mitchell	C1887/23	2019-06-27
Norma Murdoch	Claire McDade	C1887/51	2019-06-18
Ken Murray	Clive Carr	C1887/1129	2019-04-24
Sylvia Newman	Sandra Barlow	C1887/1193	Multiple
Barbara O'Donnell	Linda Mezaks	C1887/1046	2020-03-07
Sarah Oldnall	James McSharry	C1887/903	Multiple
David Owen	Stephanie Snow	C1887/622	2019-12-04
Wendy Parker	Terri Sweeney	C1887/972	Multiple
Natalie Parr	James McSharry	C1887/940	Multiple
Amit Pawa	Andrew Morley	C1887/714	2020-05-30
Patricia	Gwen Crossley	C1887/101	2018-01-31
Joan Pearton	Zoe Harewood	C1887/92	2017-12-30
Linda Pepper	Patrick Cornwell	C1887/1138	Multiple
Patrick Peters	Stephanie Snow		2022-08-23
Lisa Petryszyn-Edwards	Jennet Jumayeva	C1887/276	2019-05-13

Interviewee	Interviewer/s	URN	Interview date
Andrew Pollard	Stephanie Snow		2022-04-11
Philip Prosser	James McSharry	C1887/67	2018-02-21
Peter Rice	Wendy Hewitson	C1887/193	2019-07-30
June Rosen	Stephanie Snow	C1887/666	2019-04-25
David Rothberg	Sartaj ul Haque	C1887/1060	2019-12-17
Alfred Samuels	Gwen Crossley	C1887/880	2018-03-14
Norman Sharp	Debra Hearne	C1887/294	2019-06-12
Pat Sheehan	Stephanie Snow	C1887/686	2019-11-27
Dennis Singson	Peter Mitchell	C1887/874	2019-07-03
Derrick Stevens	Maya Pieris	C1887/338	2020-01-06
Joan Stevenson	Peter Mitchell	C1887/01	2019-01-09
Terry Stoodley	Phil Ringer	C1887/407	2020-03-10
Grainne Teggart	Stephanie Snow	C1887/641	2020-02-05
Katie Tomkins	James McSharry	C1887/886	2022-04-14
Deb Troops	Patrick Cornwell	C1887/1063	2022-03-22
Yvonne Ugarte	Patrick Cornwell	C1887/1205	Multiple
Klarissa Velasco	Stephanie Snow	C1887/827	2020-12-02
Gill Wakely	Karen Waters	C1887/18	2017-12-07
Marion Waters	Karen Waters	C1887/80	2018-01-14
Marion & Ceri Waters	Karen Waters	C1887/81	2018-01-14
Paula Wigg	Peter Mitchell/ Raveena Barjwa	C1887/690	Multiple
Lalith Wijedoru	Jon Hammond	C1887/1135	Multiple
Alice Wiseman	Debra Hearne	C1887/1039	Multiple

Notes

1   Appendix 1 lists the interviews used in the book, including details of how to access the collection at the British Library.

2   'Birth and Death Rates for 1936 in England', *Nature* 30 January 1937, p.189

3   Bevan, Aneurin, *In Place of Fear*, William Heinemann, London, 1952, p.75.

4   National Health Service Act 1946 (c.81) [Online]. London: The Stationery Office. Accessed 13 April 2023. Available from https://www.legislation.gov.uk/

5   *Daily Telegraph and Morning Post*, 6 July 1948.

6   See Further Reading for a list of sources drawn on in this book.

7   British Dental Association. *The Story of NHS Dentistry*. [Online]. Accessed 12 April 2023. Available from http://www.bda.org.uk

8   The National Health Service: Memorandum by the Minister of Health. C.P. (48)302, 13 December 1948.

9   Cutler, Tony. 2003. 'Dangerous Yardstick? Early Cost Estimates and the Politics of Financial Management in the First Decade of the National Health Service'. Medical History, 47(2), 217–238. doi:10.1017/S0025727300056726

10 Appleby, John. 2008. *Data Briefing: Why NHS budgets have always been a bugbear*. [Online]. Accessed 13 April 2023. Available from https://kingsfund.org.uk

11 *Report of the Committee of Enquiry into the Cost of the National Health Service*, Guillebaud Committee, Cmd. 9663, 1956, Parliamentary Papers (PP) 1955–56.

12 Hansard HC Deb. Vol.592 cols.1383–1506, 30 July 1958.

13 Department of Health and Social Security. 1968. Report of the Twentieth Anniversary Conference of the NHS. London: HMSO.

14 Baxter, Carol. *The Black Nurse: An endangered species – a case for equal opportunities in nursing*, National Extension College Trust Ltd, 1988.

15 Geoffrey Rivett. *The history of the NHS website. Chapter 2008–2017: An uncertain path ahead*. [Online]. Accessed 12 April 2023. Available from https://nuffield trust.org.uk.

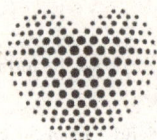

IN SUPPORT OF
NHS CHARITIES TOGETHER

NHS Charities Together is the national charity caring for the NHS, providing the extra support that's needed to care for staff, patients and communities. Working with over 230 NHS charities across the UK, representing hospitals, ambulance trusts, mental health trusts and community health services – we are here to help raise the profile of NHS charities and ensure that money raised nationally reaches the people that need support most.

Find out more at nhscharitiestogether.co.uk